LECTURE NOTES ON UROLOGY

Lecture Notes on Urology

JOHN BLANDY DM, MCh, FRCS
Professor of Urology in The University of London
at The London Hospital Medical College,
Consultant Urologist, St Peter's Hospital, London

SECOND EDITION

BLACKWELL SCIENTIFIC PUBLICATIONS
OXFORD LONDON EDINBURGH MELBOURNE

First published 1976
Second edition 1977

British Library Cataloguing in Publication Data

Blandy, John Peter
    Lecture notes on urology.—2nd ed.
    1. Genito-urinary organs—Diseases
    I. Title
    616.6   RC871

    ISBN 0-632-0045-7

Distributed in the United States of America by
J.B. Lippincott Company, Philadelphia
and in Canada by
J.B. Lippincott Company of Canada Ltd, Toronto.

Printed in Great Britain at
the Alden Press, Oxford

Contents

Preface

This book has been written for the undergraduate medical student. About a quarter of all the operations of surgery concern the genitourinary system: about 15% of all doctors suffer at some time or other from a stone in the urinary tract: one in ten of all males have to have an operation on their prostate before they reach the end of their days. The management of haematuria, of impotence, of infertility, and of urinary tract infections: the investigation of hypertension, and the evaluation of albuminuria—no doctor, however recondite his speciality—is not at some time touched by one or other of these common problems. Of all diseases in the world, in prevalence second only to malaria, schistosomiasis affects more human beings, and those more miserably, than any other. The author makes no apology therefore for the claim that the speciality of urology encompasses some of the most important, and arguably the most fascinating of all the topics of medicine and surgery. My object has been to communicate my own interest and enthusiasm to my students, for unlike some topics which they have to learn, there ought to be nothing boring or dull in this, the oldest and most vigorous of all the specialities. It is for this reason that the solemn minded reader may not approve of some of my pictures, or my omission of the customary protracted dissertation about body fluids and electrolytes for which he will have to consult those other of his textbooks which deal with them in a way which I could not imitate even if I understood. Sexually transmitted diseases are not covered in this book, not because I find them tedious, but because they are too important to be dealt with by other than an expert. On the other hand I found it impossible not to trespass from time to time on the ground normally and correctly assigned to my colleagues in nephrology from whom I crave forgiveness if, in an attempt to make an understandable and unified presentation of the subject, my ignorance has led me into too many and too barbarous errors concerning the esoteric mysteries of nephritis and hypertension. The last chapter about the operations of urology is there simply to make the students' visits to the operating theatre more interesting: they should not attempt to learn surgical technique—though I hope they may find watching operations helps in the understanding of living pathology. For the same reason the little glossary, of jargon, eponyms and gobbledygook is added for fun, not because students need learn any of it.

Preface to Second Edition

The need for a second edition so soon after the first gives me an opportunity to revise it thoroughly, to correct some mistakes, to bring the text and references up to date, and to try to improve some of my sketches in order to make them more clear.

J.P.B.

Chapter 1
The Urological History

You will find it helpful to begin at the beginning. How old is your patient, and what is his or her occupation? If he is retired, what did he do before? Make sure you ascertain any possible contact with rubber, chemicals, plastics, pitch, tar, or any other occupational hazard known to concern the urinary tract. Do not rest content if the patient tells you he is a 'company director': he may be director of Imported Carcinogens Limited. Be careful of the terms 'Process worker', and 'Engineer': the process may be the making of rubber mix containing naphthylamine, and the engines may be churning out toxic chemicals.

If the patient is a woman, begin by finding out when she was married, and how many and how old are her children: did she have trouble in her pregnancy? Was a catheter passed? Were forceps used (and inevitably a catheter passed)? Was her perineum sutured?

Then turn to the trouble which took your patient to the doctor. In urinary tract disorders there is often a long run-up to the incident which brings them to your surgery, or your outpatients. Try to find out when the prostatism began, or when the patient had her first episode of cystitis. Try to make out clearly how the pattern of the disease has changed over the years.

Always make quite certain what it is that bothers the patient right now.

End by asking the direct question—has the patient ever had *haematuria*? This one symptom is the most important in the whole of urology.

Note-taking

Although you must set down all the relevant facts in your history, it is no good writing down a host of irrelevant twaddle in the hope that someone, someday, may be able to make sense of it. Keep your notes as brief as possible, and as close to the point as you can (fig. 1.1). A drawing saves lines of prose: thus, if the patient has pain, do not merely write 'backache': make a sketch recording what the pain is like (e.g. sharp, colicky, a dull ache or burning). Note what brings the pain on, and what relieves it (e.g. exercise, passing water, making love, bending over). Show on your sketch if the pain radiates anywhere else.

Certain terms should be avoided, because they are ambiguous. *Dysuria* can mean pain, or difficulty, or both. It is better to write down *pain*, or *difficulty*. Similarly with frequency of urination, it is simple to write down $D = 5: N = 3$ if he voids five times in the day and thrice at night. Avoid the confusing terms *polyuria* and *nocturia*. *Pollakiuria* is less meaningful than 'passes urine very often': and *micturition* is a tiresome euphemism for passing water, which for all but the most prudish can be expressed very easily and clearly by the letter p. Even *'void'* is preferable to *'micturate'*.

Haematuria is of crucial importance: the patient will be able to say what colour his urine was, and whether there were clots in it. Was the urine mixed up with the blood, or did the blood just appear at the

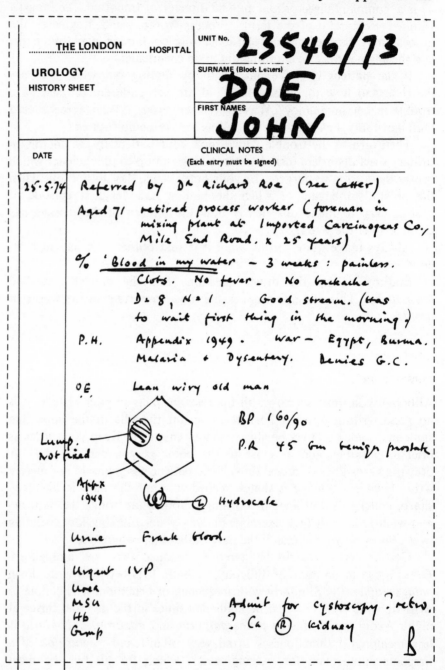

Fig. 1.1. Keep your notes as brief as possible. . . .

Chapter 1/Urological History

beginning or the end of the stream? If the blood oozes from the urethra in between urination it probably comes from the urethra itself.

Previous history

Students often feel awkward in asking about the possibility of their patient having previously had venereal disease. Since every man is flattered at the suggestion that he might have been a gay dog in his youth, you will offend few men if you enquire whether they could ever have had any venereal trouble in their younger days.

Do not forget to ask if your patient has served in a hot climate, with reference to the possibility of having developed a calculus, or of having picked up schistosomiasis from bathing almost anywhere in Africa.

In women you must enquire about the menstrual history. Apart from the obvious confusion between menstrual loss and haematuria, it is necessary to make certain that you do not inadvertently order a pyelogram in the early days of pregnancy. Always note down the date of the last menstrual period, and refer to it on the X-ray request form.

Do not waste time

While you are taking the history, you will begin to realize that certain investigations are relevant: if you start to fill in the appropriate laboratory forms as you are listening, it will not only save time, but will prevent you from writing down too much irrelevant detail.

THE UROLOGICAL EXAMINATION

General examination

In an ideal world, where every doctor had as much time at his disposal as he could wish for, and no patient was ever in a hurry to get back to his work or her children, you could make a thorough and comprehensive physical examination of every system in every case. In patients admitted for major surgical procedures this will of course be your routine practice. In your surgery or outpatient department, such a method of working would be cruelly slow. Strive to confine your attention to what matters. At the same time there are certain general features which should not escape your attention. Does the patient look ill, has he lost weight, is he anxious, depressed, anaemic, or in pain? A stink of urine may mean uraemia or merely wet trousers. Watch carefully how he comes into your consulting room: does he have Parkinsonism, or does he limp because a metastasis in his pelvis hurts?

To shake your patient's hand as he comes in is not mere politeness—it also yields useful information. Never forget that you are a doctor first, and a urologist second.

If any of these features draws attention to a disorder in some other system, then by all means examine that system as well. In any case, do not return to your desk until you have measured the blood pressure.

Abdominal examination

1   You are looking for evidence of enlargement of the kidneys or the bladder.

2   You must examine the inguinal region so as not to miss inguinal or femoral herniae, a varicocele, a saphena varix, or enlarged lymph nodes.

3   In every male, you must carefully examine each testis, epididymis, vas and spermatic cord.

4   In all patients, you should do a rectal examination. In men this will tell you about the prostate, seminal vesicles, and the ampullae of the vasa, as well as the membranous urethra and the base of the bladder.

5   In women, you must examine the vulva, urethra and vagina, preferably with a speculum as well as by palpation.

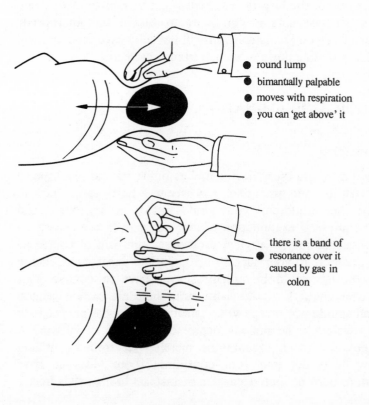

round lump
bimanually palpable
moves with respiration
you can 'get above' it

there is a band of resonance over it caused by gas in colon

Fig. 1.2. The physical signs of an enlarged kidney.

An enlarged kidney is classically supposed to give you:
1   A rounded lump in the loin
2   which moves on respiration
3   above which you can get your hand
4   and over which there is a band of resonance caused by gas in the ascending colon on the right and the descending colon on the left.

These four classical signs are notoriously misleading. Never put much trust in clinical signs, for your clinical hunch is often wrong. The 'enlarged kidney' may turn out to be liver (you are supposed to be able to get above the kidney, but you can easily be mistaken). On the left side, the 'kidney' may turn out to be the spleen, (though one cannot usually get the hand between the spleen and the costal margin, and you ought to be able to feel the notch on its anterior border). One may make a mistake over an enlarged gall bladder, which ought to be stuck to the underside of the liver, and should not have any overlying resonance. Lumps in the colon on the left or the right side may closely mimic an enlarged kidney. The moral is not to trust your physical signs, and always to confirm your clinical hunch by an excretion urogram.

The notorious kidney punch—bashing the patient over the 12th rib with the closed fist—is supposed to make an inflamed kidney hurt. Kind doctors do not need to strike their patients, and you will find gentle palpation a good deal more informative (fig. 1.3).

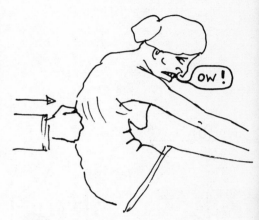

Fig.1.3. The notorious kidney punch —gentle palpation is just as informative.

PHYSICAL SIGNS OF AN ENLARGED BLADDER (fig. 1.4)

Classically the bladder is
1   a rounded lump in the lower abdomen
2   which is dull to percussion.

In practice there are certain practical snags: first, if the bladder is atonic and floppy, it may be very hard to feel. Secondly, it may not rise in the midline but to one or other side (fig. 1.4b).

The most useful physical sign is that the 'bladder' disappears after you let the urine out with a catheter.

Examination of the groins (fig. 1.5)

Never finish your examination without having examined the groins both in the standing-up and lying-down position. Remember that there are three orifices on each side, and each one must be checked.

Inguinal herniae

Indirect herniae push out lateral to the inferior epigastric vessels, and

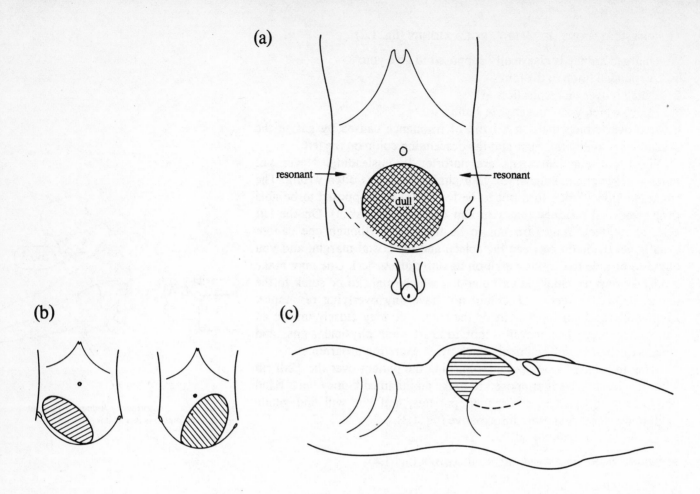

(a)

resonant →   ← resonant

dull

(b)   (c)

Fig. 1.4. The physical signs of an enlarged bladder.

follow the course of the spermatic cord down towards and eventually into the scrotum. *Direct herniae* bulge out medial to the inferior epigastric vessels, and very seldom end up in the scrotum. Of course some patients have sacs in both orifices—the so-called pantaloon herniae, and others have such huge swellings that until the hernia is

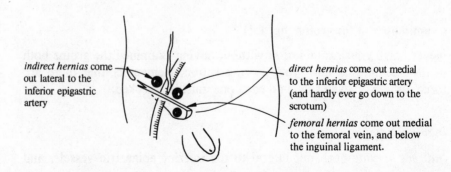

indirect hernias come out lateral to the inferior epigastric artery

direct hernias come out medial to the inferior epigastric artery (and hardly ever go down to the scrotum)

femoral hernias come out medial to the femoral vein, and below the inguinal ligament.

Fig. 1.5. Examination of the groins.

Chapter 1/Urological History

exposed at operation nobody can be sure exactly where the neck of the sac is situated.

Femoral herniae

Femoral herniae appear inferior to the inguinal ligament and, as they emerge, they bulge out through the defect in the deep fascia of the thigh through which passes the long saphenous vein to join the femoral vein. Once the femoral hernia has come out through this defect, it tends to ride upwards and laterally. Since a femoral hernia is nearly always surrounded, like an onion, by layer upon layer of fat, the lump often feels like a lipoma, and you may find it difficult if not impossible to feel any cough impulse or the gurgle of bowel. It should be enough for you to make a diagnosis of a femoral hernia if you find a 'lipoma' in the right position.

Saphena varix

A saphena varix is a dilatation of the junction of the long saphenous vein and the femoral vein. It is often quite large, and appears only when the patient is standing up. As a rule there are other varicose veins in the long saphenous system, but if these are not obvious, you may mistake the lump for a femoral hernia until you lie the patient down. When the man lies down the lump disappears entirely. It has a marked cough impulse.

The scrotum and its contents (fig. 1.6)

1 If there is a swelling in the scrotum your first step is to see if you can 'get above' it. If you can, it is in the testicle; if you cannot, then it is probably a hernia.
2 If you can get above it, the next step is to decide whether the lump is fluctuant or solid: if it is fluctuant then it is either a hydrocele or a collection of cysts of the epididymis.
3 Then determine where the testis is situated: if the testis is in front of the fluid-filled lump, it is a collection of cysts of the epididymis. If the testis is posterior to the swelling, or appears to be surrounded by it, it is a hydrocele.
4 If the lump is solid, determine whether it is in the epididymis or the testis. If it is in the epididymis, the swelling is almost certainly inflammatory, perhaps tuberculosis, more likely non-specific epididymitis. If the lump is in the testis it is probably a tumour, and malignant at that. If you are not sure, then it must be explored on that supposition.

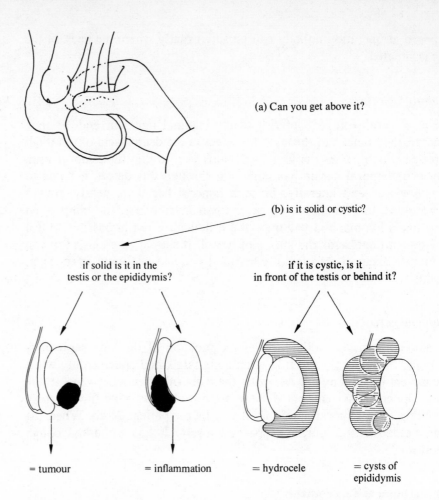

(a) Can you get above it?

(b) is it solid or cystic?

if solid is it in the testis or the epididymis?

if it is cystic, is it in front of the testis or behind it?

= tumour

= inflammation

= hydrocele

= cysts of epididymis

Fig. 1.6. The scrotum and its contents.

The spermatic cord (fig. 1.7)

A varicocele appears in the upright position, and feels like a 'bag of worms'. Like the reader, the author has never actually felt a bag of worms, but that does not stop this from being the most apt description of a varicocele. The swelling goes away when the patient lies down.

Swellings like knots, along the course of the vas deferens, may represent tuberculosis, and will be associated with a more or less craggy swelling of the epididymis.

Rectal examination (fig. 1.8)

The patient may be examined in the left or right lateral position, on his back with his legs parted or drawn up, or in a kneeling position. It is customary and probably most easy to perform it in the left lateral position with the knees drawn up, but not so tightly as to make the patient uncomfortable. Use a glove, and water-soluble lubricant so as not to leave grease on the patient's underwear. Insert your finger slowly and gently, and ask the patient to tell you if the examination is anything other than just unpleasant. It should not be painful.

Feel the wall of the rectum all round: remember that once or twice you will detect an unsuspected rectal cancer. Feel the prostate and the base of the bladder, but also remember that you cannot distinguish a small prostate with a bladder containing residual urine, from a large benign gland. Any swelling which is hard and craggy has a 50% chance of being a prostatic cancer. Try to estimate the size of the gland—expressing its weight in grams—the normal male has a gland about the size of half a spanish chestnut and weighs about 15 grams. Over the age of 50 most men have some benign nodular hyperplasia, and their prostate gland is correspondingly enlarged. This is seldom of any consequence (see Chapter 21).

FURTHER READING

BAILEY HAMILTON (1973) *Demonstrations of Physical Signs in Clinical Surgery*, 15th edn, ed. Clain A. Wright, Bristol.
BLANDY J.P. (ed.) (1976) *Urology*. Blackwell Scientific Publications, Oxford.
CAMPBELL M.F. & HARRISON J.H. (eds.) (1970) *Urology*, 3rd edn. Saunders, Philadelphia.
HENDRY W.F. (ed.) (1976) *Recent Advances in Urology—2*. Churchill Livingstone.
KIPLING M.D. (1976) Occupational considerations in carcinoma of the urogenital tract. *Brit. J. Hosp. Med.*, **15**, 465.
WILLIAMS D.I. & CHISHOLM G.D. (eds.) (1976) *Scientific Foundations of Urology*. Heinemann, London.

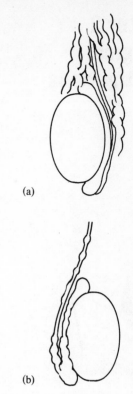

(a)

(b)

Fig. 1.7. The spermatic cord.

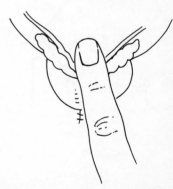

Fig. 1.8. Rectal examination allows you to feel the prostate, the seminal vesicles and the ampullae of the vasa. It also allows you to feel the base of the bladder.

Chapter 2
Urological Investigations

TESTING THE URINE

The appearance of the urine will reveal blood, clots and debris. Its smell may be very useful in detecting infection before the laboratory does. But certain routine tests are applied with which one should be familiar.

1. *pH*

Measured with pH paper or indicator on a test strip.

2. *Protein*

In urine within the normal pH range paper impregnated with bromphenol blue will go blue: protein alters this, causing it to go increasingly yellow. Very acid or very alkaline pH alters its usefulness, and an alternative screening method is the cloudy precipitate thrown down on adding 25% salicylsulphonic acid. If the urine is diluted, this may still fail to detect significant proteinuria. If there is doubt, have 24 hours' worth of urine measured for protein loss: anything more than 150 mgm per 24 hours demands further investigation.

3. *Reducing substances*

Stix tests which give colour reactions after specific enzymatic hydrolysis of glucose are available, and have replaced the use of Fehling's or Benedict's solution, when glucose and other reducing substances cause precipitation of varying amounts of orange copper oxide.

4. *Microscopic examination of the urinary sediment* (fig. 2.1)

Urate crystals are typically diamond shaped.

Pus cells are to be distinguished from red cells, and desquamated cancer cells. To isolate and identify cancer cells, the urine should be fixed with an equal volume of 10% formalin, before being centrifuged and then stained with the Papanicolaou method.

Casts are of two types: granular casts are formed from desquamation of cells lining the collecting tubules which are stuck together by protein. Hyaline casts appear when there is heavy loss of protein, and are extruded 'worms' of protein from the tubules. Heavy haematuria may similarly give red cell casts. To detect any of these it is

calcium oxalate

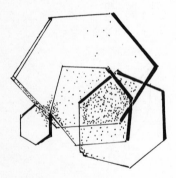

cystine

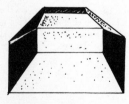

triple phosphate

Fig. 2.1. Shapes of crystals in the urinary sediment.

Chapter 2/*Urological Investigations*

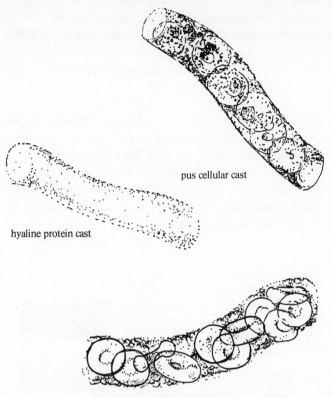

pus cellular cast

hyaline protein cast

red blood cell cast

Fig. 2.2. Casts from centrifuged urine.

important not to centrifuge the urine too rapidly or the casts may be broken up (fig. 2.2).

Ova of *Schistosoma haematobium* have a spine at one end of the egg: *S. mansoni* a spine at the side (fig. 2.3).

A gram film of the spun deposit is helpful in determining whether there are many bacteria present in the urine. If the deposit is stained with acid fuchsin, heated, washed with alcohol and acid, and counterstained with malachite green, tubercle bacilli retain the pink stain in their waxy cell membranes: this is the Ziehl–Neelsen test. Acid fast bacilli which are not *Mycobacterium tuberculosis* also occur from smegma and metal taps; do not accept the presence of AFB in the urine as proof of tuberculosis unsupported by other evidence.

BACTERIOLOGICAL EXAMINATION OF THE URINE

When urine is contaminated, from the skin of the penis or vulva, or from the air in the clinic, because it is a good culture medium, these

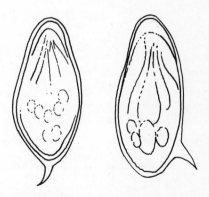

S. haematobium   S. mansoni

Fig. 2.3. Ova of Schistosoma.

contaminants will grow even at room temperature. Hence any specimen of urine to be examined bacteriologically must either be cultured at once, or put into a refrigerator (at 4°C) to inhibit multiplication of stray contaminants.

Immediate culture

A plastic slide or spoon coated with culture medium is dipped in the urine as soon as it has been voided. The spoon is put into an incubator then, or later on: a sample may even be sent through the mail to a laboratory. The slide read 12 hours later will give a sufficiently accurate idea of the numbers of colonies (i.e. the numbers of bacteria originally present in the urine) to indicate whether the urine was infected, or merely contaminated as it left the urethra (fig. 2.4).

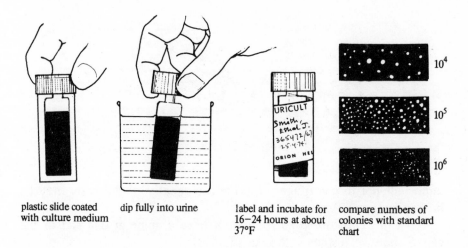

Fig. 2.4. Use of the dip inoculum slide.

plastic slide coated with culture medium

dip fully into urine

label and incubate for 16–24 hours at about 37°F

compare numbers of colonies with standard chart

In the laboratory the freshly voided urine, or the urine stored overnight in the refrigerator, is plated onto suitable media, using techniques which allow the numbers of bacterial colonies which subsequently grow to be accurately counted.

Quantitative examination of bacteriuria

It has been shown that contamination rarely yields a colony count of more than 10^5 colonies per ml, whereas true urinary infection yields a colony count which greatly exceeds this figure (fig. 2.5). Because of this, if the laboratory can provide even a semi-quantitative culture technique, there is seldom any need to obtain urine directly from the bladder.

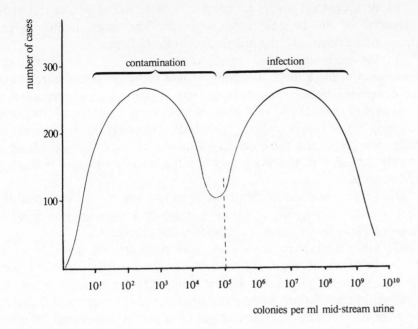

Fig. 2.5. Quantitative differences between urinary contamination and infection.

Bladder urine

Nevertheless occasions still crop up when it is necessary to get urine from the bladder. The traditional method used to be to introduce a catheter through the urethra into the bladder: but this carried the hazard of pushing organisms from the urethral mucus into the bladder, so that the test for diagnosis of infection may have caused it.

For this reason there are advantages in inserting a needle directly into the bladder just above the pubis. This may sound disagreeable, but it is virtually painless, and many patients prefer it to being catheterized. The skin is cleansed over the symphysis; a little local anaesthetic is inserted and a lumbar puncture needle is pushed downwards and backwards. Suprapubic aspiration should only be attempted when the bladder is known to be full.

RADIOLOGICAL EXAMINATIONS

Excretion urogram (the I.V.U.)

An intravenous injection of a solution of iodine-containing compound is given. The contrast medium is filtered in the glomerulus, concentrated in the renal tubule, and finally delivered through the pelvis and ureter to the bladder.

Modern contrast media all consist of three iodine atoms linked to variations of the benzoic acid molecule. The more iodine in the injection, the denser the shadow thrown in the radiograph.

In the beginning, when small doses of iodine were given, the delineation of the kidney collecting system depended upon secretion of the compound by the renal tubules, and in physiological discussion a good deal of controversy was concerned with the handling of 'diodrast' (an early iodine compound) by the tubule. Today far larger amounts of iodine are given, and the capacity of tubules to excrete the contrast is grossly exceeded, so that what gets into the urine has mainly reached it by filtration.

However, once the contrast medium has got past the glomerular filter, whether it is going to throw a dense or a pale shadow depends largely on how much water is absorbed in the tubule.

To make the tubular urine even more concentrated, one may assist the investigation by depriving the patient of water for 12 hours before the test. However, this is of marginal value; it is dangerous if applied to a patient in renal failure who cannot concentrate his urine, and it should never be accepted as an excuse to put off a pyelogram needed on other grounds.

There are two phases in the urogram which have special significance:

1. *Nephrogram* (fig. 2.6)

As soon as the first part of the injected contrast medium is carried from the vein, round the lungs, and down the aorta to the renal arteries, some of the contrast is immediately filtered off. At this stage one sees diffuse opacification of the parenchyma. The density of the nephrogram reflects the ability of the proximal tubule to reabsorb water. The early

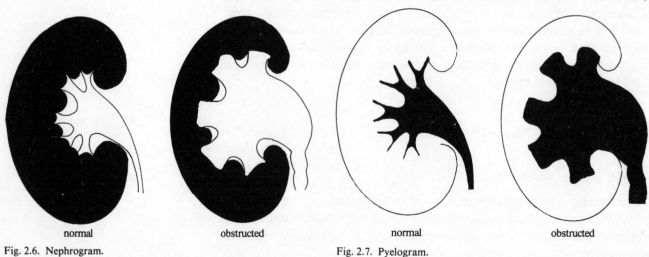

normal   obstructed   normal   obstructed

Fig. 2.6. Nephrogram.   Fig. 2.7. Pyelogram.

Chapter 2/*Urological Investigations*

nephrogram films are exceedingly useful: they show the outline of the parenchyma, and reveal scars and translucencies in its substance. Tomography—a method of producing 'slices' which are in focus, the remaining soft tissues being deliberately allowed to be blurred, is often used to supplement straightforward radiographs in the nephrogram phase.

In obstruction, there is persisting filtration combined with reabsorption of the filtered urine, so the nephrogram tends to persist even hours after the dye has been injected.

2. Pyelogram (fig. 2.7)

As the contrast enters and fills the calices and the renal pelvis, it gives useful information about their architecture and their function. The ureter is soon outlined from top to bottom, and finally the bladder. After the last radiograph—usually 25 minutes after injection—has been taken, the patient empties his bladder, and a further picture is taken which gives an accurate measurement of the quantity of residual urine remaining in the bladder.

DANGERS OF EXCRETION UROGRAPHY

Many patients get a feeling of nausea, and a few develop minor urticarial eruptions. Very occasionally (less than 1:100,000) the patient may develop severe laryngeal oedema, anaphylactic shock, and cardiac arrest. Unfortunately a history of hay fever or previous asthma is no guide to the incidence of either major or minor reactions: skin testing is useless, nor does the routine administration of antihistamines make any difference though it is customary to give them. In the event of a major reaction full resuscitative measures may save the patient.

If a patient has previously suffered a major reaction, he must not be given any more of the same contrast medium, and probably none of the other, closely related ones, since there is evidence that they cross-react.

Ureterography and retrograde pyelography

If a fine catheter is introduced through the bladder at cystoscopy, it can be passed without much difficulty up and through the ureteric orifice into the ureter, as high as the renal pelvis. Contrast medium may then be injected, which will delineate the pelvis in those cases where filtration or concentration of intravenous medium is for some reason particularly poor. For years it was customary to perform retrograde pyelograms on most kidney cases, because the pyelogram was so faint. Today, thanks to the use of large doses of the contrast medium, the definition afforded by retrograde pyelography is seldom any better than that which may be obtained by excretion urography save when the kidney function is seriously impaired.

However, the advent of the image intensifier has changed the situation, and the possibility of being able to watch the ascent of the contrast medium on the television monitor makes it much more easy to evaluate the motility of the ureter and to distinguish a carcinoma, say, from a radiolucent calculus in its lumen. To take most advantage of this new technique, a bulb-ended catheter is stuffed into the ureteric orifice at cystoscopy, and the contrast is injected up slowly, under the control of the image intensifier. Ureterography has virtually replaced retrograde pyelography in contemporary urological practice (fig. 2.8).

Cystography

Sodium iodide or intravenous contrast medium is instilled into the bladder through a catheter. Then films are taken in various ways, according to what diagnosis is suspected. In incontinence, special

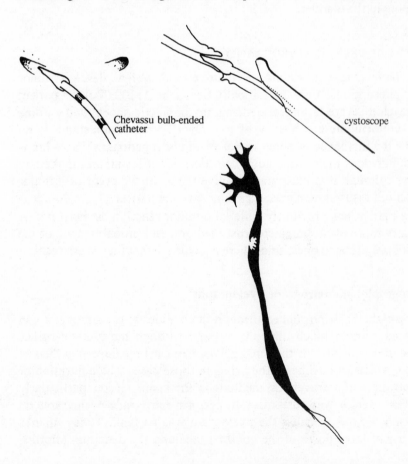

Chevassu bulb-ended catheter

cystoscope

Fig. 2.8. Ureterography using a bulb-ended catheter.

Chapter 2/*Urological Investigations*

attention is paid to the bladder outflow as the patient strains. In children with recurrent urinary infection, special attention is paid to whether or not the urine runs up the ureters towards the kidneys—vesicoureteric reflux. If the intention is to delineate a diverticulum in the bladder, the radiologist takes oblique films, and may introduce gas into the bladder in addition to contrast medium, to outline coexisting carcinoma of the lining of the diverticulum.

Urethrography

Viscous gel contrast medium is introduced through a conical rubber nozzle inserted into the penile meatus. Oblique and lateral films are taken to delineate strictures of the urethra.

Renal angiography

In patients thought to have stenosis of a renal artery, or patients found to have a soft-tissue mass in the renal parenchyma, more information is obtained by introducing a curved catheter (as used in cardiac catheterization) on a Seldinger wire, up and into the renal artery orifice. Contrast is then injected and a series of films rapidly exposed. The diagnosis may be helped by introducing very small amounts of nor-adrenaline just before the contrast is injected, since these have the effect of shrinking the vessels which go to the normal renal parenchyma, but not those belonging to a carcinoma.

Ultrasound

Sound waves emitted by a transducer at a very high frequency pass through the soft tissues of the body, like sonar or Asdic passing through the waters of the sea. If the sound waves strike an interface (like the surface of a submarine) they bounce back. These echoes are displayed on an oscilloscope whose image fades very slowly. Ultrasound can usually distinguish an echo-free fluid-filled cyst from a fleshy tumour which casts many echoes, but mistakes do occur, particularly from echoes in multilocular cysts (fig. 2.9—see over).

Lymphangiography

To find the lymphatics a little patent blue violet dye is injected intradermally into the first two web spaces of each foot. An hour later subcutaneous lymphatics can be seen as bright blue lines running up the foot, these are cut down upon and cannulated, and an oily contrast medium is injected over a long period of time. If a lymph node contains

ultrasound

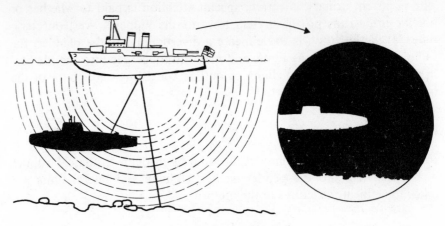

echoes detect submarine on ships Asdic

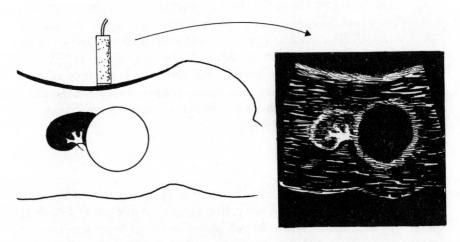

Fig. 2.9. Ultrasound.

renal cyst is seen in sonar scan as a trans-sonic mass without echoes

a metastatic deposit (fig. 2.10), there is a characteristic punched out filling defect: lymphangiography is used to assess the stage to which a testicular tumour has spread, and is being used increasingly in the assessment and staging of other cancers in the urinary tract.

CYSTOSCOPY AND URETHROSCOPY

Modern urological surgery really began with the electric cystoscope, an invention barely 70 years old. Essentially it is a long telescope and a light (fig. 2.11). The telescope which is used today owes its design to

Chapter 2/*Urological Investigations*

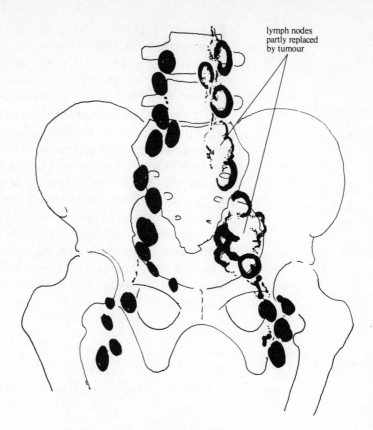

Fig. 2.10. Lymphangiography.

Fig. 2.11. (a) Conventional and (b) Hopkins' cystoscopes.

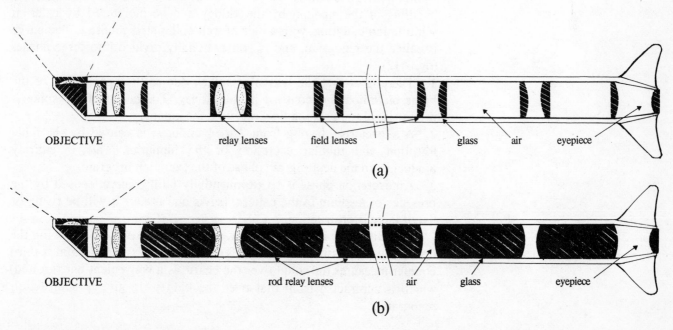

OBJECTIVE   relay lenses   field lenses   glass   air   eyepiece

(a)

OBJECTIVE   rod relay lenses   air   glass   eyepiece

(b)

Professor Hopkins of Reading University. Instead of a row of glass lenses in the tube, Hopkins uses air spaces, with glass rods as spacers. It is possible to mount and grind the ends of the glass rods with great precision, so the optical performance of a Hopkins telescope is similar to that of a first class microscope. For this reason, it is equally expensive, and must be handled with great care.

All the accessory equipment used in modern urological surgery is built up around the telescope and light: catheterizing slides permit the surgeon to pass a fine catheter up the ureters, or manipulate an electrode within the bladder to coagulate small tumours. Other modifications allow one to crush stones, cut tissues, take a biopsy, and perform the piecemeal removal of growths of the bladder or the prostate.

For the first half century the only way to illuminate the bladder was with a tiny filament bulb on the end of the cystoscope. Today the light source is kept outside the patient, and light fed down the instrument by fibres of glass, coated and bloomed to afford total internal reflection of light.

INVESTIGATIONS USING RADIOACTIVE ISOTOPES

The I^{131} hippuran renogram

If hippuran is labelled with I^{131}, which emits gamma radiation, the handling of the medium by the kidney can be monitored by external scintillation counting, with a pair of well-collimated counters. The curve is called the renogram, and is conventionally divided into three phases (fig. 2.12).

1   There is at first the 'vascular spike', due to the appearance of the bolus of radioactive contrast in the kidney. The height of the spike is proportional to the blood flow reaching the kidney.

2   A slower rise, lasting from 2 to 4 minutes, is caused by the local filtration and tubular excretion of the hippuran. This is entirely analogous to the nephrogram phase of the excretion urogram.

3   An excretion phase is an exponentially falling curve, caused by the presence of medium in the calices, pelvis and ureter. It will be rising or flat, if there is obstruction.

One difficulty in interpreting renograms has been to allow for the uptake by soft tissues of the loin. To allow for this background a third counter measures the count over the heart (as a convenient background) which is subtracted from that over the kidney, to give a 'subtraction renogram'.

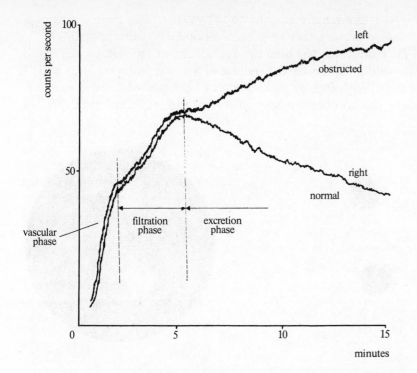

Fig. 2.12. Diagram of I^{131} hippuran renogram showing effect of obstruction on the
left side.

Wisely interpreted, and viewed against the other information which
is available, the radioactive renogram can be useful, especially when
there is doubt as to whether renal failure is caused by obstruction. The
reader should however be critical of some of the claims made for this
test, which in practice has a rather limited application.

In recent years other isotopes have however been found to give very
valuable information about the structure and function of the kidney.

Renal scanning

The structure of the kidneys may be studied using the relatively slow
scanning methods in which a collimated scintillation counter moves to
and fro over the kidneys, or using the gamma camera, whereby a battery
of little counters feeds a pointilliste picture to a television screen. By
means of these techniques one may get useful information about the
architecture of the kidney, if an isotope is given which is taken up by,
and lingers in, the renal tubules. Such isotopes are Hg^{197}-labelled-
radioactive chlormerodrin, which is bound to plasma proteins, and gets
held up in the distal tubules, and $Technetium^{99}$ -labelled iron-
ascorbic acid complex, which is partly filtered, but tends to be fixed in
the kidney. In time the use of these isotopes may spare patients the need

to undergo arteriography in order to tell whether they have a cyst or a tumour, but at present, they have been unreliable and disappointing.

Of far more value has been the application of the gamma camera to dynamic studies of the renal handling of various isotopes, such as I[131] Hippuran, which, often by making use of very sophisticated computers, may allow one to obtain measurements of the individual renal plasma flow.

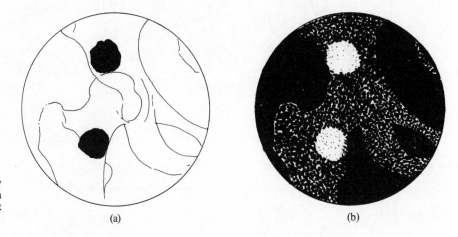

Fig. 2.13. (a) Radiograph reveals bony metastases. (b) Gamma camera reveals area of uptake of isotope by metastasis as 'hot spots'.

(a)   (b)

Bone scanning

The uptake by bony metastases of isotopes such as radioactive Technetium[99] or Fluorine[18] proves to be most useful in the detection of metastases of carcinoma of the prostate in bones which seem normal on radiology, picking up as many as one in four which would otherwise be missed.

RENAL FUNCTION TESTS

Glomerular filtration rate

Although inulin clearance is the ideal method, it is too time consuming to be of practical value. For clinical purposes endogenous *creatinine clearance* provides a sufficiently accurate method of measuring glomerular filtration rate, provided that a large volume of urine (i.e. 24 hours' output) is collected and measured accurately. The chief source of error arises from failure of collection of the whole of the 24-hour specimen. The plasma creatinine is measured at some convenient time during the period of urine collection. Clearance is given by the formula UV/P where U = urine creatinine mgm/100 ml, V = urine volume ml/minute and P = plasma creatinine mgm/100 ml, and is expressed in ml per minute.

^{51}Cr *EDTA clearance.* Ethylene diamine tetra acetate is handled like inulin, and entirely cleared by glomerular filtration. It is conveniently labelled with the radioactive isotope ^{51}Cr, and so its disappearance from the blood measures glomerular filtration without the necessity for collecting urine. This makes it particularly useful for measuring renal function in children and in adults with fistulae.

Tests of tubular function

Response to acid load mainly measures the function of the distal tubule. After taking two control collections of urine over a period of 2 hours, the patient is given 0.1 gram per Kg body weight of NH_4Cl in the form of gelatin capsules taken slowly with a litre of water over a period of one hour. An hour's collection of urine is taken 3 to 4 hours later. The healthy tubules should respond to this acid load by secreting urine with a pH less than 5.3, a titratable acidity more than 25 mEq/minute and ammonium more than 35 mEq/minute.

Urine concentration test. The normal kidney will respond to a period of water deprivation by secreting more concentrated urine, but since the response is mediated by the antidiuretic hormone, one can achieve the same result more simply, and without such discomfort for the patient, by giving him a dose of posterior pituitary extract containing the antidiuretic hormone. Ideally one would wish to measure the osmolality of the urine (reflecting the number of molecules per kilogram of urine) but in practice careful measurement of the specific gravity is sufficiently exact for clinical purposes. If the S.G. starts off greater than 1.018 then there is not likely to be much wrong with the patient's concentrating ability. The patient is given no fluid to drink after 6 p.m., an injection of pitressin tannate in oil (5 units subcutaneously) is given at 8 p.m. and the bladder emptied at 10 p.m. The specific gravity is measured on all samples of urine passed thereafter until 10 a.m. the following morning, by which time the test may be discontinued. Care is needed in making sure that the pitressin is all mixed up in the oil before injection.

FURTHER READING

ASSCHER A.W. (1976) The detection and natural history of urinary infection. *Urology*, ed. Blandy J.P., p. 167. Blackwell Scientific Publications, Oxford.
BARRATT T.M. (1976) Fundamentals of renal physiology. *Scientific Foundations of Urology*, eds. Williams D.I. and Chisholm G.D., p. 19. Heinemann, London.

BLACK D.A.K. (ed.) (1976) *Renal Disease*, 3rd edn. Blackwell Scientific Publications, Oxford.

BUCK A.C., CHISHOLM G.D., MERRICK M.V. & LAVENDER J.P. (1975) Serial Fluorine[18] bone scans in the follow-up of carcinoma of the prostate. *Brit. J. Urol.*, **47,** 287.

DAVIES E.R. (1976) Radioisotope studies of the kidney. *Urology*, ed. Blandy J.P., p. 117. Blackwell Scientific Publications, Oxford.

DE WARDENER H.E. (1973) *The Kidney*, 4th edn. Churchill Livingstone, Edinburgh.

GRAINGER R.G. (1975) Adverse reactions to radiological contrast media. *Proc. Roy. Soc. Med.*, **68,** 765.

GOW J.G. (1976) Urological Technology. *Urology*, ed. Blandy J.P., p. 3. Blackwell Scientific Publications, Oxford.

GOW J.G. (1976) The cystoscope. *Brit. J. Hosp. Med.*, **16,** 16.

HATELY W. (1976) Angiography, Sonography and Cyst Puncture. *Urology*, ed. Blandy J.P., p. 44. Blackwell Scientific Publications, Oxford.

JOEKES A.M. (1976) Investigation of the kidney: nuclear medical methods. *Scientific Foundations of Urology*, eds. Williams D.I. and Chisholm G.D., p. 39. Heinemann, London.

JONES N.F. (1975) *Recent Advances in Renal Disease*. 1. Churchill Livingstone, Edinburgh.

KERR, D.N.S. & DAVISON J.M. (1975) The assessment of renal function. *Brit. J. Hosp. Med.*, **14,** 360.

MITCHELL J.P. (1974) Optical Criteria of Urological Endoscopes. *Proc. Roy. Soc. Med.*, **67,** 803.

MITCHELL J.P. (1976) Endoscopes in Use. *Scientific Foundations of Urology*, eds. Williams D.I. and Chisholm G.D., p. 421. Heinemann, London.

SCHLEGEL J.U. & HAMWAY S.A. (1976) Individual renal plasma flow determination in 2 minutes. *J. Urol.*, **116,** 282.

SECKER-WALKER R.H. & COLEMAN R.E. (1976) Estimating relative renal function. *J. Urol.*, **115,** 621.

SHERWOOD T. (1976) Intravenous urography. *Urology*, ed. Blandy J.P., p. 31. Blackwell Scientific Publications, Oxford.

THOMPSON F.D. (1976) Investigation of the kidney: laboratory and biochemical tests. *Scientific Foundations of Urology*, eds. Williams D.I. and Chisholm G.D., p. 28. Heinemann, London.

The left kidney

1. POSTERIOR RELATIONS (fig. 3.1)

Behind the left kidney lies the 12th rib, diaphragm, pleura and the lower edge of the lung. The quadratus lumborum muscle spans the gap between rib and iliac crest, and medial to this is the psoas muscle covered with a tough layer of fascia, which takes origin from the tips of the transverse processes of the lumbar vertebrae.

2. ANTERIOR RELATIONS (fig. 3.2)

The kidney nestles behind the spleen and the tail of the pancreas, which can get damaged during a rough nephrectomy. In front of the kidney are the descending colon and splenic flexure, the fourth part of the duodenum and the duodenojejunal flexure. In exposing the kidney from the anterior approach, as is necessary for many tumours, these viscera must be mobilized and drawn medially (fig. 3.3).

3. MEDIAL RELATIONS

The aorta, and the adrenal.

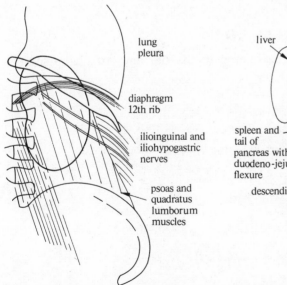

Fig. 3.1. Posterior relations of left kidney.   Fig. 3.2. Anterior relations of left kidney.

Chapter 3/*Kidney: Structure and Function*

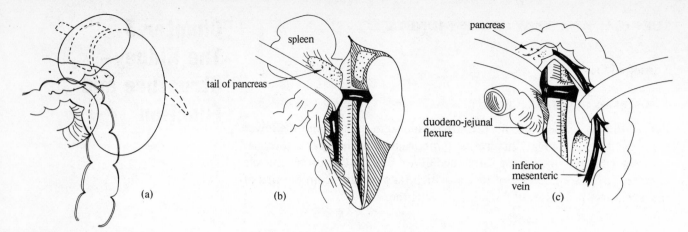

(a)

spleen

tail of pancreas

(b)

pancreas

duodeno-jejunal
flexure

inferior
mesenteric
vein

(c)

Fig. 3.3. (a) Anterior and medial relations of left kidney.

(b) Anterior surgical approach to the left kidney.

(c) Useful keyhole approach to left kidney when it is necessary to control the bleeding before you start to remove both the kidney and the colon in an invading carcinoma.

4. LATERAL RELATIONS

Quadratus lumborum and abdominal muscles.

The right kidney

1. POSTERIOR RELATIONS

Just the same as those on the left (fig. 3.4).

2. ANTERIOR RELATIONS (fig. 3.5)

On the right side the kidney is overlain by the ascending colon and hepatic flexure, and by the second part of the duodenum.

3. MEDIAL RELATIONS (figs 3.6, 3.7)

The duodenum used to be injured in the old days of clamp-and-cut

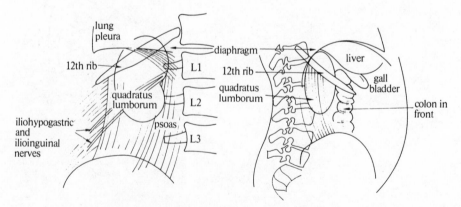

lung
pleura

12th rib

quadratus
lumborum

iliohypogastric
and
ilioinguinal
nerves

psoas

L1

L2

L3

diaphragm

12th rib

quadratus
lumborum

liver

gall
bladder

colon in
front

Fig. 3.4. Posterior relations of right kidney.

Fig. 3.5. Anterior relations of right kidney.

Chapter 3/*Kidney: Structure and Function*

nephrectomy, and duodenal fistulae were then, as now, lethal. At risk too was the inferior vena cava.

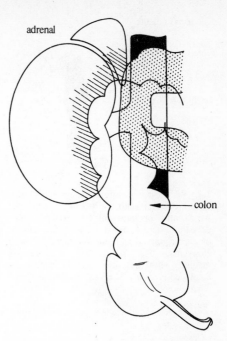

Fig. 3.6. Medial and anterior relations of the right kidney.

4. LATERAL RELATIONS

As for the left kidney.

There are certain tiresome facts about the gross anatomy of the kidney which determine how one approaches it in surgical operations.

1 The renal veins lie anterior to the arteries. This makes it more difficult when approaching a kidney from the front, since it is safer to ligate the artery first (because it curtails unnecessary loss of blood). To do this the vein must be carefully retracted and the artery underrun. For this reason many surgeons prefer to approach their renal cancers from behind.

2 The right renal vein is very short: this makes it dangerous when performing nephrectomy, since it is very easy to tear a long split in the side of the vena cava.

3 Note the nuisance of having the renal vessels coursing in front of the renal pelvis. This means that to get a large stone out, it is better to approach the renal pelvis from behind.

4 The proximity of the pleura and lung mean that they are easily cut or torn during the surgical approach to the kidney from behind.

Incisions used in approaching the kidney

A. ANTERIOR APPROACH (fig. 3.7)

Through a transverse muscle cutting abdominal wall incision, or a long midline or paramedian incision (according to the build of the patient), the peritoneum is opened. Then on the right side the ascending colon and duodenum are reflected medially, and on the left side, the descending colon and duodenojejunal flexure reflected medially.

B. LOIN INCISION (fig. 3.8)

Although there are numerous modifications of the lumbar approach, the incision the author uses as a routine strips the periosteum off the top and front of the 12th rib. The rib is pushed downwards, the peritoneum pushed forwards, and the pleura and diaphragm gently retracted upwards. Many surgeons resect the rib—but this is probably unnecessary nowadays.

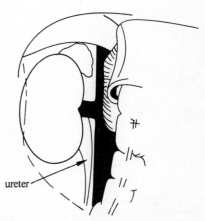

Fig. 3.7. The anterior approach to the kidney which is used in the removal of tumours.

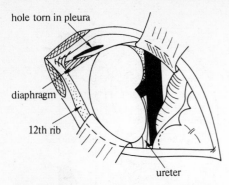

Fig. 3.8. Posterior surgical approach to the right kidney through the bed of the 12th rib, which may or may not be resected. Note how the pleura is easily torn—hence danger of post-operative pneumothorax, even empyema. The peritoneum is reflected medially with the colon, and the duodenum displaced medially to reveal the inferior vena cava.

For less extensive dissections, as used in operations to correct deformities at the pelviureteric junction, a similar anterior approach can be made without entering the peritoneal cavity, if the peritoneum is carefully stripped forward.

Complications common to operations on the kidney

Just as its surgical anatomy and relations determine how one can get to the kidney, so its position leads to certain common post-operative complications.

A. ATELECTASIS OF THE LUNG BASE

Because the incision injures the diaphragm, and because it hurts to cough, the patient tends not to expand the basal segments of his lung on the operated side: hence collapse, infection, and pneumonitis.

B. ILEUS

Because leakage of urine or blood into the retroperitoneal tissues occurs after many renal operations, it gives rise to temporary dilatation and disturbance of peristalsis—'paralytic ileus'.

MACROSCOPIC STRUCTURE OF THE KIDNEY (fig. 3.9)

Each kidney is made up of two elements: the nephrons, and the pelvicalicine collecting system. The nephrons together form the parenchyma, and are separated from the pelvis, except at the conical

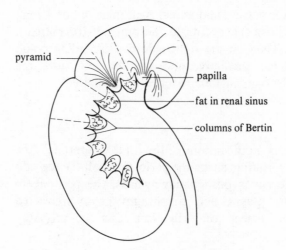

Fig. 3.9. Structure of the kidney.

Chapter 3/*Kidney: Structure and Function*

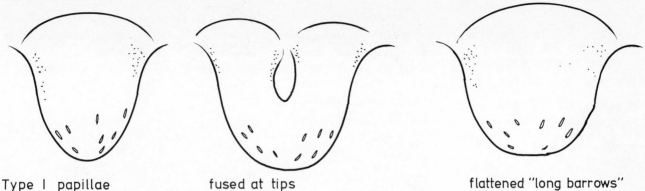

Type I papillae   fused at tips   flattened "long barrows"

entry of the collecting ducts in the renal papillae, by a plane of cleavage. This plane of cleavage can easily be opened up, and allows bloodless surgical access to the necks of the calices (p. 277).

Each papilla collects the urine from some 70,000 nephrons whose collecting tubules join up to form about eight 'ducts of Bellini' opening on to the cribriform area on the tip of the papilla. The way these ducts open on the papilla depends to some extent on the structure of the papilla, which may take the form of a conical nipple, or a pair of nipples joined together (Type I of Ransley, fig. 3.10). In this form all the ducts of Bellini are slit shaped and valvular, so that when the pressure rises inside the calix they are shut off, and urine does not get forced up the collecting ducts and threaten the parenchyma with an injection of urine or perhaps micro-organisms if the urine is infected. Sometimes the tip of the papilla forms the confluence of several papillae, and its cribriform area becomes cup-shaped as in Type II of Ransley (fig. 3.11) or in Type III where the fused papillae form a long hog's back ridge (fig. 3.12). If the ducts of Bellini open on to the hollow of the Type II volcano-shaped papilla or the flattened crest of the Type III ridge, they gape, and so when the pressure rises inside the pelvis, urine and infected material can run up into the parenchyma (fig. 3.13).

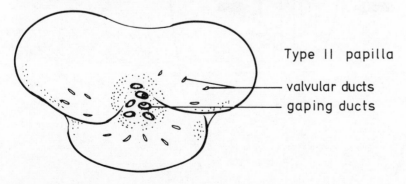

Type II papilla

— valvular ducts
— gaping ducts

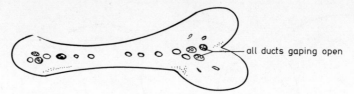

Type III ridge-shaped papillae

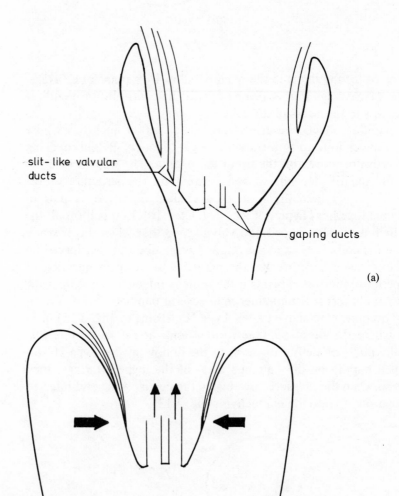

(a)

(b)

Fig. 3.13 (a & b). Showing how slit-like ducts opening on the side of the papilla are open under low pressure (a) and closed when pressure rises in calix (b).

Chapter 3/*Kidney: Structure and Function*

BLOOD SUPPLY

The renal artery on each side divides into a main anterior and posterior branch. The anterior branch then divides into four. The posterior branch supplies the middle part of the back of the kidney (fig. 3.14).

These renal arteries are end-arteries, and there are no anastomoses between them. Unfortunately the territory they supply does not correspond in any straightforward and easily understood way with the wedges of parenchyma drained by the individual papillae.

Any or either of these five renal arteries may come off the aorta directly, a situation which has given rise to the notion of 'aberrant renal arteries' (fig. 3.15).

In cases where there is an obstruction at the junction of the renal pelvis and the ureter, the bulging pelvis may balloon out in the gap between the main leash of renal arteries and the one going to the lower pole (fig. 3.16). Perhaps this artery may make things worse, perhaps not, but this is the origin of the idea that an 'aberrant lower pole artery' is the cause of idiopathic hydronephrosis. (This is one of those how-many-angels-can-stand-on-the-point-of-a-needle controversies which cause

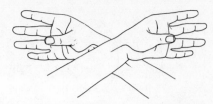

Fig. 3.14. To remember the branches of the renal arteries cross your hands in front of you: the thumbs remind you of the single posterior segmental branch, the four fingers represent the four main anterior segmental arteries.

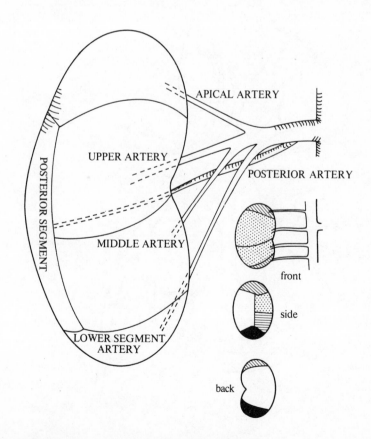

Fig. 3.15. Each of the renal arteries is an end-artery and there is no anastomosis between the territory supplied by each segmental artery. The main branches may come off the aorta separately.

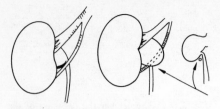

Fig. 3.16. If the lower segment (lower pole artery) branches off early it may kink the pelviureteric junction and cause or at least add to hydronephrosis.

folk to hold opinions with vehemence inversely proportional to evidence.)

Smaller branches of the renal arteries

The individual segmental arteries branch and rebranch within the kidney on their way to the cortex, but there is no anastomosis between the smaller branches of one segment and those of another. Here we encounter a very curious thing: textbook after textbook tells of 'arcuate' or 'arciform' arteries, as if these formed loops within the parenchyma at the junction between cortex and medulla. There are no such things. The finest endings of the segmental arteries end up between the individual 'corn-cobs' of glomeruli, and run peripherally to form so-called 'interlobular' arteries (fig. 3.17).

From these interlobular end branches of the segmental vessels individual arterioles pass to each glomerulus, entering the glomerulus as

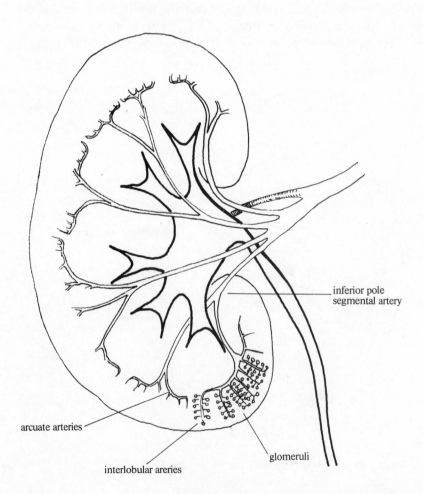

inferior pole segmental artery

arcuate arteries

interlobular areries

glomeruli

Fig. 3.17. Arrangement of the renal arteries.

Chapter 3/*Kidney: Structure and Function*

the afferent artery of the glomerulus, leaving its capillary cluster as the efferent arteriole of the glomerulus, and then breaking up into the capillary plexus which surrounds the proximal and distal convoluted tubules. Just before the efferent arteriole breaks up into this capillary plexus, if it belongs to centrally placed glomerulus which borders on the medulla, it gives off a straight branch which flows centrally, down towards the apex of the papilla, which is called the vas rectum.

In contrast to this pattern of end-arteries, the renal veins are formed in a series of intercommunicating arcades, with free anastomoses between them. These arcades are arranged like a perpendicular Gothic window in parallel systems, one on top of the other (fig. 3.18).

THE GLOMERULUS (fig. 3.19)

The entry of the afferent artery into the glomerulus has been the object of much study, and is rich in fascinating detail. Just before the afferent artery dives down into the glomerulus, one can identify in its wall certain smooth muscle cells with conspicuous cytoplasmic granules in them, which, from various lines of enquiry, seem to be the precursors of renin—these are the *juxtaglomerular cells.*

These special granular cells are in contact with the intima of the artery on one side, and their outer side touches the *macula densa*—the darkly staining segment where the ascending limb of the loop of Henle turns into the distal convoluted tubule.

Just exactly what goes on here is not precisely known: but there seems little doubt that the granular juxtaglomerular cells of the afferent arteriole, and the special length of tubule of the macula densa, work together, and so they are generally termed the '*juxtaglomerular apparatus*'.

One suggestion is that in circumstances where the blood pressure falls, or there is a diminution in blood volume, renin is secreted by the juxtaglomerular cells from their granules. Renin appears to be an enzyme which splits a plasma protein to form Angiotensin I, which in turn is modified (probably in the lung) to Angiotensin II. Angiotensin II makes the adrenal cortex secrete aldosterone and so increase tubular conservation of sodium, and at the same time angiotensin acts as a peripheral vasoconstrictor to keep up the blood pressure. The close proximity of JG cells and the critical macula densa on the gateway to the distal tubule suggests that there may well be a more direct, or 'backdoor' mechanism which achieves the same ends without so much confusion.

After it enters the glomerular capsule, the afferent arteriole splits up into the knot of capillaries which forms the glomerulus proper. These

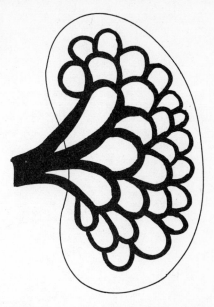

Fig. 3.18. Arcades of veins within the kidney (based on Graves (1971) *The Arterial Anatomy of the Kidney*).

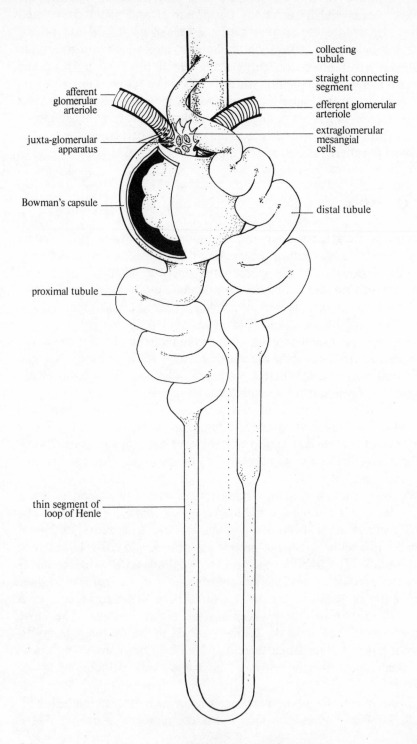

collecting tubule

straight connecting segment

afferent glomerular arteriole

efferent glomerular arteriole

extraglomerular mesangial cells

juxta-glomerular apparatus

Bowman's capsule

distal tubule

proximal tubule

thin segment of loop of Henle

Fig. 3.19. A nephron.

Chapter 3/*Kidney: Structure and Function*

are suspended, like a cherry on a stalk, within the capsule: the knot of capillaries is covered with a visceral layer of cells belonging to Bowman's capsule. Then there is a space, like a water jacket, separating the visceral layer from the parietal layer of cells which leads down to the proximal convoluted tubule.

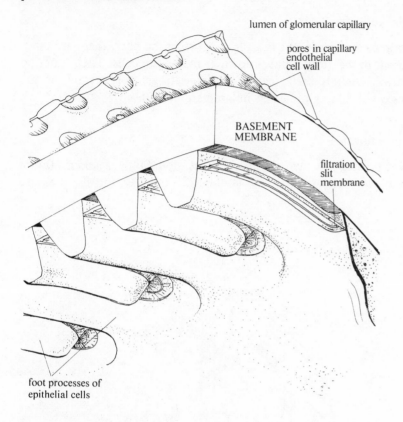

lumen of glomerular capillary

pores in capillary endothelial cell wall

BASEMENT MEMBRANE

filtration slit membrane

foot processes of epithelial cells

Fig. 3.20. Glomerular filter.

The glomerular filter (fig. 3.20)

The most interesting thing about the glomerulus is the structure of its filter. The filter proper is the *basement membrane*. This is made up of a feltwork of short filaments rather like filter paper. The filter is about 1200 Å in thickness. On either side, the filter is supported by a meshwork. On the capillary side, the endothelial cells are stamped with a regular pattern of circular dimples where the thickness of the endothelial cell is reduced to no more than 70 Å. On the Bowman's capsule side, the mesh which supports the filter is made up of interlacing struts, each with a wedge-shaped cross section. These struts are the so-called foot processes of the cells of Bowman's capsule. The foot processes of one cell fit between those of the next, like putting two combs together. The gap between one tooth and the next is about 400 Å.

These gaps are known as the 'slit pores'. It has been shown by studying the way peroxidases of known molecular size penetrate into Bowman's capsule, that these slit pores will let through protein molecules of about 40,000 mol. wt, but not those of 160,000 mol. wt.

Mesangial cells (fig. 3.21)

In addition to the two layers of cells supporting the filter, there are other cells present in the glomerulus, known as mesangial cells. Their function is unknown, though they seem to be the target for certain of the processes involved in glomerular inflammatory disease.

Glomerular filtrate

The blood pressure in the capillaries of the glomerulus is about 60 mm Hg. The plasma oncotic pressure is about 25 mm Hg and the pressure

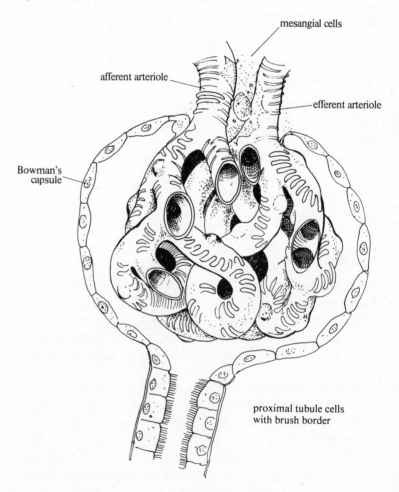

Fig. 3.21. Glomerulus

Chapter 3/*Kidney: Structure and Function*

inside Bowman's capsule about 10 mm Hg; hence there is a filtration pressure squeezing fluid out of the blood of about $60-(25+10)=25$ mm Hg. With the tremendous surface area of the basement membrane and its slit pores, it is not surprising that there is a large glomerular filtration rate, amounting to about 120 ml/minute, or 170 litres per 24 hours. The GFR is measured by the clearance of creatinine, which is not wholly accurate, since a trivial amount of creatinine is added to the urine in the tubules; by inulin clearance since inulin slips through the glomerular filter and is not subsequently reabsorbed; or by the rate of disappearance from the blood of filtered substances such as EDTA labelled with [51]Cr.

THE TUBULES (fig. 3.22)

Leading out of Bowman's capsule is the proximal convoluted tubule. This is made up of thick active cells, with interdigitating borders like pieces of a jig-saw puzzle, and a luminal surface raised to increase its surface area by innumerable long bristles like a brush. Rich in vacuoles and mitochondria, the cells of the proximal tubule show all the electron microscopical signs of active metabolic work. It is here in the proximal tubule that 80% of the filtered sodium in the glomerular filtrate is retained, and where 80% of the filtered water is sucked back.

The loop of Henle

Seven out of eight nephrons have only a very short loop of Henle, and it

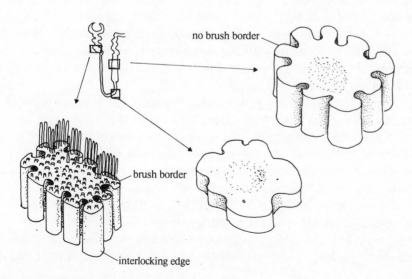

no brush border

brush border

interlocking edge

Fig. 3.22. The cells lining the proximal tubule have a brush border: those in the loop of Henle are flat and plain, and those in the distal loop thicker, but without a brush border.

is only the eighth, which belongs to the inner circle of glomeruli near the corticomedullary junction, which contributes the very long loop which dips like a hairpin right down into the renal papilla. Each loop of Henle is made up of two different kinds of cell: the descending loop is made of thin cells, the ascending part of thick cells. The thin cells seem to have a rather simple structure in electron micrographs which is in accord with the concept that in this part of the loop of Henle not much happens to the glomerular filtrate except that water and salt is withdrawn from it by osmosis, and the urine in the lumen becomes more concentrated.

The ascending limb of the loop of Henle, on the other hand, is made up of active, fat cells, with electron microscopic features suggesting much enzymatic activity. There is no brush border. The different histological structure of the distal convoluted tubule and the ascending loop of Henle may be related to their different physiological role. It is here—it is believed—that ion exchange is carried out, and sodium absorbed in exchange for potassium and hydrogen ions, a metabolic process calling for the expenditure of energy.

Collecting tubules

Finally the urine enters the collecting tubules through a short straight part of the distal convoluted tubule. The collecting tubule, the stalk of the corn-cob, becomes gradually wider in bore as it nears the renal papilla. Throughout its entire length it is lined by cuboidal epithelium, which becomes taller and more columnar near the papilla. This epithelium spreads out over the papilla itself, which is not lined by transitional epithelium, as is the rest of the renal pelvis and calices.

It is believed that these collecting ducts are influenced by pituitary antidiuretic hormone to become permeable to water, allowing it to escape from the lumen into the high osmolarity of the renal papilla. Hence water is absorbed and the urine becomes concentrated. Without the antidiuretic hormone's influence the collecting tubules appear to be waterproof, allowing no escape back of water from the urine which flows, dilute, into the renal pelvis.

The collecting tubules join together, within a few millimetres of the tips of each papilla, to form the larger ducts of Bellini which open on the cribriform area at the summit of the papilla. In addition to the bundles of collecting ducts, the papillae contain the hair-pin loops of Henle belonging to the innermost or 'juxtamedullary' glomeruli' and a very profuse and peculiar arrangement of blood vessels.

This complex arrangement is believed to have great importance in the so-called counter-current mechanism, by which the urine from the proximal tubule runs the gauntlet of an increasingly concentrated tissue osmolarity, losing water to the tissues, and becoming more concentrated, as a result of osmosis through the thin and functionless cells of the long loops of Henle. As the urine rises up in the active thick distal tubules sodium is actively pumped out of the urine. It is here that the most important metabolic work is done, and without this part of the kidney the glomerular filtrate cannot be adequately concentrated or acidified, nor sodium be conserved.

Such a mechanism is peculiarly vulnerable. Not only are physiological solutes excessively concentrated in the papillae, but so also may be toxic chemicals, for example phenacetin, which can injure the vasa recta, while an increase in pressure may squeeze the corkscrew-shaped arteries which supply the very tip of the papilla (fig. 3.23 below). Either process may cause the papilla ischaemic damage and result in necrosis. According to the prevailing counter-current hypothesis, the urine from the proximal tubule runs the gauntlet of this increasiongly concentrated tissue osmolarity, losing water to it, and becoming more concentrated itself, by simple osmosis through the thin and rather functionless descending loop of Henle. As the urine rises up in the thick, actively metabolizing loop of Henle and through the distal convoluted tubule, sodium is pumped out of the urine. It is here that the most important metabolic work is done to the urine, and here that the final processing of the urine is carried out. Without renal papillae, the glomerular filtrate leaves the proximal tubule dilute, rich in sodium, and unacidified.

In practical terms it is most important to note the importance of the renal papilla. It bears the brunt of urinary infection, it is atrophied in hydronephrosis, and it may slough right away as a result of chemical or therapeutic insults. Any kidney thus shorn of its papillae is functionally crippled.

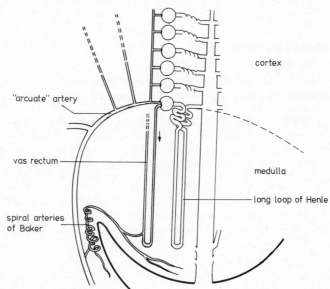

THE CALICES AND RENAL PELVIS (fig. 3.24)

The calix is made up of smooth muscle, and lined with the same urothelium (transitional cell epithelium) which lines the rest of the urinary tract from top to bottom. There is active contraction of the calix, and this active contraction is propagated down to the renal pelvis, and so down the ureter, in a series of peristaltic waves.

It is believed that the stimulus to this contraction is distension by urine. The contraction is of such a form that the urine is cut up into boluses, and fed down the urinary tract in a series of compartments. In diseases which result in dilatation of the calices to such an extent that their walls no longer touch each other, there can be no compartmentation of the urine, and no onward peristalsis. In such circumstances the force which carries the urine down to the bladder must be filtration pressure or gravity, not peristalsis.

The calices, pelvis, and ureter are part of the same collecting system. Its motility is thought to be governed not by ganglia or nerve cells, but by the interconnections between one smooth muscle cell and the next, which are rather like the connections which join one heart muscle cell to the next, and which were formerly thought to represent a syncytium. If ganglion blocking agents or adrenergic or cholinergic agents act on the smooth muscle of the pelvis or ureter at all (and it is doubtful if they do) their effect is probably mediated rather by the blood vessels to which the parasympathetic fibres run, than by any effect upon the muscle cells themselves.

Large veins and branches of the segmental arteries of the kidney are found in the sleeve of fat which surrounds the neck of the calix.

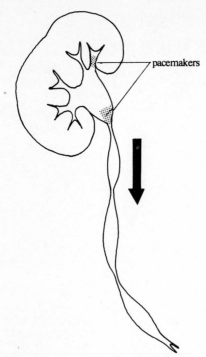

Fig. 3.24. Coordinated peristalsis passing discrete compartments full of urine down ureter.

FURTHER READING

BAKER S.B. DE C. (1959) The blood supply of the renal papilla. *Brit. J. Urol.*, **41,** 53.

BLOOM W. & FAWCETT D.W. (1968) *A textbook of Histology*, 9th edn. W. B. Saunders Co., Philadelphia.

GRAVES F.T. (1976) The kidney: the vascular tree. *Scientific Foundations of Urology*, eds. Williams D.I. and Chisholm G.D., p. 1. Heinemann, London.

NOTLEY R.G. (1976) Anatomy and physiology of the ureter. *Urology*, ed. Blandy J.P., p. 568. Blackwell Scientific Publications, Oxford.

RANSLEY P.G. (1976) The renal papilla and intrarenal reflux. *Scientific Foundations of Urology*, eds. Williams D.I. and Chisholm G.D., p. 79. Heinemann, London.

TIGHE J.R. (1976) The kidney: histology and ultrastructure. *Scientific Foundations of Urology*, eds. Williams D.I. and Chisholm G.D., p. 9. Heinemann, London.

WEISS R.M. (1976) Initiation and organisation of ureteral peristalsis. *Urological Survey*, **26.** 2.

EMBRYOLOGY

In primitive vertebrates, there is a set of nephrons to every somite of the body. One can conveniently regard them in three groups. Most cranial of all—the *pronephros* (fig. 4.1) never appears at any stage in man's embryological recapitulation of his pedigree. The next set, midway down the body, would, if it persisted in man, cause us to keep our kidneys in our chest; this is the *mesonephros*. It too disappears. It is only the most caudal group of nephrons of all which persists—the *metanephros*.

In the most primitive of our ancestors, each nephron emptied into a common drain, the Wolffian duct, which ran the whole length of the animal. We retain only the part of the duct belonging to the meso-nephros, which plays a key part in the elaboration of nephrons, somite by somite, and no duct means no kidney. One may encounter patients

Fig. 4.1. Embryological development of the kidney.

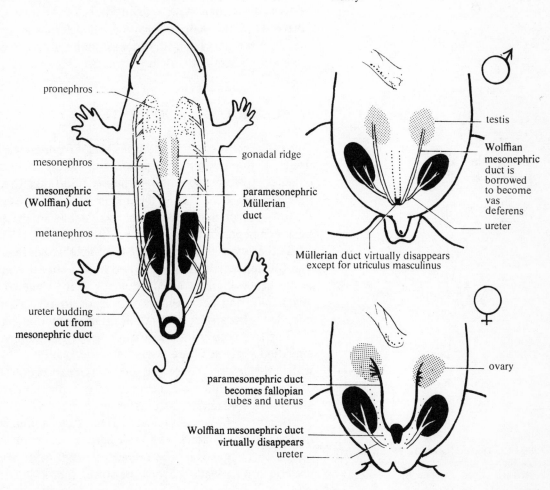

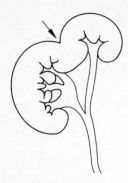

Fig. 4.2. Exaggerated column of Bertin (arrow). This gets mistaken for a renal tumour and may lead to unnecessary nephrectomy.

who have no identifiable renal tissue whatever on one side, presumably from failure of development of the mesonephric duct—(renal agenesis).

The second batch of tubules, the mesonephros, makes only a brief appearance in the embryo, and then vanishes, but not before it has led to the formation of an additional duct—the paramesonephric or Müllerian duct. This additional duct would be merely an embryological whim, were it not for the fact that later on it is borrowed by the gonad in the female to become the Fallopian tube. In males, all that one can find of the Müllerian paramesonephric duct is the little pit on the top of the verumontanum (sometimes glorified as the 'utriculus masculinus'), and a few tiresome little cysts which sometimes undergo torsion as they sit on the top of the testis or epididymis.

The kidneys proper arise from the most caudal group of nephrons, the *metanephros*. The large branch of the mesonephric Wolffian duct which drains them is retained as the ureter in both sexes. The rest of the mesonephric Wolffian duct is discarded in the female (except for tiny vestiges discernible with a strong light in the ovarian ligament)—but is borrowed by the male to form the vas deferens and seminal vesicle. It is therefore not surprising that occasionally a boy is born whose ureter is joined to his seminal vesicle.

DUPLEX KIDNEY AND URETER

One of the most common oddities arises from an 'early' branching of the ureter. If this occurs up near the kidney, one may see the two kidneys either completely separated, or nearly fused together. When nearly fused together this gives rise to the appearance of an exaggerated column of Bertin—a common appearance which has in the past led to many a mistaken nephrectomy for cancer. (fig. 4.2)

If the two half-kidneys are completely separated, one always finds that the upper half-kidney has two main caliceal elements, the lower one three: hence there is a tendency for more urine to be secreted by the lower half, and occasionally this leads to see-saw reflux distension or infection—because it does not drain properly (fig. 4.3).

The two ureters may fuse anywhere from kidney to bladder, or they may find their separate ways into the bladder. Owing to the way in which the lower end of the ureter is reabsorbed into the developing trigone of the bladder, the ureter from the uppermost half-kidney is always situated nearer the bladder neck (fig. 4.4).

Because of this, the lower ureter runs a longer course under the mucosa of the trigone, and may even be covered by a balloon-shaped dilatation of mucosa—the ureterocele (fig. 4.5). In contrast, the upper ureteric orifice leading from the lower half-kidney runs a short direct

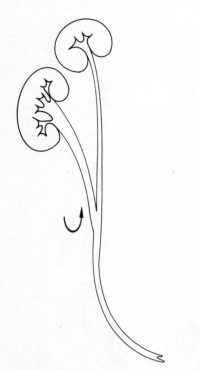

Fig. 4.3. Duplex. Rarely the urine runs from one limb up to the other and causes pain and persistent urinary infection.

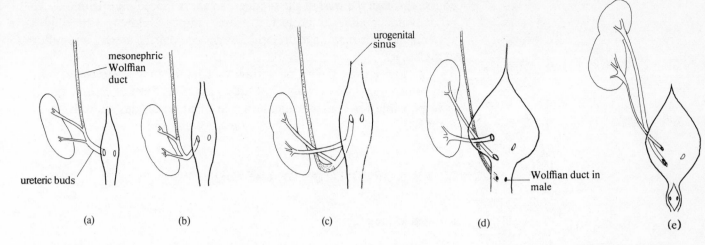

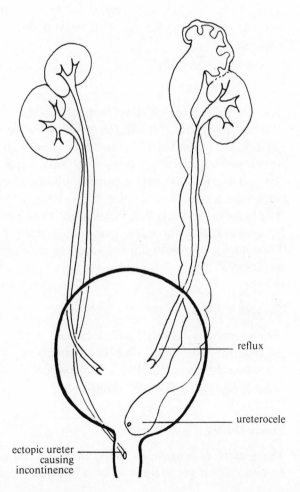

Fig. 4.4. (a) Ureters bud out from Wolffian duct.

(b) Note 'elbow' on Wolffian duct.

(c) As the urogenital sinus elongates, it loops up the Wolffian duct and ureters which now cross each other.

(d) Lateral expansion of the trigone incorporates the ends of the ureters.

(e) The kidneys now move upwards.

Fig. 4.5. Duplex with separate entry of the ureters. Note that the upper half-kidney always drains into the lower of the two ureteric orifices.

The short tunnel of the upper ureter leads to reflux to the lower half-kidney.

The lower ureter often ends in a ureterocele and is sometimes so low down that it enters in the vagina in girls or the prostatic urethra in boys.

course through the wall of the bladder, so short indeed that there may be no valvular action to protect it from reflux. Children with duplex systems like this may have ureteroceles on one pair of ureters and reflux in the other.

The lower ureter, with or without a complicating ureterocele, may also be taken up into the vagina of little girls. This form of ectopic ureter is responsible for constant incontinence of urine by day as well as by night.

ERRORS OF POSITION OF THE KIDNEY

Rotated kidney (fig. 4.6)

Not uncommonly one or other kidney sits in the loin facing forwards rather than sideways. It is not known why this comes about. The pyelogram will reveal a calix or two pointing medially, and not uncommonly the lower pole of each kidney is inclined towards the midline.

Horseshoe kidney (fig. 4.7)

The extreme form of this anomaly occurs when there is bilateral rotation of the kidneys, and the lower poles are fused together in front of the aorta. Associated with this 'horseshoe' kidney there are often other abnormalities, including congenital narrowing of the junction between the ureter and renal pelvis causing hydronephrosis. Hydronephrosis in horseshoe kidney has nothing to do with the isthmus between the two half-kidneys, and dividing the isthmus does not do anything to help the hydronephrosis. Horseshoe kidneys are easily palpable in the abdomen. They may give rise to difficulty during operations on the aorta, e.g. for aneurysms.

Ectopia (fig. 4.8)

If one kidney is entirely fused to the one on the opposite side, it is called *crossed renal ectopia*. This is a condition which is seldom of any consequence, except that in a slim patient the finding of an abdominal lump gives rise to consternation.

Pelvic kidney (fig. 4.9a)

The kidney is sometimes found in the pelvis or iliac fossa. Curiously seldom does it get in the way of a baby at childbirth and most mothers

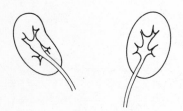
Fig. 4.6. Rotation of kidneys.

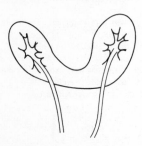
Fig. 4.7. Horseshoe kidney, a common oddity. Odd vessels may cause PUJ obstruction; the isthmus does not cause the obstruction.

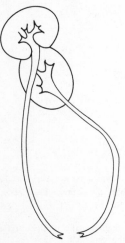
Fig. 4.8. Crossed renal ectopia, the so-called 'cake kidney' (gives rise to a confusing lump on abdominal palpation and surprise at laparotomy for the ignorant or the unwary).

with this anomaly can successfully get through a trial of labour. These pelvic kidneys are slightly more likely to become infected than normal ones, and if encountered at laparotomy by the unwary surgeon, they can turn out to be a very sanguinary pitfall. They get their five renal segmental arteries from the adjacent vessels—the bifurcation of the aorta and the common iliacs. There is seldom any need to meddle with them.

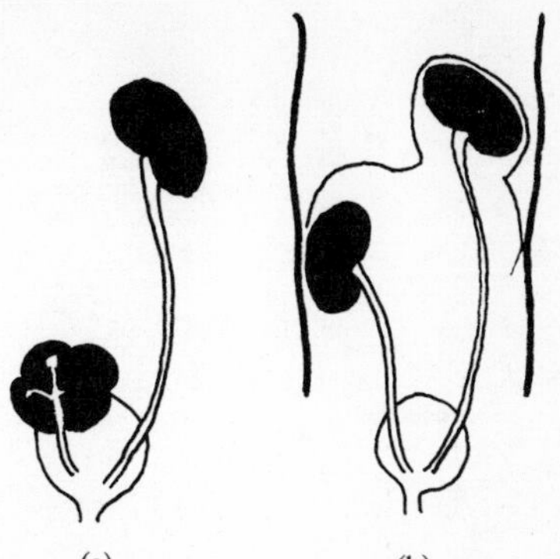

Thoracic kidney (fig. 4.9b)

In babies with a congenital diaphragmatic hernia the kidney may find its way into the chest along with other viscera. More rarely a thoracic kidney is picked up in a routine chest radiograph. The kidney is not really in the thorax, for it is always covered by a thin layer of eventrated diaphragm. Apart from its interest to collectors of surgical curiosities, it is of no importance, unless it gets explored by a surgeon who mistakes it for a tumour of the lung.

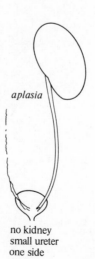

(a) (b)

Fig. 4.9 (a) Pelvic and (b) Thoracic kidney with eventration of diaphragm.

AGENESIS, APLASIA, DYSPLASIA AND HYPOPLASIA

If there is no mesonephric Wolffian duct, there is no trigone, no ureter, and no kidney on that side. It is not uncommon, is perfectly compatible with a normal life expectancy, and is called *agenesis* (fig. 4.10).

If the ureteric bud has started to develop, but the nephrons have not differentiated in the metanephros, one finds a trigone, and a ureteric orifice, but the ureter is usually very narrow, and ends in a little nubbin of tissue in which not a single glomerulus can be identified. This is called *aplasia* (fig. 4.11).

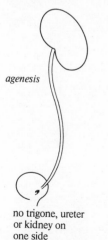

agenesis

no trigone, ureter
or kidney on
one side

Fig. 4.10. Agenesis.

aplasia

no kidney
small ureter
one side

Fig. 4.11. Aplasia.

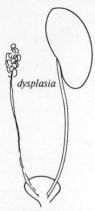

dysplasia

odd kidney
with cartilage
etc.

Fig. 4.12. Dysplasia.

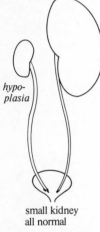

*hypo-
plasia*

small kidney
all normal

Fig. 4.13. Hypoplasia.

If the same thing occurs, but there is partial, or abnormal development of the renal tissue, the condition is called *dysplasia* (fig. 4.12): in the nubbin of tissue one finds a few nephrons, some odd tubules resembling vas deferens and epididymis, pieces of cartilage and sometimes bone. Numerous little cysts are common, and thought to represent secreting nephrons whose urine cannot get out.

Hypoplasia is a term to be wary of. It is defined as a small but normal kidney. Most of the kidneys put down as being hypoplastic are shrivelled up from scarring, or show evidence of dysplasia (fig. 4.13).

CYSTIC DISEASES OF THE KIDNEY

Cysts in the kidney are very common: hardly any elderly person's kidney is examined at post mortem without one or two little cysts being found. Attempts to attribute some simple embryological explanation to the different kinds of cysts which are encountered adds nothing but confusion to an already confused picture. The following represents a working classification.

Medullary sponge kidney (fig. 4.14)

In this condition the whole kidney may be affected, or only a part of it. It usually appears in young adult life, and gradually becomes more

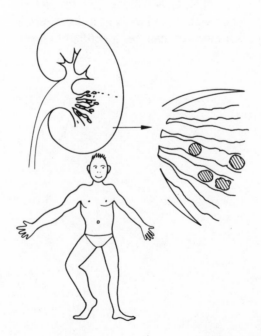

Fig. 4.14. *Medullary sponge kidney*. Congenital 'ectasis' of the collecting tubules which lead to stone formation. Eventually to renal failure. Associated with unilateral hemi-hypertrophy of the limbs—so ask about odd sizes of shoes and gloves!

Chapter 4/*Kidney: Congenital Disorders*

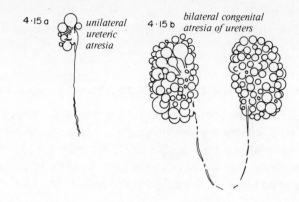

4.15a unilateral ureteric atresia

4.15b bilateral congenital atresia of ureters

Fig. 4.15 (a) Unilateral ureteric atresia. (b) Bilateral congenital atresia of ureters. Sometimes called 'congenital multicystic sponge kidneys'.

pronounced, and more complicated. Essentially the disorder is a dilatation of the collecting tubes within the renal papilla. The kidney (or its affected part) is swollen, because the medulla is distended owing to the dilatation of the ducts. The ducts become infected, and usually form multiple little calculi. These in turn lead to obstruction, and make matters even worse. The condition may be bilateral or unilateral, and is associated quite often with other anomalies, including hemihypertrophy of the body. So ask about odd sizes in shoes or gloves.

Cysts caused by obstruction

1. WITH CONGENITAL URETERIC DYSPLASIA (fig. 4.15)

In children with a narrow ill-formed ureter, there is often a collection of cysts in the dysplastic kidney tissue attached to it. These are thought to result from intrauterine functioning of obstructed nephrons. Rarely a child may be born with both ureters thus obstructed, and both kidneys converted into large sponge-like organs. Such children have never passed urine *in utero*, and so there is no amniotic fluid. Compressed against the uterus during his development the child's face has a flat nose and crumpled ears. The condition is not compatible with life. Other congenital abnormalities are also present. The kidneys show other evidence of dysplasia e.g. the presence of tissues such as cartilage.

2. DUE TO OBSTRUCTION OF THE CALIX (fig. 4.16)

If the calix alone is obstructed, either by scarring or from some disorder of motility about which one can only speculate, urine distends the calix

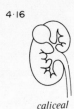

4·16

caliceal

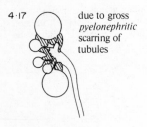

4·17   due to gross
pyelonephritic
scarring of
tubules

Figs. 4.16 and 4.17. Cysts caused by obstruction.

to form a cystic swelling. It is generally only noticed because of infection, or sometimes because stones form in the cyst. They occur at any age.

3. DUE TO SCARRING OF THE COLLECTING TUBULES (fig. 4.17)

A not uncommon consequence in the terminal stages of acquired scarring of a kidney by pyelonephritis, is the occlusion of collecting ducts in the scarred renal papillae or what remains of them. Proximal to these obstructed tubules large cysts may develop. In extreme cases the kidney may be mistaken for a polycystic or dysplastic kidney.

Cystic diverticula of the collecting ducts—'Polycystic disease' (fig. 4.18)

There are two, probably separate, entities here. A baby born with the Potter's facies and oligohydraminios may be found to have huge sponge-like kidneys. Cut section shows them to be composed of innumerable cysts, which microdissection proves to be formed from diverticula of the collecting ducts. Unfortunately other siblings may be affected too, and it is thought that the condition may be caused by a recessive gene, which is associated also with progressive fibrosis of the liver, coming on at a slightly later age.

The second form of the disease is the common adult '*polycystic disease*' which every medical student will undoubtedly encounter if not in the urological wards, then in his final examinations. Microdissection shows the cysts to be composed of diverticula of the collecting tubules. Family studies show that the disease is transmitted by a Mendelian dominant gene. It may show itself at different ages, but as a rule causes a palpable lump, or evidence of renal failure in middle life—about 45 to 50. Histologically the cysts are separated by what seems to be healthy renal parenchyma squashed thin (fig. 4.19). For a long time function remains reasonably good: eventually hypertension, uraemia, and

DIVERTICULA OF COLLECTING TUBULES

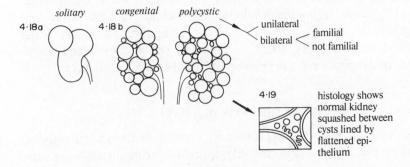

4·18a   *solitary*   4·18b   *congenital*   *polycystic*   unilateral
                                                                bilateral ⟨ familial
                                                                            not familial

4·19   histology shows
normal kidney
squashed between
cysts lined by
flattened epi-
thelium

Fig. 4.18. (a) and (b) Diverticula of collecting tubules.
Fig. 4.19. Histology shows normal kidney squashed between cysts lined by flattened epithelium.

Chapter 4/*Kidney: Congenital Disorders*

sometimes infection, supervene. These patients may have associated cystic changes in their liver and pancreas, and are prone to subarachnoid haemorrhage from berry aneurysms. They are of particular importance in modern urology since they have a very slow rate of deterioration, and form a most rewarding group of patients to be dealt with by dietary means, by dialysis, or ultimately by transplantation.

In former days it was the custom to pop these cysts at operation. Today this procedure (Rovsing's operation) is no longer performed except when the cysts are painful, become infected or occlude a renal calix, because it makes renal function if anything, worse

CONGENITAL DISORDERS OF THE RENAL TUBULES

Certain disorders of tubular function occur congenitally. It is convenient—if somewhat oversimple—to try to classify them according to the segment of tubule which is involved.

Proximal tubular disorders

1. CYSTINURIA

Here there is a defect in the transport of dibasic amino acids, lysine, ornithine, arginine and cystine across the proximal tubule as well as the small bowel. It is inherited as a Mendelian dominant, and there is an interesting quantitative relationship between the genetic pattern and the amount of cystine in the urine. If the gene is present in both chromosomes (homozygous) the patient may put out as much as 1000 mgm of cystine per 24 hours; if heterozygous, only half as much. Since cystine is virtually insoluble, stones readily form in the supersaturated urine. Penicillamine reacts with cysteine to form a soluble penicillamine-cysteine disulphide, and may be used to treat patients who cannot keep their cystine in solution by drinking enough water.

2. HARTNUP DISEASE

A whole group of amino acids are here involved in a similar transport defect in the proximal tubule and the jejunum. Dietary tryptophane is the most important item, since it is not absorbed, and the patient gets pellagra and cerebellar ataxia from deficiency of nicotinamide of which tryptophane is a precursor. It responds to a low protein diet and administration of oral neomycin, but unfortunately mental deficiency afflicts about a quarter of its sufferers.

3. FANCONI'S SYNDROME

Poor reabsorption of another group of amino acids, together with failure to reabsorb phosphate, and proximal tubular acidosis, goes along with proteinuria. Microdissection shows deformity of the proximal tubule.

4. PHOSPHATURIA

This disorder is sometimes called vitamin-D-resistant rickets. Something is wrong with the reabsorption of phosphate in the tubule, making these patients require enormous doses of vitamin D.

5. RENAL GLYCOSURIA

If the proximal tubules fail to reabsorb glucose from the glomerular filtrate glucose will appear in the urine even though the blood glucose is normal. Fortunately it seems to do no harm, but it must be distinguished from diabetes mellitus.

Distal tubular disorders

1. RENAL TUBULAR ACIDOSIS

Unable to pump out hydrogen ions in the distal tubule, the kidney cannot form an acid urine. In the presence of the resulting metabolic acidosis there is an increase in the amount of calcium not bound to protein, so more calcium gets into the glomerular filtrate, and because the urine remains alkaline, calcium salts are precipitated, leading to the appearance of speckled calcification in the renal medulla—'nephrocalcinosis'.

2. NEPHROGENIC DIABETES INSIPIDUS

Here something is wrong with the way in which the lining of the collecting tubule responds to the antidiuretic hormone, as a result of a sex-linked Mendelian recessive gene occurring in males. The ill effects are those of dehydration, which, unremedied, may lead to brain damage in the child.

FURTHER READING

DARMADY E.F., OFFER J. & WOODHOUSE M.A. (1970) Toxic metabolic defect in polycystic disease of the kidney. *Lancet*, **1**, 547.
DE WARDENER H.E. (1973) *The Kidney*, 4th edn. Churchill Livingstone, Edinburgh.

FINE H. & KEEN E.N. (1976) Some observations on the medulla of the kidney. *Brit. J. Urol.*, **48**, 161.

JOHNSTON J.H. (1976) Congenital anomalies of the Calices, pelvis and ureter. *Urology*, ed. Blandy J.F., p. 521. Blackwell Scientific Publications, Oxford.

JOHNSTON J.H. (1972) Problems in the diagnosis and management of ectopic ureters and ureteroceles. Chap. 2, *Problems of Paediatric Urology*, eds. Johnston J.H. and Scholtmeijer R.J. Excerpta Medica, Amsterdam.

JOHNSTON J.H. & GOODWIN W.E. (1975) *Reviews in Paediatric Urology*. Excerpta Medica, Amsterdam.

PITTS W.R. & MUECKE E.C. (1975) Horseshoe kidneys: a 40 year experience. *J. Urol.*, **113**, 743.

POTTER E.L. (1973) *Normal and abnormal development of the kidney*. Lloyd-Luke Medical Books, London.

RANSLEY P.G. (1976) The renal papilla and intrarenal reflux. *Scientific Foundations of Urology*, eds. Williams D.I. and Chisholm G.D., p. 79. Heinemann, London.

SPENCE H.M. & SINGLETON R. (1971) What is sponge kidney and where does it fit in the spectrum of cystic disorders? *Trans. Amer. Assoc. G.U. Surg.*, **63**, 37.

WATTS R.W.E. (1976) Xanthinuria and xanthine stone disease, and Cystinuria and cystine stone disease. *Scientific Foundations of Urology*, eds. Williams D.I. and Chisholm G.D., pp. 302 and 310.

ZELCH J., LALLI A.F., STEWART B.H. & DAUGHTRY J.D. (1976) Complications of renal cyst exploration versus renal mass aspiration. *Urology*, **7**, 244.

Chapter 5
The Kidney—
Trauma

CLASSIFICATION

Injuries of the kidney may be either open or closed.

Open injuries

These may be caused by bullet and other missile wounds, or penetrating wounds caused by a knife. In either case the surgeon will not be able to tell, from the situation of the entry wound, how much or how little damage has been done to the abdominal contents. The injury to the kidney will be detected in the course of the abdominal exploration. If possible, lacerations will be repaired, and detached portions of kidney removed. Today, with the extensive blast injury caused by very high velocity bullet injuries, if the kidney has been involved, the surgeon is virtually obliged to perform a nephrectomy, since the penalty for not doing so may be a massive secondary haemorrhage some days later.

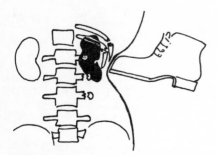

Fig. 5.1. Closed injuries to the kidney commonly also have fractures of lower ribs and lumbar transverse processes.

Closed injuries (fig. 5.1)

Whatever causes a closed injury of the kidney is likely to fracture the lower ribs or transverse processes on the same side, so that the lung and spleen (on the left side) and liver may be injured in the same accident. A common cause of closed injury of the kidney is sport, e.g. skiing or football. There is usually not much pain when the injury occurs, but later there is aching in the loin, pain on breathing and blood in the urine.

Pathology

The usual lesion is a split in the parenchyma (fig. 5.2), which enters one or two calices. Left to itself the bleeding soon stops and the kidney heals without appreciable scarring. Because it heals with a clot, and the clot may dissolve with urinary fibrinolysins, the patient should be considered at risk for a secondary haemorrhage.

If the injury fragments the kidney (fig. 5.3), and lacerates the renal artery, its branches, or the vein, the loss of blood may be exsanguinating. In such a case the initial injury which lacerated the artery may have caused its edges to retract and temporarily stop the bleeding. Hence the rule is to admit every such patient, in case of later, massive reactionary haemorrhage.

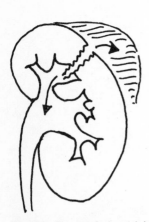

Fig. 5.2. The usual closed injury lesion is a split in the parenchyma, with a tear into a calix (which will heal perfectly well on its own). There is seldom much of a peri-renal haematoma.

CLINICAL FEATURES

Following the injury, there may be pleuritic pain, from the associated injury to the ribs.

Before long he notices blood in his urine. At this stage there may be no physical signs other than some local discomfort in the loin or lower chest. Every patient with this story must be admitted to hospital.

On admission a careful examination must be performed with a view to detecting other closed injury to the liver spleen or bowel. A radiograph of the chest will be taken as an emergency, as well as an excretion urogram. The purpose of the emergency IVP is to show whether or not the other kidney is all right, should an emergency operation become necessary later during the night on the injured side.

All specimens of urine will be saved for your inspection: most cases improve spontaneously over the 12 hours after admission, and the urine becomes progressively less bloodstained and the colour of the blood less fresh.

A pulse and blood pressure chart is kept at half-hour intervals to detect internal bleeding. The patient is re-examined from time to time with a view to detecting any swelling (due to haematoma) in the loin, or any evidence of adjacent visceral damage e.g. by the disappearance of bowel sounds.

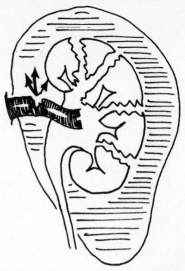

Fig. 5.3. If the injury fragments the kidney, there is often laceration of the renal vein or artery or both. Bleeding is profuse, but blood may be limited at first by the fascia of Gerota.

MANAGEMENT

Realizing that most of these injuries will be parenchymal lacerations which heal on their own, there are only two early indications for interfering:
1   if there is evidence of internal bleeding: e.g. a rise in pulse rate or fall in blood pressure, and/or an increasing swelling due to an enlarging haematoma in the loin;
2   if the patient becomes hypertensive.

If the patient develops either of these features, and if his general condition allows it, an angiogram should be performed, in order to determine with precision the nature and extent of the injury to the kidney, and allow the exploration to be planned in advance with due precautions. Of course, if the condition of the patient rapidly gets worse, there is no time for this delay and an operation must be done at once. Sometimes injection of fibrin or minced muscle into one of the bleeding injured vessels can stop the bleeding and save the need for an operation.

OPERATION FOR RUPTURED KIDNEY

The kidney is approached through the anterior transabdominal route, in order to allow control of the renal pedicle before the fascia of Gerota is opened and all the tense haematoma inside it spills out. Once haemorrhage is controlled, the fascia is opened, clot removed, and a decision made whether or not it is going to be possible to save all or part of the kidney. It is in a situation such as this that it is comforting for the surgeon to know that the other kidney is all right.

RECOVERY AND FOLLOW UP

Most cases get better simply with time and rest in bed. After two or three days hardly any bloodstaining remains in the urine. There is a temptation to send the patient home, but this should be avoided, for there is a risk that secondary haemorrhage with massive loss of blood may occur up to and after the tenth day. If the urine is infected, the appropriate antibiotic should be given.

In following up these patients three late sequelae need to be kept in mind.

1. Late renal artery stenosis (fig. 5.4)

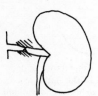

Fig. 5.4. Renal artery stenosis may follow scarring of small tears in the artery.

Delayed onset of hypertension has been recorded from time to time, and it is wise to determine the patient's blood pressure at intervals over the next few months.

2. Hydronephrosis (fig. 5.5)

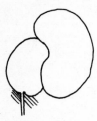

Fig. 5.5. Hydronephrosis may follow injury or be brought to light by it.

This may follow injury—or perhaps be brought to light because of the injury: in either event it may need to be treated on its own merit by means of an appropriate pyeloplasty.

3. Pseudocyst (fig. 5.6)

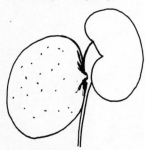

Fig. 5.6. A pseudocyst may be formed by a collection of urine which has leaked from a hole in the renal pelvis.

If there has been the collection of a large volume of extravasated urine around the kidney it may develop a thick fibrous wall, with a partly calcified shell, which may obstruct the ureter. This kind of pseudocyst can also displace and obstruct the colon or duodenum. It is not common.

For these two reasons the patient should be followed at intervals for the first year, with an excretion urogram at 1, 3 and 12 months.

FURTHER READING

ANGORN I.B. (1977) Segmental dearterialization in penetrating renal trauma. *Brit. J. Surg.*, **64,** 59.
COCKETT A.T.K., FRANK I.N., DAVIS R.S. & LINKE C.A. (1975) Recent advances in the diagnosis and management of blunt renal trauma. *J. Urol.*, **113,** 750.
PRYOR J.P. & WILLIAMS J.P. (1975) A study of 137 cases of renal trauma. *Brit. J. Urol.* **47,** 45.
WHITNEY R.F. & PETERSON N.E. (1976) Penetrating renal injuries. *Urology,* **7,** 7.

Chapter 5/*Kidney: Trauma*

GLOMERULONEPHRITIS

Although by tradition the diseases to be described in this section are called *glomerulonephritis* because the brunt and the distinctive features of the inflammation are seen in the glomerulus, it is probable that the entire nephron is involved. Nevertheless it is convenient and useful to think of them as being mainly diseases of the glomerulus. Today, thanks to electron microscopic study of these diseases, it is no longer possible to draw up a satisfactory classification, which does not have to be so hedged about with ifs and buts that it becomes almost incomprehensible. The following is an attempt to make an orderly scheme out of what is at present somewhat ill-understood: inevitably therefore, it is an oversimplification and almost certainly will in time be proved to be wrong.

Aetiology

Inherited predisposition may render some races more susceptible to certain antigens, or antigen–antibody complexes, and more resistant to others: e.g. the sickle-cell trait makes some Africans less likely to develop blackwater fever after malaria.

Pathology

At the risk of oversimplifying the causes of these diseases, it is possible to identify four pathological processes:

1 *Antibodies against basement membrane* are a very rare cause of glomerulonephritis, for example Goodpasture's syndrome (p. 61).

2 *Antigen–antibody soluble complexes* account for most forms of glomerulonephritis. They may be already attached to complement, or they may fix complement after they have got stuck in the filter, in which case an inflammatory reaction is set up to add to the damage (fig. 6.1). There are innumerable antigens which may be responsible.

3 *Vascular damage* may result from the action of certain antigen–antibody reactions, for example polyarteritis nodosa, serum sickness, allergy to butazolidine: here a dominant feature is the damage to the afferent arteries of the glomeruli which leads to infarction of the glomerular tuft.

4 *Infiltration* of the tissues of the glomerulus is seen in diabetes and in amyloid. In diabetes a hyaline material may involve the glomerular arteries in a diffuse way, or may be set down in irregular lumps within the glomerulus (Kimmelsteil and Wilson's disease).

In the first two of these disease processes, as the result of the appearance on the basement membrane of antigen–antibody complex, two types of reaction may occur. In the first, the lumps of complex get held up in the basement membrane filter, clogging it and destroying its efficiency. But in the second reaction, complement is fixed, attracts platelets, coagulates blood in the capillaries, liberates Factor XII, frees the kinins which increase vascular permeability and fibrinolysis, and summons white cells to the scene which digest the basement membrane and wreak havoc (fig. 6.1).

The antigens which have been incriminated as a cause of glomerulonephritis are legion: they include viruses, and bacteria notably streptococci, sometimes staphylococci, and occasionally

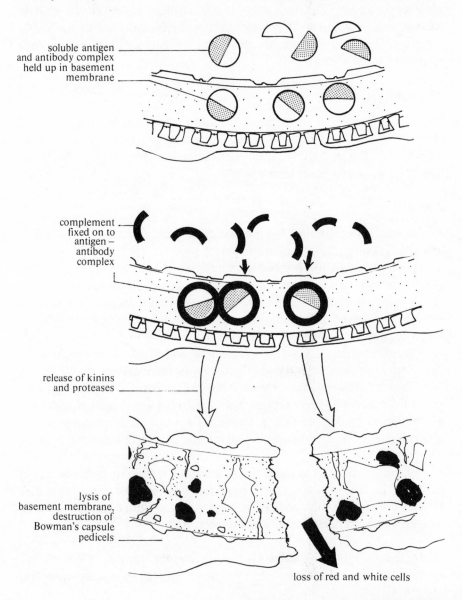

soluble antigen and antibody complex held up in basement membrane

complement fixed on to antigen – antibody complex

release of kinins and proteases

lysis of basement membrane, destruction of Bowman's capsule pedicels

loss of red and white cells

Fig. 6.1. Pathological processes of glomerulonephritis.

Chapter 6/*Kidney: Acute Inflammation*

Treponema pallidum. Protozoa include *Plasmodium malariae*; and even the worm *Schistosoma mansoni* can cause this pattern of disease. Indeed almost any allergen acting by itself or as a hapten will suffice: e.g. drugs such as tridione and penicillamine, pollen, bee-stings, poison ivy, butazolidine: the list is endless and growing. In systemic lupus even the patient's own DNA acts as an allergen.

The duration of the attack

It appears that many attacks are mild, evanescent, and succeeded as in other types of inflammation, by spontaneous and complete *resolution*. This is the state of affairs which occurs in most cases of 'acute nephritis'.

As in other inflammations however, it can continue if there is continual bombardment by antigen or antigen–antibody complex, or if the original attack damages enough basement membrane for this in turn to act as an antigen, and so set up a vicious cycle of autoimmune changes. In such circumstances the sequel of inflammation is *scarring*.

If either the first attack, or the later repeated attacks end up by damaging the arteries of the glomerulus, then *infarction* of the glomerulus will add its own measure of irreversible damage to the pathological picture.

Histopathological changes

1. THE 'MINIMAL LESION' (fig. 6.2)

To be truthful, there is no evidence at present to prove that this is an immunological disorder at all, though it ought to be. It occurs mainly in

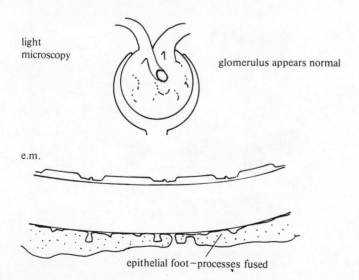

light microscopy

glomerulus appears normal

e.m.

epithelial foot–processes fused

Fig. 6.2. Minimal lesion glomerulonephritis. There is a loss of small protein molecules through the basement membrane and so a relatively greater loss of albumin than globulin, producing 'selective proteinuria'.

babies, and is characterized clinically by tremendous loss of protein across the filter. Light microscopy shows nothing amiss, but when the glomerulus is examined with the higher resolution of the electron microscope it is possible to see that the foot processes of the supporting grid of Bowman's capsule are congealed and fused together, as if to try to hold back the protein which is otherwise leaking through the filter. Functionally it is possible to detect this early damage to the filter, because albumen is retained, while globulin (which is a larger molecule), is held back, and the urinary albumen:globulin ratio is increased.

2. MEMBRANE GLOMERULONEPHRITIS (fig. 6.3)

Even by light microscopy it is now possible to discern damage to the glomerulus. The relatively enormous swelling of the basement membrane all but obliterates the lumen of the capillary. Under the electron microscope the thick, swollen, distorted filter membrane, now filled with irregular lumps and bumps of densely staining material, is obviously diseased. But still the damage is mainly limited to the filter and its supporting grid of Bowman's capsule, where the foot processes are fused and distorted. On the capillary side the endothelial cells appear as yet little affected.

But the severity of the damage is not only characterized by the poor state of the basement membrane: fibrosis all around the glomerulus shows that scarring has already begun.

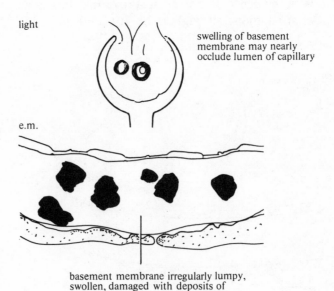

light

swelling of basement
membrane may nearly
occlude lumen of capillary

e.m.

basement membrane irregularly lumpy,
swollen, damaged with deposits of
soluble antigen–antibody complex

Fig. 6.3. Membranous glomerulonephritis—the filter is more damaged than in minimal lesion glomerulonephritis and larger molecules escape with greater globulin loss producing 'unselective proteinuria'.

The function of the glomerulus in membranous glomerulonephritis is even more severely damaged than in the minimal lesion illness: now the filter is so badly damaged that both albumen and globulin are lost in equal amounts, and the urine no longer contains a disproportion of albumen.

3. PROLIFERATIVE GLOMERULONEPHRITIS (fig. 6.4)

Here the difference is that the antigen-antibody complexes have fixed complement, and in addition to the damage brought about by the clogging effect of the complexes in the filter, there is the added damage brought about by the inflammatory process. Diapedesis of cells has led to an accumulation of debris within the space of Bowman's capsule: protein, white cells and red cells congregate together as 'crescents' more or less occluding the lumen of the capsule. Around the damaged glomerulus more and more fibrosis can be seen.

Clinical features

It would be very convenient if one could find a nice clinical syndrome to

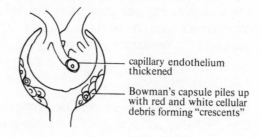

capillary endothelium thickened

Bowman's capsule piles up with red and white cellular debris forming "crescents"

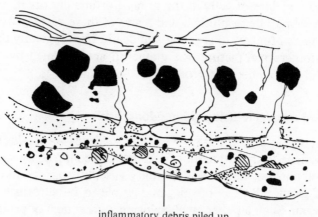

inflammatory debris piled up on Bowman's capsule cells

Fig. 6.4. Proliferative glomerulonephritis with all layers of the membrane damaged. The urine contains red and white cell casts and shows unselective proteinuria.

suit each of these histological patterns, but such is not the case. Nevertheless one can distinguish two main clinical syndromes:

1. THE NEPHROTIC SYNDROME

This results from damage to the filter. Protein and lipid pour out from the plasma. When the filter is minimally damaged, it is mainly albumen which is lost along with lipid. When the filter is more severely injured, the albumen and globulin are equally wasted. As a result of the loss of plasma proteins, the plasma oncotic pressure can no longer keep the plasma water within the vascular compartment, and oedema occurs in every tissue of the body (including the kidney) whence the old adage about the 'large pale kidney in the large pale child'. The tubules do their best to reabsorb the lipid which is leaking through the membrane along with the protein, and so there is hypercholesterolaemia, and in the kidneys one may see streaks of lipid in the parenchyma. The oedematous, swollen kidneys do not work well: there is uraemia, and some hypertension. In children this clinical picture is usually the result of the 'minimal lesion', from which the membrane usually makes a good recovery, and so the prognosis is excellent. In adults, the lesion in the membrane is usually caused by the lumps and bumps of antibody–antigen complex, and the outlook is not so good because sooner or later complement tends to be fixed, and the far more sinister state of affairs due to the inflammatory process may wreak havoc in the glomeruli.

2. ACUTE NEPHRITIS

This is much more dangerous. Antigen–antibody complexes in the filter are fixing complement. (The antigen is usually a streptococcal one.) With the attack of the inflammatory process upon the glomerulus there is hypertension, renal failure—even oliguria or anuria—haematuria and massive loss of cells in the urine. Fortunately (as in all inflammations) there may be resolution, and many of these cases get completely better. Others progress to scarring and death. Histologically there is always the 'proliferative' picture: the glomeruli are occupied by cellular crescents and surrounded by fibrosis.

End-stage sclerosing glomerulonephritis

At the end of the day, when the evidence as to the site of the initial damage to the glomerulus is hopelessly confused by subsequent scarring and fibrosis, and when secondary vasculitis has led to death and fibrosis of glomeruli, it is no longer possible to be sure just where the illness began. Such a patient will be losing a great deal of protein, and may also have developed hypertension. The entire kidney, scarred and contracted symmetrically, offers the histopathologist an impossible puzzle to unravel. This is end-stage kidney disease, and it is sometimes impossible to distinguish a hopelessly damaged kidney which has arrived at this stage because of immunological damage from one which has reached this stage in consequence of interstitial fibrosis secondary to bacterial inflammation.

It must be emphasized that the scheme set forth here is an oversimplification. The wise nephrologist who can assess both clinical features and microscopical evidence, comes to a reasonably accurate working diagnosis, and gives a reasonably accurate prognosis, even though the exact relationship between the histological and clinical changes remains a mystery. Some of these inflammatory processes can be halted or subdued by steroids: others are not improved at all. Much of the physician's skill depends on the pattern-recognition of certain clinical syndromes. Some of these should be noted.

Henoch–Schönlein purpura

Here there is a sudden onset of acute nephritis in a child with joint and abdominal pains, and perhaps gastro-intestinal bleeding. Microscopy shows proliferative changes, with cellular exudates and gross membrane damage: but despite this, the outlook is good in children though bad in adults.

Goodpasture's syndrome

Thought to be the result of a cross-reacting antigen common to the basement membrane of both the lung and the glomerulus, the patient develops a pulmonary infection, becomes sensitized to antigen liberated from the damaged lung, and his antibodies then attack his own glomerular membranes. A rapid and fatal glomerulonephritis follows.

Alport's syndrome

An autosomal dominant gene gives rise to a hereditary nephritis of uncertain cause: there is nerve deafness and proteinuria, with recurrent bouts of haematuria precipitated by infection and perhaps by diet.

SLE (systemic lupus erythematosus)

Ten times more common in women than in men, this autoimmune disease, in which the patient makes antibodies to her own cellular DNA, leads to renal damage in half the cases, thanks to deposition of the soluble complex on the filter. This usually gives rise to the nephrotic syndrome, and only rarely to an acute nephritis. Crescent formation may occur and there may be, in time, scarring and hyalinization of the glomeruli.

Diseases due to deposition of 'foreign' material in the kidney

DIABETES

In diabetes there are two elements of damage. The glomeruli are characteristically scarred, with marked vascular changes. In addition, there is a deposit of hyaline material in the mesangium and the basement membrane. Damage to the filter gives rise to the nephrotic syndrome, and the vascular damage leads to hypertension.

AMYLOIDOSIS

Usually this is a complication of chronic sepsis or rheumatoid arthritis. Some of the light-chain components of immunoglobulin are deposited in the tissues of the kidney, clogging the basement membrane, and causing loss of protein and the nephrotic syndrome.

BACTERIAL INFLAMMATION OF THE KIDNEY

Aetiology

Acute bacterial infection of the kidney is exceedingly common and very important, but is surrounded by unsolved problems. In the West, it attacks women many times more than men, affecting them at different ages: at the time girls first go to school (around 5 or 6); at the age of onset of menstruation (around 12 to 14); then at the age when intercourse begins (honeymoon cystitis); again it may plague them through their married life, or it may only attack them after childbirth. Finally, the woman who has escaped all these perils, may develop intractable urinary infection with the onset of the menopause. At all ages and in all sexes, infection in the kidney is specially apt to occur when the ureter has been obstructed on that side, or when there is reflux of urine from the bladder to the kidney. There is no doubt that some bacterial infection leads to the formation of interstitial scars in the kidney: but this is difficult to distinguish from the other causes of scarring which may give an identical appearance in the kidney. Infection is certainly one cause of 'pyelonephritis' but not the only cause.

Because of the suggestion that unchecked infection in the kidney in little girls may be followed by scarring if not prevented by chemotherapy, many areas have set up schemes for examining the urine of school girls in order to detect significant numbers of organisms (bacteriuria) in the urine before the child has any symptoms. It may well prove to be a useful measure of preventative medicine: but it is worth pointing out that, at the time of writing, it is no more than an unproven hypothesis. There is at least a possibility that other causes of scarring may act upon little girl's kidneys, and that by focusing our attention too much on the presence of infection in the urine we may be contemplating not the chicken, but the egg.

For in the last decade we have become more and more aware of these other influences which can damage the kidney, giving rise to scars in its parenchyma which are indistinguishable from scars produced by infection. Of these *analgesic overconsumption* is the most easy to detect, and is still grossly underdiagnosed. Being aware of the possibility of other causes of renal scarring means we ought always to wonder why the kidney has become infected, not merely what organism has taken up its temporary sojourn there; for most of the clinical, and all of the experimental evidence shows that organisms only take a hold in a kidney if it has been injured.

Pathology—1. Ascending infection

ORGANISMS

The common organisms which cause ascending pyelonephritis are *Escherichia coli*, *Klebsiella* species, or *Streptococcus faecalis*. If the patient has been in hospital, or has had a stone, *Proteus morgani* and *Pseudomonas pyocyanea* will be found, the latter the more often the patient has been given antibiotics.

It should be noted that these organisms are commonly found in the patient's own intestinal flora, and it has been shown that successive attacks of acute infection are due as often to attacks by new strains of organism as to recurrence of old strains.

ROUTE OF ENTRY OF INFECTION

Since the urethra opens into the unsterile vagina, which is populated by coliform organisms from the bowel, it seems likely that most infections in women occur by upward migration of faecal organisms into the urethra and bladder. Attempts to imitate this invasion by deliberately inoculating the trigone with organisms has always failed in the healthy volunteer. Here, as elsewhere in microbiology, there is always a disorder of the soil as well as of the seed. Why some women are more susceptible to recurrent infections is simply not known.

Examination of the bladder early in the disease is seldom performed (because it hurts) but if done, inadvertently, it shows oedema and inflammation of the lining urothelium (see page 169). Similarly, one must suppose that the lining of the ureter is usually involved, though for want of an appropriate endoscope, it is not examined.

In acute pyelonephritis the entire kidney is swollen, oedematous and painful (fig. 6.5). The pelvis is particularly oedematous, red and swollen, and histological features of acute inflammation are most marked in the renal pelvis, where the urothelium is oedematous and infiltrated with polymorphs. In the kidney itself there are more or less large wedge-shaped areas with oedema and white cell infiltration stretching out from the fornices of the calices into the parenchyma.

Functional changes in the acutely inflamed kidney are important, though one seldom measures them carefully. An excretion urogram will show the whole kidney to be enlarged in the nephrogram, oedema may obscure the edge of the psoas shadow, and the calices may seem thinner and more 'spidery' than normal, because of oedema of their lining urothelium.

The glomerular filtration is reduced on the acutely infected side, as is tubular function. Chlormerodrin may be taken up hardly at all on the acutely inflamed side. This is of importance when one is dealing with acute infection in a solitary kidney or a renal transplant, where infection may produce a reversible but frightening fall-off in renal function.

THE SEQUELAE OF ACUTE INFECTION

Acute inflammation in the kidney, as elsewhere in the body, may either *resolve* completely, or *suppurate*, or heal by *scarring*: in addition there may be *papillary necrosis* and *calculus* formation (fig. 6.6).

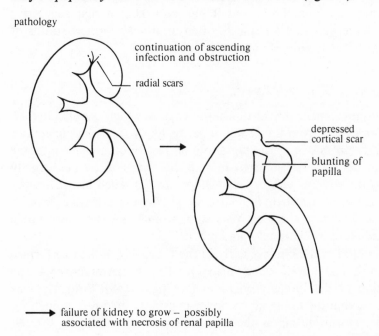

pathology

continuation of ascending infection and obstruction

radial scars

depressed cortical scar

blunting of papilla

failure of kidney to grow – possibly associated with necrosis of renal papilla

Fig. 6.5. Inflammatory changes in the kidney.

Chapter 6/*Kidney: Acute Inflammation*

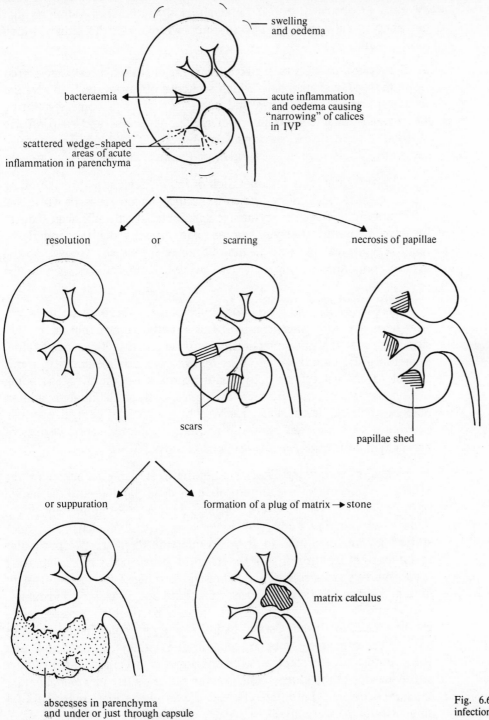

swelling
and oedema

bacteraemia

acute inflammation
and oedema causing
"narrowing" of calices
in IVP

scattered wedge-shaped
areas of acute
inflammation in parenchyma

resolution   or   scarring   necrosis of papillae

scars

papillae shed

or suppuration   formation of a plug of matrix → stone

matrix calculus

abscesses in parenchyma
and under or just through capsule

Fig. 6.6 The sequelae of acute bacterial
infection of the kidney.

1 *Resolution* is the rule in most cases of acute ascending pyelonephritis, where there is no continuing cause for the infection such as reflux or obstruction to the ureter or kidney. Neither radiologically, nor histologically can one see anything wrong with the kidney which has been affected.

2 If *suppuration* occurs, it takes the form of little abscesses scattered along the wedge-shaped area which stretches out from the fornix of the calix. Minute abscesses form and coalesce. If they become very large they extend out to the periphery of the kidney, raise and strip off the capsule, and form a subcapsular abscess. This may secondarily perforate and give rise to one form of perinephric abscess.

3 *Scarring* after acute inflammation of the kidney caused by ascending infection takes place along the same wedge-shaped areas in which the inflammation had been most intense. Characteristically the scar ends up by drawing in the overlying cortex, and drawing out the underlying renal papilla, leaving a pit in the outline of the kidney (shown on the nephrogram) and a dimple in the outline of the calix (shown in the pyelogram).

4 *Necrosis of the renal papilla.* Unfortunately the damage does not stop here. By what means is still not exactly known, but in certain situations scarring after infection leads to necrosis of the renal papilla. Sometimes the papilla quietly dies *in situ*: in other instances it seems almost to be cast off, as if by acute necrosis. Suppurative ascending pyelonephritis, as may be seen in the very ill or debilitated, and in diabetes mellitus, is typically followed by necrosis of several papillae. Section of such a kidney shows in addition to the red septic wedges of parenchymal infection, yellow necrosis of the papillae.

5 *Calculus formation.* The last aftermath of acute infection in the kidney is the result of shedding protein or dead papillae into the lumen of the collecting system, where it acts as a nucleus for stone deposition. Almost any foreign body will serve as a crystal nucleus, and once started, a stone continues to grow. In infection there are two particular and important features: first, if the infection is caused by a urea-splitting organism such as *Proteus*, the ammonia produced by metabolism of urea makes the pH rise, and causes precipitation of urinary phosphates on the nucleus already formed. Secondly, a particularly dense protein can be precipitated when certain bacterial antigens come in contact with antibodies formed by tubular cells in the kidney: these dense and virtually insoluble proteins are thrown down as a kind of glue-like cast of the interior of the kidney which serves as the matrix in which calcium salts are deposited. Fortunately stones are an uncommon aftermath of a single straightforward attack of urinary infection.

CLINICAL FEATURES

The red, oedematous, swollen kidney causes pain in the loin, which may be worse when the patient takes a deep breath or moves around. Palpation over the loin is uncomfortable. Fever is often high, and accompanied by rigors, indicating accompanying bacteraemia (which may be confirmed by blood culture).

Since many of these infections originate in the bladder, it is not uncommon for the patient to have associated symptoms of cystitis—though not always are these present. In children in particular, they seem to be often absent or unnoticed.

INVESTIGATION

In a condition which is so common, it is difficult to know where to draw the line between needless investigation of trivia and neglect of the important. Certain guidelines may be found helpful: first, all males with evidence of upper tract infection should be thoroughly investigated since the incidence of structural damage or underlying pathology is high in this group. In females, the third (and possibly the second) attack deserves to be investigated. Investigations will consist of meticulous quantitative microbiological investigation of the urine excretion urography: micturating cystography to rule out reflux in children: and—eventually—when the acute infection has died down, cystoscopy if there has been haematuria at any stage of the disease.

DIFFERENT DIAGNOSIS

Two common conditions pose a surgical difficulty: in children discomfort and tenderness in the right loin may closely imitate appendicitis: examination of the urine for pus cells is the most simple method of settling the matter, but it may still be wise to remove the appendix if there is any doubt. The penalty for leaving an acute appendix can be death.

In adult women acute salpingitis may be difficult to distinguish from pyelitis until the urine has been microscoped.

TREATMENT

Having obtained urine for culture and microscopy (see page 10) the patient should be put to bed and encouraged to drink a large amount of fluid. There is no special reason to prefer one form of water to another. (Traditionally barley water is given to most English women with pyelitis but there is no therapeutic reason behind it. The prescription probably antedates modern medicine by centuries, and is based on the magical idea that if it looks like infected urine it ought to do it good.)

The antibacterial substance most likely to be effective should then be given: nowadays most hospitalized patients are infected with organisms which are resistant to sulphonamides by themselves, so that ampicillin or trimethoprim-sulphonamide should be given.

When the patient is better, then he or she ought to be investigated on the lines described above.

RELAPSES

If the patient gets attack after attack without any good reason being discovered by routine investigations, the choice is between waiting for the next attack and treating it when it comes, or giving the patient a low dose of some suitable chemotherapeutic agent in the hope of preventing attacks. There is so far no evidence upon which to choose between these two alternative lines of treatment. In theory the former is more sound, since the strains which invade the urinary tract tend to be different ones, and there is no reason to suppose that a long-term low dose of nitrofurantoin or sulphonamide will deal with the next strain of organism even if it cured the first one. But in practice when attacks follow immediately upon discontinuing a course of antibiotics it is better to keep the patient on a low dose of medication for 6 to 12 months at a time.

At the same time there are certain measures which may be found useful. First, the patient ought to get into the habit of voiding often in order to keep the residual volume in the bladder as small as possible. If one thinks of the urinary tract rather like a dustbin, it is no good pouring lysol on top of the rubbish, when what is really necessary is for the bin to be emptied out.

If the patient is to get her bladder emptied out every 2 hours or so, it is necessary that she should drink an appropriately large amount of fluid. I do not believe it matters a jot what the fluid consists of so long as it is mainly water, and I see no reason why patients should not make it tea, coffee, soup or even beer (in moderation) if that is how they find their water tastes best. But the volume needs to be very considerable i.e. about a glass of water per hour.

If the attacks always follow sexual intercourse, there seems to be wisdom in the advice to the woman to empty her bladder afterwards (if she can remember to do so). Local antibiotic creams have been advised, but on no controlled evidence. A little tactful enquiry as to whether the parts are being adequately lubricated, and whether there is any possibility of an allergy to condom or contraceptive cap may also save a lot of worry. (Stinging after intercourse by no means always signifies infection.)

Chapter 6/*Kidney: Acute Inflammation*

Pathology—2. Haematogenous infection (fig. 6.7)

In the laboratory animal it is possible to produce all the features of 'ascending pyelonephritis' by giving the organisms intravenously, so long as the kidney itself has been traumatized or obstructed in some way.

In the human patient we sometimes can recognize acute haematogenous infection when it follows staphylococcal infection elsewhere, leading to staphylococcal bacteraemia which settles in the kidney; or in very debilitated patients such as drug addicts or patients on immunosuppressive therapy, where the organism responsible may be of an unusual type.

At first there are multiple embolic septicaemic abscesses scattered throughout the renal cortex just where one would expect them to form knowing the pattern of arterial blood supply to the kidney.

As a rule, in the patient who survives, most of these miliary abscesses heal up, and only one or two remain, grow, coalesce and enlarge. A feature of staphylococcal infection in the kidney (as in other situations) is its tendency to produce massive necrosis of tissue. Large areas of the cortex may slough, and here, as in the more classical subcutaneous infective sloughing which is the mark of the staphylococcal carbuncle, it is massive necrosis of tissue which makes renal carbuncle such a distinct entity.

Renal carbuncle

CLINICAL FEATURES

Today this is an uncommon condition, found among ill diabetics, or drug addicts who are debilitated and given to more or less dirty intravenous injections. There is toxaemia out of all proportion to the

Fig. 6.7. Haematogenous infection of the kidney.
    (a) Multiple embolic septicaemic abscesses scattered through the renal cortex.
    (b) Renal carbuncle
    (c) Peri-renal abscess

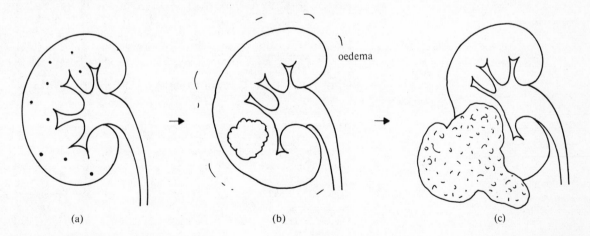

(a)   (b)   (c)

oedema

size of the local lesion. The kidney is tender and painful, and there may be local swelling. The urine is not infected because the organisms are in the cortex and away from the collecting system. The kidney is displaced by a soft tissue mass in the urogram, and the psoas muscle shadow is obscured by oedema. Often the lumbar spine is bent over by spasm.

Differential diagnosis has to be made nowadays from a tumour and is not easy, since most cases have received chemotherapy, often not for long enough or in high enough dosage to cure the infection, but just enough to make the diagnosis difficult. Hence the problem may be one of a patient with a soft tissue mass in the kidney with some inflammatory features. Since this is a well-known presentation of a carcinoma of the kidney, carcinoma is diagnosed.

The angiogram is said to be characteristic.

TREATMENT

If the diagnosis has been made correctly, then a high dose of antibiotics, given for a sufficient period of time, together with treatment of the underlying cause of debility (e.g. diabetes) will make the inflammatory mass resolve completely and the urogram return to normal.

There is seldom any need to drain the mass or remove it.

FURTHER READING

Glomerulonephritis
BLACK D.A.K. (1973) *Renal Disease*, 3rd edn. Blackwell Scientific Publications, Oxford.
CAMERON J.S. (1972) Bright's Disease Today—The pathogenesis and treatment of glomerulo-nephritis. *Brit. Med. J.*, **4**, 87, 160 and 217.
GLASGOW E.F., MONCRIEFF M.W. & WHITE R.H.R. (1970) Symptomless haematuria in childhood. *Brit. Med. J.*, **2**, 687.
Goodpasture's Syndrome (Editorial) (1970) *Lancet* Oct. 31, **2**, 916.
KINCAID-SMITH P., MATHEW T.H. & LOVELL BECKER E. (1973) (eds.) *Glomerulonephritis: Morphology, Natural History and Treatment*. Wiley, New York.
PETERS D.K. (1973) The immunological basis of nephritis. *Brit. J. Hosp. Med.*, **9**, 63.
Prognosis and pathology in acute glomerulonephritis. (Editorial) (1974) *Lancet* **1**, 787.
STRAUSS M.B. & WELT L.G. (1972) (eds.) *Diseases of the Kidney*, 2nd edn. Little Brown and Co., Massachusetts.
WHITE R.H.R. (1970) Glomerulonephritis in children. *Brit. J. Hosp. Med.*, **3**, 746.

Bacterial infections
ASSCHER A.W. (1976) The natural history of urinary infection Chap. 9, *Urology*, ed. Blandy J.P. Blackwell Scientific Publications, Oxford.
Bacteraemic shock. (Editorial) (1974) *Lancet* Feb. 23, **1**, 296.
DODGE W.F., WEST E.F. & TRAVIS L.B. (1974) Bacteriuria in schoolchildren. *Amer. J. Dis. Child*, **127**, 364.
KUNIN C.M. (1975) New developments in the diagnosis and management of urinary tract infection. *J. Urol.*, **113**, 585.
LEWIS J.G. (1972) Gram-negative bacteraemia. *Brit. J. Hosp. Med.*, **8**, 308.

MARSH F.P. (1976) Natural and therapeutic defences against urinary infection. Chap. 10, *Urology*, ed. Blandy J.P. Blackwell Scientific Publications, Oxford.

PARKER J., & KUNIN C. (1973) Pyelonephritis in young women: a 10 to 20 year follow up. *J. Amer. Med. Ass.*, **224,** 585.

Carbuncle

CRAVEN J.D., HARDY B., STANLEY P., ORECKLIN J.R. & GOODWIN W.E. (1974) Acute renal carbuncle: the importance of preoperative angiography. *J. Urol.*, **111,** 727.

GADRINAB N.M., LOMA L.G. & PRESMAN D. (1973) Renal abscess: role of renal arteriography. *Urology*, **2,** 39.

Chapter 7
The Kidney—Chronic Inflammation

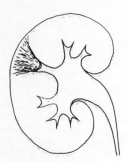

Fig. 7.1. Wedge-shaped scars of pyelo-nephritis.

INTERSTITIAL NEPHRITIS—PYELONEPHRITIS (fig. 7.1)

At the time of writing we are in a quandary. We know that following acute pyelonephritis caused by bacteria the wedge-shaped areas of acute septic infection in the kidney may heal by characteristic wedge-shaped scars, and sometimes these scars are accompanied by sloughing of the renal papilla. Unfortunately an identical end-result occurs after a host of other conditions which we know about, and possibly an even larger list of aetiological agents about which we are still ignorant. Obstruction alone may cause these changes: so many analgesic overconsumption though we do not know for sure whether it is the aspirin, phenacetin, or codeine which is the culprit—or perhaps all three. The list of causes of 'interstitial nephritis'—i.e. wedge-shaped scarring, is legion. Since it is seldom that we find a patient who has not taken some analgesics as well as having some infection, and since we know that infection is apt to occur in a kidney already damaged by interstitial scarring, we ought to be asking ourselves in any given case—Are we dealing with the cause or the effect?

Table 7.1. Causes of chronic pyelonephritis, interstitial nephritis, and papillary necrosis

Mechanical
    obstruction*
Vascular
    hypertension
    diffuse intravascular coagulation
    result of acute tubular necrosis
    old age
    anoxaemia*
Physical
    radiotherapy
Metabolic
    diabetes*
    nephrocalcinosis
    potassium depletion
    hyperuricaemia
    choline deficiency
    hyperphosphataemia
    sickle cell anaemia*
Infective
    leptospirosis
    bacterial infection*
Drugs and toxins
    sulphonamides
    analgesics*
    anticonvulsants
    balkan nephropathy*
    lead
    cadmium

* = known cause of papillary necrosis as well as interstitial scarring.

Bacterial chronic pyelonephritis

Clinical information suggests that this is an illness with its onset in childhood, seen more often in girls than boys and often associated with dysplasia in the kidney parenchyma, and reflux or ectopia affecting the ureters. *Reflux* of uninfected urine by itself seems seldom to lead to scarring in the child's kidney, and infection in the urine in the absence of reflux or obstruction seems equally innocuous. The combination of reflux or obstruction with an infected urine causes havoc in the kidney. In the child one not only finds the typical depressed cortical scar and punched out papilla, but there may be failure of the kidney to grow, as judged by nephrograms taken year after year.

In the adult, we see a similar picture appearing for the first time very seldom, unless the patient has recently undergone obstruction to the ureter. A calculus passing down the ureter, especially if the urine has become infected, may leave in its wake a seriously scarred and contracted kidney. A rather similar picture occurs as a sequel of pregnancy, and although there is still a good deal of argument as to exactly what the agent is which causes ureteric obstruction in pregnancy—whether the engorged ovarian veins squash the ureter, or whether the baby butts it with its head against the rim of the

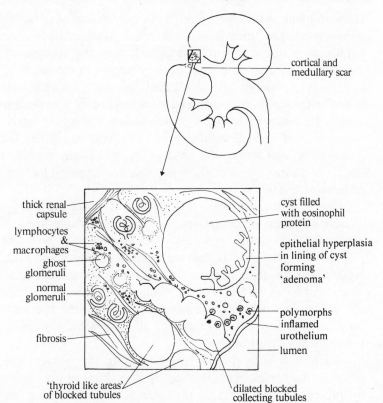

Fig. 7.2. Pyelonephritis—diagram of histological changes.

pelvis—there is no doubt that ureters do get obstructed in pregnancy, especially the right one, and if infection complicates the picture the kidney may be badly damaged as a result.

Once the kidney has developed scars, the process may be self perpetuating. The reason is found in the histology of the damaged kidney (fig. 7.2). Not only is scar tissue deposited in the radiating streaks from papilla to capsule, but this scar tissue obstructs, distorts, and obliterates some of the collecting tubules, which become distended and full of inspissated debris. Sometimes this clear eosinophil material looks like thyroid colloid, and these areas have been likened to the thyroid. There is little doubt that these obstructed scarred zones in the kidney parenchyma harbour organisms, so that relapse of infection is common.

Again, once scarring has occurred in the kidney, it is often accompanied by formation of stones in the calices or renal pelvis. These stones harbour organisms, and are coated with a 'butter' of slime which is full of bacteria. It is small wonder that it is virtually impossible to eradicate infection from a kidney which bears scars or stones.

Papillary necrosis (fig. 7.3)

Hand-in-hand with whatever it is which causes scarring in the parenchyma goes necrosis of the renal papilla. Sometimes the renal papilla becomes completely detached, and the slough, at a line of demarcation, passes down the urinary stream to get stuck in the ureter. Here it gives rise to all the clinical features of a calculus: i.e. colic, pyrexia (if there is infection), and hydronephrosis. The dead papillae can usually be removed with a Dormia basket, when they have the typical appearance of a bit of yellowish jelly. In Australia where the condition is common, and where the oysters are somewhat smaller than those from Colchester, the sloughed papillae are known to every urological resident as 'oysters'.

One of the most important causes of renal papillary necrosis is overconsumption of analgesics. In Sweden a whole town developed a craze for analgesic powders; in Switzerland watch-makers eat phenacetin-containing tablets to keep their sweating fingers dry; in Australia ladies pass round analgesic tablets with their morning coffee as a social habit. In England the public are inundated by promised cures for colds, lumbago, indigestion, and hangover; the advertisements promise 'fast fast fast pain relief'; slow slow slow papillary necrosis would be more truthful.

Analgesics give rise to two lesions in the kidney: the first is a lesion in the cortex accompanied by interstitial fibrosis and manifested by proteinuria. In the second, there is a lesion in the renal papilla

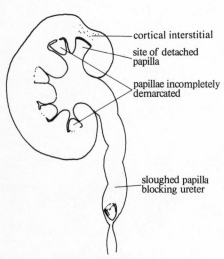

cortical interstitial

site of detached papilla

papillae incompletely demarcated

sloughed papilla blocking ureter

Fig. 7.3. Papillary necrosis.

Chapter 7/*Kidney: Chronic Inflammation*

which takes a wide spectrum of forms from deposition of calcium near the tip of the papilla to frank sloughing.

Hypertension follows in a proportion of these patients: the sloughed papillae may form the nidus for subsequent calculus formation: bacterial infection follows almost inevitably sooner or later: and worst of all, there is evidence that those who suffer from papillary changes have an increased risk of urothelial cancer.

CHRONIC GRANULOMATA OF THE KIDNEY

Far the most important of these is *tuberculosis*, which still gives rise to a steady toll of new patients even in the advanced countries of the West, while in underdeveloped areas tuberculosis causes disease in upwards of three million people every year. Of these about 2 or 3% will develop tuberculosis in the urinary tract. It is a curious paradox that in Britain, while tuberculosis of the lungs continues to wane year by year, the notification of new cases of tuberculosis of the genitourinary tract remains virtually unchanged in the last 30 years. It arises secondarily to blood-borne infection from a distant focus, often in the lungs, sometimes in the bone. Any age may be affected.

In Britain today the infecting organism is usually the human strain of *Mycobacterium tuberculosis*.

Pathology

Miliary tubercles form after blood-borne spread, and affect both kidneys in the peripheral cortex. Of the many tiny abscesses which form, most heal up completely, and very often one kidney only is left with a localized focus (fig. 7.4).

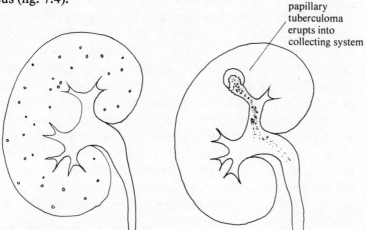

papillary tuberculoma erupts into collecting system

Fig. 7.4. Miliary spread of tuberculosis to kidney.
Fig. 7.5. Papillary tuberculoma erupts into collecting system.

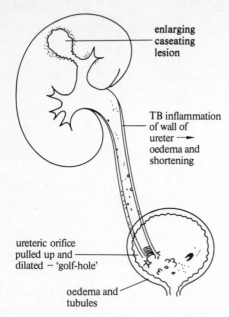

enlarging
caseating
lesion

TB inflammation
of wall of
ureter →
oedema and
shortening

ureteric orifice
pulled up and
dilated – 'golf-hole'

oedema and
tubules

Fig. 7.6. Tuberculous granuloma spreads
down ureter to bladder.

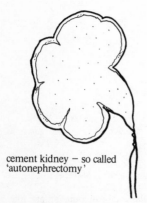

cement kidney – so called
'autonephrectomy'

Fig. 7.7. Late stage.

The small cortical tubercle grows, and eventually bursts into a papilla, discharging its contents into the calix and down the collecting system (fig. 7.5).

Progressing, the infection now involves the wall of the calix and pelvis, the ureter, and the bladder, at first causing superficial inflammation and oedema, later leading to more deep seated granulomata, with ulceration, caseation and fibrosis (fig. 7.6).

In the kidney, if the disease is unchecked, it slowly spreads through the renal cortex, until the entire kidney is replaced by a caseating bag, partly calcified and functionless, but not sterile. The wall of the 'cement kidney' still contains viable organisms. (fig. 7.7).

Clinical features

1   It may be entirely symptomless, the kidney quietly becoming calcified and replaced without giving rise to local pain or urinary symptoms.

2   The typical early case is seen at the stage when the papillary abscess has discharged its contents into the collecting system. Pus and debris pass down the ureter. Inflammatory oedema has affected the ureter and the urothelium of the bladder, and the symptoms are those of increased frequency and discomfort on voiding. There may be haematuria from the granulations in the eroded calix.

At this stage one has no other infecting organisms in the urine, so there is no reason for it to alter its pH. Pus is present in quantities, but the urine is sterile on routine culture. Hence the adage that there is 'sterile pyuria in an acid urine'.

There are two other common causes for sterile pyuria: the first is a bladder carcinoma, the other a treated cystitis. When there is the least doubt a cystoscopy ought to be done to exclude the former.

3   The late case. Here the tubercles have involved the wall of the ureter, making it thickened, oedematous, and shorter. The ureteric orifice is as if pulled up from outside, giving a curious appearance, likened to a golf-hole, in the bladder. The bladder wall is also involved, and may show tubercles, ulcers, or generalized redness and oedema. Because its wall is oedematous and inflamed, its capacity seems to be reduced. Now the patient complains of intense frequency, passing small volumes of urine at a time with discomfort whenever the bladder is full. Urography shows more or less calcification, due to the caseation up in the kidneys, the ureter is straight and may be dilated from fibrosis here and there, and the bladder wall is spherical and small. The urine teems with pus cells, and acid-fast bacilli may be found in them with the Ziehl–Neelsen stain.

Investigations

The most important single test is to culture the tubercle bacilli. This is most easily done by examining a series—at least three, preferably six—early morning specimens of urine. The freshly voided urine is centrifuged, and cultured on Loewenstein–Jensen medium, a culture medium containing a detergent which inhibits the growth of *Escherichia coli* and other contaminants. If positive, the slope will show tubercle bacilli after two to three weeks. A negative result is declared if no growth occurs after six.

Guinea pig inoculation is a valuable adjunct to the L–J culture but, because of the hazards it entails for laboratory staff, is rarely used unless there is some specific need for it.

Demonstration of acid-fast bacilli in the urine by the ZN stain (see page 11) is helpful, but not conclusive, unless confirmed by culture of *M. tuberculosis*.

Urography

In the earliest stages there may be little to see. A fleck or two of calcification near a renal papilla, and the tell-tale erosion of its tip, may be all that one can find. It is at this stage that one wants to make the diagnosis, for at this stage, with treatment, one can expect a complete cure (fig. 7.8).

Later on there will be more obvious patches of calcified caseation up in the kidneys, and more obvious erosions and deformities of the calices. A note of caution must be raised here: Africans rarely calcify their tuberculous lesions and you may be badly misled in interpreting an African patient's radiograph if you are relying on calcification. It is not known why this is so: African patients are relatively immune from renal calculi, and the two phenomena may be related.

Cystoscopy

Although one should expect to see miliary tubercles under the mucosa (and one may see them from time to time) most of the speckles which resemble tubercles turn out to be collections of sub-urothelial lymphocytes, which occur in any non-specific form of cystitis.

Ulcers occur late in the disease. Aggregations of oedema which resemble papillomata occur around the ureter, and sometimes in the vault of the bladder. These must always be biopsied as must any 'tumour' in the bladder. They will be shown to be simply chronic inflammation. True tubercles may be found and resemble tiny furuncles.

On the whole the findings on cystoscopy are not helpful: the entire

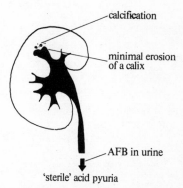

calcification

minimal erosion of a calix

AFB in urine

'sterile' acid pyuria

Fig. 7.8. When TB ought to be diagnosed.

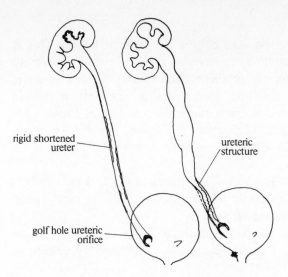

rigid shortened
ureter

ureteric
structure

golf hole ureteric
orifice

Fig. 7.9. Involvement of ureter

bladder as a rule is red and oedematous. If the ureter is drawn up and rigid—the 'golf-hole' sign—the diagnosis may be assisted (fig. 7.9).

At cystoscopy it sometimes speeds things up if a ureteric catheter is put up the suspected ureter. The fluid obtained from the kidney on that side should be examined for acid-fast bacilli, cultured and, if possible, injected into a guinea pig.

Treatment

All surgical treatment is deferred until the patient has had at least 6 weeks of anti-tuberculous therapy, and no anti-tuberculous chemotherapy is given until the diagnosis has been established by culture of the tubercle bacilli.

The standard therapy over the last decade has been:

Streptomycin 1 gm IM
Isoniazid 300 mgm orally   } Daily
Para-amino-salicyclic acid 12–15 gm orally

This 'triple therapy' was given for 3 months, after which the streptomycin was stopped, and the other two continued every day until two years had passed by.

More recently newer antituberculous drugs have been developed, including rifampicin, ethionamide, and ethambutol, all of which may be given orally. These are given as an initial regime of rifampicin 450 mgm, INAH 300 mgm, and ethambutol 800 mgm daily for the first 3 months, followed by rifampicin and INAH in the same dose for a further 3–6 months.

In practice the surgeon treating the patient with genitourinary

Chapter 7/*Kidney: Chronic Inflammation*

tuberculosis must appreciate that his patient is only suffering from one manifestation of a systemic disease. Every other system at risk, particularly the lungs, must be checked, and the family and place of work must be looked into. In practice too in England the patient is best cared for by a physician interested in tuberculosis in collaboration with the community physician and general practitioner. Not least is the surgeon responsible for keeping these other doctors informed of the patient's diagnosis, and he should bear in mind his medicolegal responsibility to notify the patient, since failure to notify the disease may result in some other member of the family failing to have the disease diagnosed: such a failure has been held to be negligent by the courts.

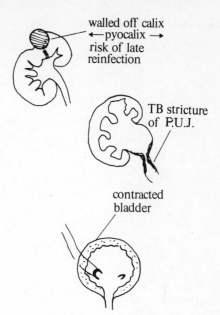

Fig. 7.10. Healing of granuloma may cause stenosis.

Follow up

One month after the start of effective treatment the patient undergoes another urogram: this is done in order to detect healing in calices, pelvis, or ureter which might result in obstruction (fig. 7.10). At this stage areas of unsuspected granuloma in the caliceal neck or the lower end of the ureter begin to scar down, as chemotherapy kills the tubercle bacilli and healing takes place. It may be necessary to act rapidly and by performing an appropriate plastic surgical procedure, remove the obstruction and save the kidney.

Similar radiographs are performed at 6 and 12 months. Thereafter the patient is followed up with annual radiographs, and routine culture of the urine for tubercle bacilli. It is customary to follow the patient for 2 to 3 years. Relapse after this time is very uncommon.

Salvage surgery

In the kidney a calix may get dammed off, leading to a localized hydrocalix, in which infection must persist. Such a localized area of infection should be removed: one cannot expect antituberculous therapy to diffuse into the middle of a cold abscess in the kidney. The localized abscess may be drained (cavernostomy) or resected together with the adjacent healthy rim of kidney (partial nephrectomy).

If, as treatment progresses, the whole kidney is revealed to be hopelessly riddled with tuberculosis, then nephrectomy should be performed without too much delay. As modern treatment gets progressively better, so more and more cases seem to fall into two extremes: either nothing needs to be done to the kidney, or it is so hopeless that it had better be removed. Less and less is there any indication for conservative surgery—cavernostomy or partial nephrectomy.

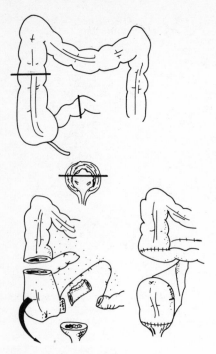

Fig. 7.11. Caecocystoplasty.

If the ureter is obstructed, it is implanted into the bladder.

If the bladder is contracted, then some form of enlargement is carried out, nowadays for preference using the caecum (fig. 7.11).

SEMINAL TUBERCULOSIS

In men, involvement of the upper tract by tuberculosis not uncommonly goes hand in hand with infection of the seminal tract—the prostate, seminal vesicle, vasa, epididymis and testis.

OTHER GRANULOMATA OF THE KIDNEY

Xanthogranulomatous pyelonephritis

In presence of a calculus together with continuing septic infection in the interstitium of the renal parenchyma, one can get a curious change in the macrophages, which become laden with fat, and give the chronic fibrous tissue in and around the kidney a startling bright yellow hue. This colour looks very like the colour of the lipid-laden 'clear cells' of a renal adenocarcinoma. It is easy for the unfortunate surgeon encountering a hard yellow lump which invades and is stuck to surrounding tissues to think he has encountered an inoperable cancer. This is xanthogranuloma, and all it needs is a local nephrectomy. Xanthogranuloma has a tendency to burrow into and form a fistula between the adjacent colon and the pus-filled kidney.

Malakoplakia

Another odd granuloma in the kidney which occurs in response to *E. coli* infections is malakoplakia. The kidney is honeycombed with abscesses, containing peculiar calcified bodies (Michaelis–Guttman bodies) which are said to be formed if *E. coli* and urine are brewed up together in suitable conditions. Clinically this, though rare, is a nightmare. Unless radically removed, the patient develops a labyrinth of fistulae through the abdominal wall and up and down the psoas from which he may eventually perish.

Brucellosis

Very like tuberculosis, infection of the kidney by *Brucella* causes a granuloma, sometimes with calcification, which ends up by destroying the kidney.

Chapter 7/*Kidney: Chronic Inflammation*

Fungus infections

Fungi grow in the kidney as a rule only when the patient's defences have been paralysed by immunosuppression, or their normal bacterial intestinal and urological flora killed by wide spectrum antibiotics. They are seen therefore in debilitated transplant patients, in heroin addicts, and patients under treatment for lymphoma. The mass of fungus may cause a soft 'calculus' which obstructs the urinary tract.

FURTHER READING

BLANDY J.P. (1976) Surgical infections of the kidney. *Urology*, ed. Blandy J.P., p. 195. Blackwell Scientific Publications, Oxford.

ELLENBOGEN P. & TALNER L.B. (1976) Uroradiology of diabetes mellitus. *Urology*, **8**, 413.

FREEDMAN L.R. (1976) Pathophysiology of pyelonephritis. *Scientific Foundations of Urology*, eds. Williams D.I. and Chisholm G.D., p. 71. Heinemann, London.

GOW J.G. (1976) Genitourinary tuberculosis. *Urology*, ed. Blandy J.P., p. 226. Blackwell Scientific Publications, Oxford.

GOW J.G. (1976) Genitourinary tuberculosis: a study of short course regimens. *J. Urol.*, **115**, 707.

IOANID P.C. & GALESANU M. (1976) New aspects of urinary tuberculosis. *Eur. Urol.*, **2**, 185.

MICHIGAN S., (1976) Genitourinary fungal infections. *J. Urol.*, **116**, 390.

MURRAY R.M. (1974) Analgesic abuse. *Brit. J. Hosp. Med.*, **11**, 772.

NOYES W.E. & PALUBINASKAS A.J. (1969) Malakoplakia of the kidney. *J. Urol.*, **84**, 231.

O'BOYLE P.J., GALLI E.M. & GOW J.G. (1976) The surgical management of tuberculous lower ureteric stricture. *Brit. J. Urol.*, **48**, 101.

PETEREIT K.M.F. (1970) Chronic renal Brucellosis: a simulator of tuberculosis. *Radiology*, **96**, 85.

PURPON I. & TAMAYO R.P. (1960) Malakoplakia of the kidney. *J. Urol.*, **84**, 231.

SHERWOOD T. (1973) Ureteric reflux 1973: chronic pyelonephritis versus reflux nephropathy. *Brit. J. Radiol.*, **46**, 653.

Chapter 8
The Kidney—
Obstruction

THE EFFECTS ON THE KIDNEY OF OBSTRUCTION (fig. 8.1)

A similar sequence of events takes place whether the obstruction to the kidney is complete or only partial. In obstruction the pressure rises inside the ureter, then the pelvis, then the calices. The rising pressure is instantly transmitted to the collecting ducts and through them to the tubules and the glomerulus. The pressure need only rise by 25 mm Hg for the filtration pressure to be equalled. When this occurs, filtration stops. The circulation in the kidney continues but there is no glomerular filtration.

This state of affairs lasts a very short time—in the experimental animal, an hour or so at most. Then a safety-valve effect takes place, and the kidney 'bursts' inwardly (fig. 8.2). Tiny cracks now appear beginning at the edge of the caliceal fornices, and entering the rich plexus of veins surrounding the papilla at this point. Urine now enters the veins and adjacent lymphatics, directly from the renal calices.

Once this has happened the pressure within the renal pelvis rapidly falls off and so does that within the glomerular capsule. Filtration starts all over again, but now instead of the urine which has been formed

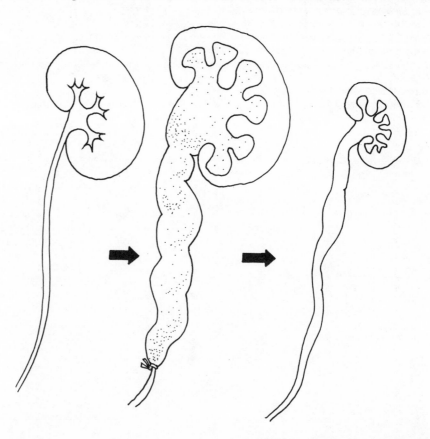

Fig. 8.1. Obstruction

Chapter 8/*Kidney: Obstruction*

passing down the ureter, it leaks back through the cracks at the neck of the fornix of the papilla into the parenchyma. Explored at this stage, one finds the entire kidney swollen and oedematous, and its surrounding tissues wet with oedema or extravasated urine. If an excretion urogram is performed at this stage one can easily distinguish the tracks made by the contrast spreading back along the line of the renal lymphatics and veins, as well as macroscopic extravasation of urine outside the kidney and its pelvis. The urograms tend to show a long-delayed nephrogram, since the flow of glomerular filtrate down the tubules is slow, and contrast is trapped in the cortex.

Thanks to this safety-valve effect, little damage occurs even when the kidney is totally obstructed—at least at first—provided there is no infection.

Later on a slow change takes place in the obstructed kidney. First there is a progressive loss of nephrons beginning with those placed most centrally, whose long loops of Henle dip down into the renal papillae. At the same time as these nephrons disappear, the renal papilla also

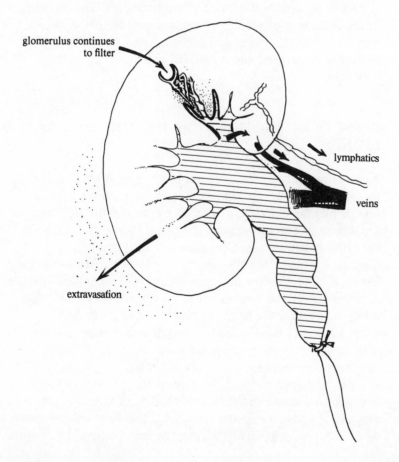

Fig. 8.2. Obstruction—intravasation to lowering of intrapelvic pressure.

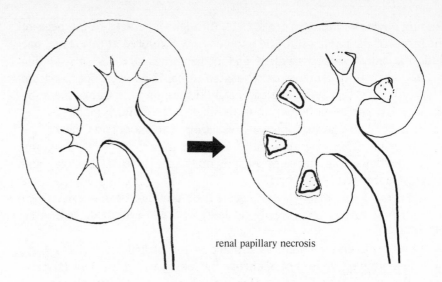

renal papillary necrosis

Fig. 8.3. Obstruction followed by death of renal papillae.

atrophies, usually slowly, but sometimes with dramatic suddenness if the papillae undergo necrosis (fig. 8.3).

As in time rank after rank of nephrons undergo atrophy, only those in the periphery of the cortex remain behind. If the obstruction is now removed, then the distended kidney may collapse like a pricked balloon, leaving a contracted and atrophied shell of renal parenchyma to carry on working.

EFFECTS OF OBSTRUCTION ON THE FUNCTION OF THE KIDNEY

At any time after the obstruction has begun, it may be relieved. At first, the only change which can be detected is that there may be a short-lived loss of tubular function, as shown by its inability to concentrate urine, for just as one would expect, the distal tubule and collecting tube bear the brunt of the increased pressure in the system. At such an early stage there is a danger that the clinician may not realize that the patient is having a large diuresis, and may fail to provide sufficient salt and water to make up for the loss which takes place. After a few days the distal tubule recovers and concentration returns to normal.

If there has been more prolonged obstruction and some degree of wasting has already taken place in the renal papilla and inner ranks of nephrons then there may be a permanent loss of renal concentrating and acidifying capacity. Such a kidney may never be able to make a concentrated urine, and the patient—if both kidneys have been affected, may always have a measure of diuresis and be unable to conserve salt or deal with an acid load. Worse, he may arrive in hospital with a

Chapter 8/*Kidney: Obstruction*

considerable clinical water and salt deficiency. Such a patient is the typical old man with chronic prostatic obstruction. If one does not recognize that he is short of salt and water he may be brought to the operating table without these deficiencies having been corrected (see page 202).

Related to obstruction there may be alterations in the renal blood flow leading to release of renin and to hypertension. Though not a common cause of systemic hypertension urinary obstruction is an important one because it can usually be put right.

In hydronephrosis there may be disturbance of the metabolism or production of erythropoietin, leading either to anaemia—as is often seen in chronic obstruction, or to polycythaemia—which is uncommon.

EFFECTS ON THE STRUCTURE OF THE COLLECTING SYSTEM

Dilatation occurs thanks to the increasing pressure within the system. If any of these tubes are dilated beyond a certain point, their walls cannot meet during peristalsis, and so peristalsis will become ineffective since a bolus of urine cannot then be milked downwards (fig. 8.4).

To compensate for the increased pressure and the need to grip the

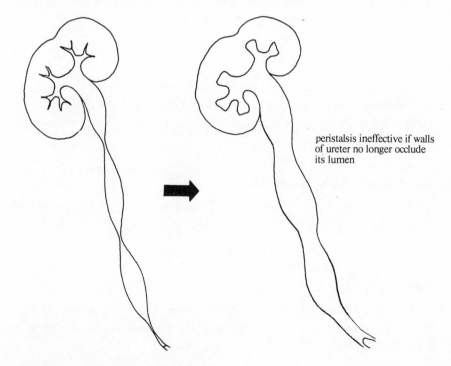

peristalsis ineffective if walls of ureter no longer occlude its lumen

Fig. 8.4. Dilatation makes peristalsis ineffective.

bolus of urine more tightly, there occurs a measure of hypertrophy in the wall of the ureter, renal pelvis, and calices.

The next stage is one of decomposition—as if the baggy muscle of the pelvis gives up. Viewed with the image intensifier on the television screen one sees hardly a ripple of activity. The kidney collecting system has deteriorated into a passive bag, incapable of helping itself. The only forces pushing the urine down to the bladder are glomerular filtration and gravity. Histologically the pelvis and ureter at this stage show infiltration by collagen among the smooth muscle fibres.

THE EFFECT OF INFECTION WHEN ADDED TO THAT OF OBSTRUCTION

1. Bacteraemia

The most dangerous consequence of infection added to obstruction is the entry of organisms into the bloodstream. It is easy to see how this can occur when urine containing bacteria is under pressure, and the dilated urinary tract, lined only by one or two layers of cells, offers a poor defence against the entry of organisms into the blood. When in addition there is a crack in the calix, then the bacteria have a direct access to the bloodstream.

2. Scarring

It seems likely that the presence of urine in the kidney parenchyma does sometimes cause scarring, but not badly. However if the urine is full of bacteria, each split soon becomes the seat of small abscesses, and the scarring which follows is devastating.

3. Stasis and relapse of infection

Without a clean flux of urine through the system bacteria remain undisturbed to re-emerge when treatment stops and to cause a clinical relapse.

4. Stone formation

Following infection in an obstructed system a calculus is apt to form especially when there is a urea-splitting organism present such as *Proteus morgani*.

5. Metaplasia of the urothelium

Prolonged infection or irritation of urothelium causes it to change into squamous epithelium. In time this may lead to squamous carcinoma—exceedingly rare in the kidney, less rare in the bladder.

FURTHER READING

GOODWIN F.J. (1976) Urinary obstruction and renal function. Chap. 22, *Urology*, ed. Blandy J.P. Blackwell Scientific Publications, Oxford.

LEWIS J.G. (1972) Gram negative bacteraemia. *Brit. J. Hosp. Med.*, **8**, 308.

ORMOND J.K. (1975) A classification of retroperitoneal fibrosis. *Urol. Survey.*, **25**, 53.

RANSLEY P.G. (1976) The renal papilla and intrarenal reflux. *Scientific Foundations of Urology*, eds. Williams D.I. and Chisholm G.D., p. 79. Heinemann, London.

WHITAKER R.H. (1976) Pathophysiology of ureteric obstruction. *Scientific foundations of Urology*, eds. Williams D.I. and Chisholm G.D., p. 18. Heinemann, London.

Chapter 9
Urinary Calculi

Cutting for the stone was perhaps the oldest operation performed as a therapeutic manoeuvre rather than a religious ritual. It also has the distinction of being the first procedure for which specialization was recognized to be an advantage—even in Hippocrates' day young physicians were enjoined to leave cutting for the stone to those who specialized in that subject (advice worth repeating today).

Until the turn of the century, 'stone' implied stone in the bladder, for throughout the ancient world as in many underdeveloped areas today,

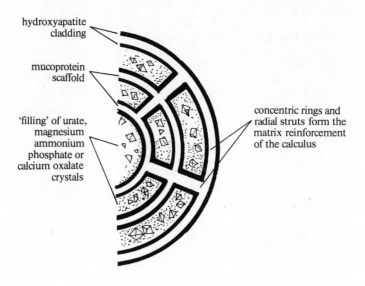

hydroxyapatite cladding

mucoprotein scaffold

'filling' of urate, magnesium ammonium phosphate or calcium oxalate crystals

concentric rings and radial struts form the matrix reinforcement of the calculus

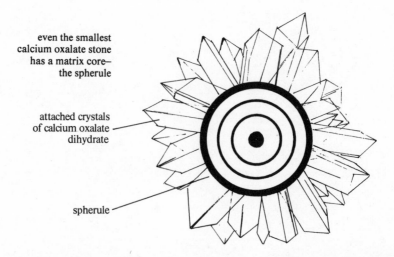

even the smallest calcium oxalate stone has a matrix core— the spherule

attached crystals of calcium oxalate dihydrate

spherule

Fig. 9.1. Structure of a stone.

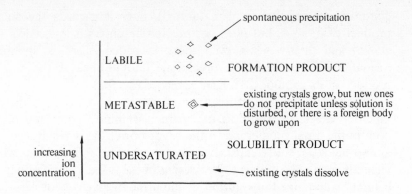

Fig. 9.2. Supersaturation.

stones in the bladder were very common. It seems likely that they originated as small calculi in the kidneys early in childhood. These small calculi would then descend the ureter to the bladder, but be unable to escape. Staying in the bladder, the stones would remain, growing year by year, until the symptoms became intolerable in later life.

At the beginning of this century, perhaps related to the improvement in sanitation throughout the civilized world, bladder stones began to disappear. But from that time onwards, there has been a steady increase in the incidence of small calculi affecting the kidney and ureter of adults, an increase whose upward trend was only, and temporarily, halted by the two world wars. Today about one in ten men in Britain may expect a ureteric calculus, and in some professions the incidence is even higher than this, e.g. in contemporary Scotland the incidence is about 20% among surgeons.

Structure of a urinary calculus

Even the smallest stone has quite an elaborate structure, (fig. 9.1) in which there is an organic scaffold, clad in apatite (rather like the iron in ferroconcrete) and a 'filling' of crystalline material. The way the layers of crystalline 'filler' are arranged suggests the growth rings of a tree, but nobody knows whether the organic matrix scaffold comes first, or whether it simply precipitates down along with the crystalline material because the proteins forming the matrix happen to be present in urine.

Factors leading to stone formation

1. SUPERSATURATION WITH COMPONENTS OF THE STONE

A solute may be present in increasing concentration in urine, at first it continues to dissolve (undersaturated), later it exceeds the solubility product of its ions, but does not precipitate unless it is 'seeded' (metastable) and finally when even more is added, there is spontaneous formation of the crystalline precipitate (labile) because the 'formation product' of its component ions is exceeded (fig. 9.2).

The purest example of this type of stone is *Cystine*. Here there is an inherited defect in transport of cystine, arginine, lysine and ornithine both in the renal tubule and in the small bowel. As a result, the filtered amino acids are not reabsorbed in the tubules, and cystine, which is virtually insoluble, comes to be present in the urine in an amount which cannot be contained in solution. If the urine output is kept very high, it may not precipitate: its solubility is greater in an alkaline urine, so it may help to keep the pH above 7: but if stones continue to form one may have to give the patient penicillamine which seizes one of the twin cysteine molecules which form cystine, and combines with it to form a soluble penicillamine cysteine disulphide (fig. 9.3).

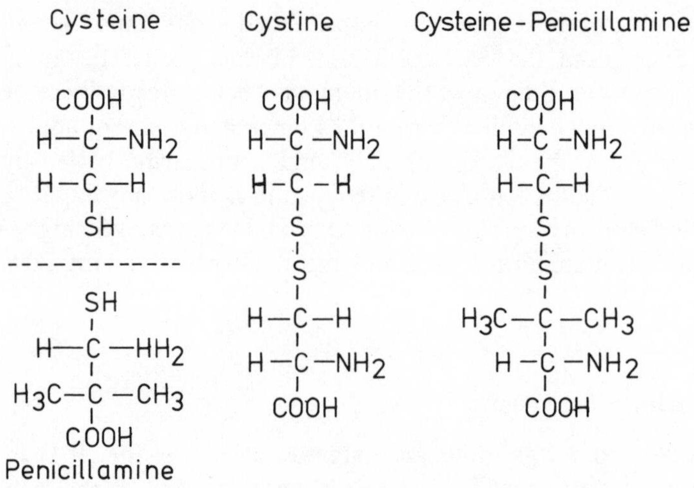

Fig. 9.3.

Another good example of supersaturation causing stones is seen in uric acid calculi. Urates are soluble in urine of pH greater than 6.8, but precipitate out in concentrated and acid urine even when the normal output of urate is present in human urine. Some people are unable to form an alkaline urine, and so produce uric acid stones whenever their urine is allowed to be concentrated. Others put out too much uric acid, either because they have gout, or because they are breaking down protein, for example when being given chemotherapy for metastases of carcinoma, or for leukaemia. In such patients it may be necessary to block the formation of uric acid by giving them allopurinol, a xanthine oxidase inhibitor, in addition to alkalis and a high fluid input.

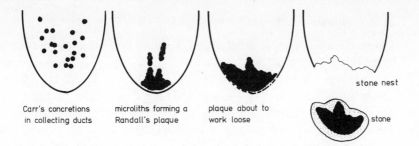

Carr's concretions in collecting ducts · microliths forming a Randall's plaque · plaque about to work loose · stone nest · stone

Fig. 9.4. Formation of a supersaturation stone in the renal papilla.

In clinical practice most stones are composed of calcium oxalate or phosphate, with or without magnesium-ammonium-phosphate. Small calculi are very often made of calcium oxalate, and so an increase in the urine output of either calcium or oxalate may be enough to precipitate the crystals which go to make the 'filler' of the stone.

An increase in urinary calcium is seen in its classical form as a result of hyperparathyroidism (see p. 98) but it may also be present in certain males for no apparent reason, hence it is called idiopathic hypercalciuria, as well as in patients with bone destruction resulting from trauma, confinement to bed, and widespread metastases from carcinoma. An increase in urinary oxalate may occur in some of the males with the idiopathic hypercalciuria and contribute to their stone recurrences, but it is also seen in people who have had the last few feet of ileum removed, for example for Crohn's disease. This is because bile acids are reabsorbed in this part of the terminal ileum, to be recycled in the liver. If the ileum no longer absorbs the bile acids, there are not enough of them secreted in the bile to allow dietary fat to be absorbed, and the unabsorbed fat forms insoluble soaps with calcium, leaving an excess of oxalate to be absorbed. One can deal with this by giving these patients an oxalate-free diet, or the ion-exchange resin cholestyramine, which binds the oxalate. Whether the oxalate in the diet is an important factor in the formation of ordinary calculi is a vexed question. Probably it is of importance in those people, for example the males with idiopathic hypercalciuria, who are particularly prone to recurrent small upper tract stones. The principal sources of oxalate in the Englishman's diet are tea, coffee, chocolate, spinach and rhubarb. Strawberries, traditional sources of oxalate, are not of importance.

In the kidneys of men with recurrent calcium stones one can detect many tiny concretions both in the collecting ducts of Bellini as well as just under the tip of the renal papillae. These were noticed by Randall as glistening plaques in kidneys at post mortem, and when the little stones grow, and separate, they leave an irregularity behind which may perhaps predispose to further stone formation, hence the idea of the 'stone nest' of Hamilton Stewart.

2. DEFICIENCY OF PROTECTIVE SUBSTANCES IN THE URINE

Urine is not a simple solution at all, but contains mucoproteins and magnesium and other ions, all of which seem to play an important role in keeping calcium salts from being precipitated even when their solubility product is well exceeded. Trace amounts of magnesium seem capable of preventing recurrence of stones, though there is controversy as to how they work, and how important they are. Similarly, the presence of amino acids may help to keep calcium salts from being precipitated, and it has been found that stone formers may be deficient in the amount of amino acids in their urine. Small amounts of protein in urine may work both ways, either tending to glue the little crystals together, or keep them apart.

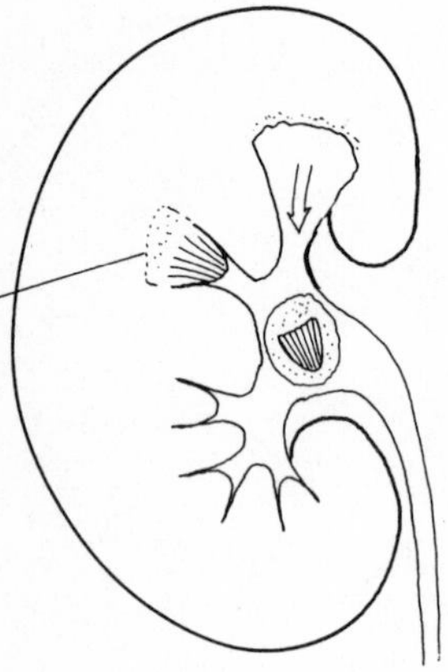

3. PAPILLARY NECROSIS (fig. 9.5)

Sometimes a section through a small stone will identify a fossilized papilla in the middle, or it can be seen in the radiograph as a radio-lucent middle within the stone. For this reason it is important to enquire carefully for any of the well known causes of papillary necrosis in any patient who has multiple or recurrent calculi (see page 72).

4. INFECTION (fig. 9.6)

Some stones are first seen shortly after an episode of upper-tract infection. Characteristically they first appear as soft lumps of matrix, which later undergo calcification. More often one cannot be sure

necrosed
papilla about
to separate

Fig. 9.5. Calculus forming on necrosed renal papilla.

infection and stone formation

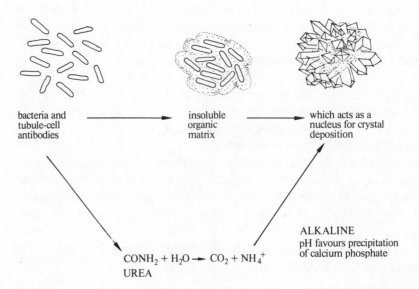

bacteria and tubule-cell antibodies → insoluble organic matrix → which acts as a nucleus for crystal deposition

$$CONH_2 + H_2O \rightarrow CO_2 + NH_4^+$$
UREA

ALKALINE
pH favours precipitation of calcium phosphate

Fig. 9.6. Infection and stone formation.

Chapter 9/Urinary Calculi

whether the stone or the infection came first. Once it is there, the stone acts as a hiding place for organisms, and a reason for relapse of the infection. If a strain of urea-splitting organisms infects the kidney, the rate of increase in the size of the stone is much accelerated.

PATHOLOGICAL EFFECTS OF CALCULI (Fig. 9.7)

1. Obstruction

A calculus may obstruct its calix, or the pelviureteric junction, or the ureter. The obstruction may be temporary or permanent. Behind the

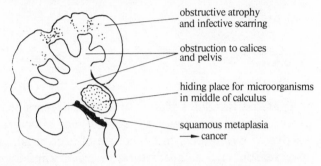

obstructive atrophy
and infective scarring

obstruction to calices
and pelvis

hiding place for microorganisms
in middle of calculus

squamous metaplasia
→ cancer

Fig. 9.7. Pathological effects of calculus.

obstruction there will be progressive atrophy made worse by scarring if there is also infection and the alteration in renal function described on page 82). If there is infection there may be a pyocalix or pyonephrosis and the pus under pressure may lead to bacteraemia and the formation of perinephric abscess.

2. Infection

Both as a hiding place for organisms in its matrix, and because it gives rise to a pool of undrained urine, a calculus may perpetuate infection. If a stone is present infection probably cannot be entirely eradicated by giving chemotherapy, since the chemotherapeutic agent cannot diffuse into the middle of the stone.

3. Metaplasia of the urothelium

Prolonged contact between the stone and the urothelium may give rise to squamous metaplasia and in time, albeit in rare instances, to squamous carcinoma.

CLINICAL FEATURES

1. Stone in a calix (fig. 9.8)

Many small stones stuck to a renal papilla and perhaps constituting an

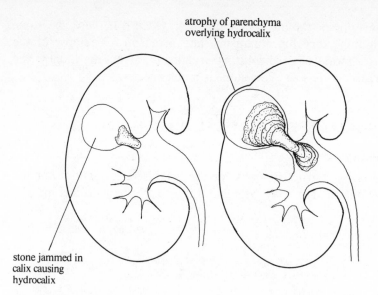

atrophy of parenchyma
overlying hydrocalix

stone jammed in
calix causing
hydrocalix

Fig. 9.8. Stone in a calix.

unseparated Randall's plaque or a partially ossified renal papilla, stay where they are and cause no trouble year after year. They tend to be discovered by accident in the course of a urogram carried out for some other reason such as haematuria or urinary infection. They can be left alone.

Sometimes they get detached, but become impacted in the neck of a calix. Now they cause obstruction. If infected, then bacteraemic episodes are common with shivering and rigors. Progressive atrophy and scarring quickly destroy the overlying parenchyma draining into that calix and lead to a pyocalix.

Such a stone may also grow progressively and gradually come to occupy more and more of the renal pelvis.

2. Stone in the renal pelvis (fig. 9.9)

Stones in the renal pelvis arise—more often than not—from stones in a calix which have got so far and can get no further. They will not go down the ureter if they are more than 0.5 cm in diameter. They are seldom entirely symptomless. They cause episodes of pain and fever if they get stuck in the pelviureteric junction. Gradually as time goes by they enlarge and the atrophy of the kidney gets worse. Such a stone should be removed as soon as it has been found.

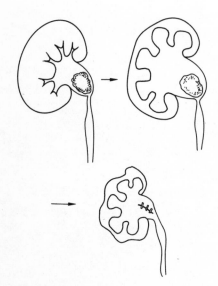

Fig. 9.9. Atrophy following obstruction from a stone impacted at the pelvi-ureteric junction.

3. Stone in the ureter (fig. 9.10)

If a stone can get into the upper end of the ureter one would expect it to go all the whole way down to the bladder, but in practice calculi which

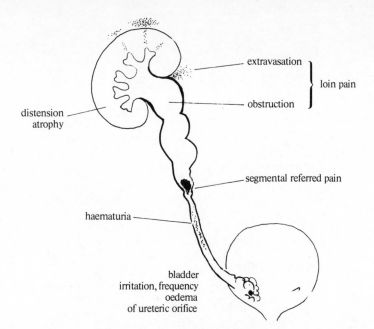

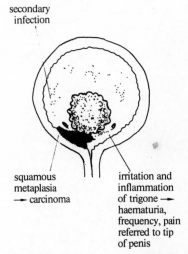

Fig. 9.10. Clinical features of stone in ureter.

are more than 0.5 cm in diameter seldom do, and nearly always have to be operated on. They give rise to colicky pain referred to the loin, to the umbilicus, groin, and scrotum. As they near the bladder, their pain is associated with discomfort on voiding, and frequency. Haematuria is a common feature of a ureteric calculus. They should be removed if they are obviously too large to descend spontaneously, e.g. if they are more than 0.5 cm in diameter, if they are accompanied by dilatation and infection of the kidney above the stone, or in a few instances, if they stick and do not budge month after month.

4. Stone in the bladder (fig. 9.11)

If the stone has reached the bladder the patient typically has pain referred to the tip of the penis, thanks to the innervation of the trigone. There is frequency, a feeling of incomplete emptying of the bladder (strangury), haematuria and pain on voiding. Once stones get into the bladder they can usually get out again, unless there is outflow obstruction. Hence they are rare in women, but more common in very small boys who tend to have a relative degree of outflow obstruction in childhood and in older men with prostatic enlargement.

5. Staghorn calculi (fig. 9.12)

Not uncommonly a calculus grows and enlarges year by year in the kidney, coming to fill not only the pelvis but several or all of the calices.

Fig. 9.11. Clinical features of stone in the bladder.

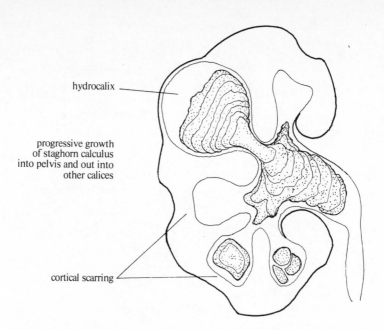

hydrocalix

progressive growth
of staghorn calculus
into pelvis and out into
other calices

cortical scarring

Fig. 9.12. Formation of typical staghorn
calculus.

The appearance is like coral, or a stag's antlers. Formerly it was
believed that these stones were 'silent' and could be safely left alone.
Careful examination of the evidence shows all too tragically that these
stones are generally followed by pyonephrosis and a perinephric abscess
if they are not removed. Newer surgical techniques allow their complete
removal with safety so that the truly conservative management of a
staghorn calculus is to remove the stone before the kidney is quite
destroyed or the life of the patient is threatened.

INVESTIGATIONS OF A PATIENT WITH A STONE

In addition to the usual complete history and physical examination, one
must pay attention to certain salient points.

History

Note whether there has been any prolonged illness requiring the patient
to lie in bed: e.g. paraplegia, fractured femur. Recumbency is associated
with an outpouring of skeletal calcium into the urine as well as with
relative stasis of the urine in the renal pelves.

Note whether the patient has served for any time in a hot climate,
and this includes working as a stoker in a boiler house.

Enquire whether there is a family history e.g. some cases of uric acid
stone disease are familial, as are all cases of cystinuria.

Has the patient had gout? Has he taken an excessive quantity of
alkalis, of milk, or of analgesics?

　　　　　　　　　　　　　　　　　　　　Chapter 9/Urinary Calculi

Physical examination

It is rare for a calculus to offer any physical signs. But you should always feel the neck carefully—one can occasionally feel a parathyroid tumour.

Investigations

1. ANALYSIS OF THE STONE

No stone should be given to the patient as a trophy. It should always be carefully analysed to see what it is made of.

2. URINE EXAMINATION

If the qualitative nitroprusside test for cystine is positive, the 24 hour urine should be collected and quantitative measurement made of the cystine passed. Filter paper chromatography will reveal the associated amino acids arginine lysine and ornithine in cases of cystinuria.

The urine must be examined bacteriologically.

Twenty-four hour collection of urine should be made, and the quantity of calcium measured per 24 hours. The normal upper limit for men is said to be 350 mgm/24 hours, for women 300 mgm/24 hours.

On the same sample of 24 hour urine one may measure uric acid (upper limit of normal 900 mgm/24 hours).

3. BLOOD

In addition to routine measurements of blood urea and creatinine, as a rough guide to overall glomerular filtration function, one should be measuring the blood uric acid to detect hyperuricaemia, and the blood calcium. Preferably the blood should be taken fasting and collected without the use of a tourniquet, which may misleadingly increase the relative amount of protein-bound calcium. This error can be allowed for if the plasma proteins are measured at the same time.

Note that the blood calcium estimation is prone to laboratory error. Any high result should be repeated and if necessary checked by another laboratory.

4. UROGRAPHY

One cannot evaluate where or what the stone is doing without excretion urography. It may have to be carried out as an emergency if the surgeon cannot tell whether the patient is passing a ureteric stone or has an acutely inflamed appendix. But these emergency 'casualty officer's pyelograms' may spread much unnecessary alarm if too much attention is paid to the somewhat terrifying appearance of the upper tract which is often seen at the height of the colic, when extravasation of urine from the kidney is particularly marked.

Stones ought to show on the preliminary film, unless they are lying in front of the sacroiliac joint, and so cannot be distinguished from the shadow of the bone, or are radiolucent. Radiolucent calculi are either made of matrix, a sloughed renal papilla, or uric acid. Cystine stones, though faintly opaque to Xrays, are not translucent, thanks to their sulphur content.

Evaluation of the stone case

1 First, you must decide whether the stone requires surgical interference: the indications for operation are whether or not the stone is likely to be able to pass spontaneously i.e. is it bigger than 0.5 cm in diameter and is it causing obstruction? The borderline cases will be the marginal-sized ureteric stones which are giving rise to temporary obstruction while they are passing down the ureter. Here one should wait and see.

2 Secondly, you must attempt to determine the likely cause of his or her stone. Very few patients have a *metabolic cause* for their stone; perhaps 1 to 5% will have a parathyroid tumour (see below). A similar proportion will have cystinuria, or the uric acid diathesis.

There will be a big group, amounting to about half the women, in whom the calculi seem to be related to urea splitting *urinary infection*, generally *Proteus morgani*.

A smaller group of patients will be found to be passing an excessive amount of calcium in the urine: only a tiny number of these will be doing this because they have a *parathyroid tumour*. Sometimes this 'hypercalciuria' stems from a taste for an excessive amount of cheese or milk in the diet, or for eating doctored white bread, loaded with chalk and other adulterants. Most often one cannot find any obvious cause for the hypercalciuria, so it is put down as 'idiopathic'.

There remains a large group of patients whose urinary calcium is within normal limits, whose blood calcium is repeatedly found to be normal, and who have nothing obviously wrong with their urinary tracts. Into this category will fall the majority of your patients.

PARATHYROID TUMOUR

The parathyroid gland secretes a hormone which probably has the task of encouraging the osteoclasts to dissolve the bony skeleton, and release calcium into the blood stream. Under normal circumstances, this office is nicely regulated by the need for calcium to be added to the blood, as indicated by the level of blood calcium.

Calcium exists in the blood as a large fraction bound to protein, and a smaller fraction in solution, part of which is ionized and part not ionized. The product $[Ca \times P]$ is kept constant.

If for any reason the level of calcium is increased, then that of [P] falls, and vice versa.

In primary hyperparathyroidism, for no good reason, the parathyroid seems to hypertrophy and secrete more parathormone than it ought to. The consequence is that more calcium salts are taken down from the bony skeleton and put into the blood stream, so elevating the plasma [Ca], and in turn there is a fall in plasma $[PO_4]$. This fall in plasma phosphate may be partly brought about by compensatory slowing of the reabsorption of phosphate in the proximal tubule, and for this reason it was once thought that the parathormone might act primarily on the tubule rather than on the bone.

The superfluous calcium in the blood is filtered in the kidney so the glomerular filtrate is charged with an excess of calcium. In severe cases of primary hyperparathyroidism precipitation of the calcium salts begins to take place in the collecting tubules, causing speckling in the plain film, scattered throughout the kidney, but most marked in the renal medulla.

To detect primary hyperparathyroidism it is possible to measure the increased amount of parathormone in the blood—preferably in the veins leaving the parathyroid glands. This can be done using radio-immunoassay techniques, but at the time of writing, they are not yet generally available. Or one can infer their overaction, by measuring an increase in the plasma [Ca]. This increase may not be present all the time but may be intermittent, and calls not only for accurate biochemical techniques to get the measurements right, but for them to be repeated several times if cases are not to be missed. The plasma phosphate will, predictably, be found to be lowered; (one can also estimate the amount of tubular phosphate which is being reabsorbed, though it is hardly worth the bother.) The total amount of calcium lost in the urine per 24 hours may also be raised.

Secondary hyperparathyroidism

In renal failure, one of the metabolic by-products which gets retained by the ailing kidney is phosphate. So the plasma phosphate increases, depressing the plasma [Ca]. The plasma calcium may be precipitated in soft tissues as heterotopic calcification, or put back in the bones.

Whatever the mechanism, down falls the level of circulating calcium. In response to this, the parathyroid may react by increasing its output of parathormone, accompanying this by hyperplasia of all four parathyroid glands. This condition is often encountered in patients undergoing treatment for renal failure. One can help matters by giving calcium either in the diet (assisting its absorption by means of vitamin D) or by increasing its concentration in the dialysate if the patient is undergoing dialysis: or one may have to remove the hyperplastic parathyroids if more simple measures fail.

Tertiary hyperparathyroidism

There may come a time when the over-zealous hyperplastic parathyroids seem not to know when their services are no longer required. Instead of pushing out just as much parathormone as is necessary to maintain a reasonable blood level of calcium, they put out an excess. Osteolysis proceeds apace even while heterotopic calcification is occurring in unwanted situations. The plasma calcium rises uncontrollably, and the only recourse must be to remove the hypertrophied glands.

Parathyroidectomy

The parathyroids are four in number, and lie at the side of and behind the lateral lobes of the thyroid gland. They are found by tracing along the main branches of the superior and inferior thyroid arteries to which they bear a more or less constant relationship. So easy is it to make a mistake, and remove a small thyroid nodule instead of a parathyroid gland, that each operation is controlled step-by-step by frozen sections. Each parathyroid is identified in turn, and all four are explored. Often there is more than one adenoma.

FURTHER READING

ANDERSON C.K. (1976) Pathology of nephrocalcinosis and stone formation. *Scientific Foundations of Urology*, eds. Williams D.I. and Chisholm G.D., p. 282. Heinemann, London.

BLACKLOCK N.J. (1976) Epidemiology of urolithiasis. *Scientific Foundations of Urology*, eds. Williams D.I. and Chisholm G.D., p. 235. Heinemann, London.

BLANDY J.P. (1976) The case for a more aggressive approach to staghorn calculi. *J. Urol.*, **115**, 505.

BOYCE W.H. & GARVEY F.K. (1956) The amount and nature of the organic matrix in urinary calculi: a review. *J. Urol.*, **76**, 213

DE VRIES A. & SPERLING O. (1976) Uric acid stone formation: basic concepts of aetiology and treatment. *Scientific Foundations of Urology*, eds. Williams D.I. and Chisholm G.D., p. 297. Heinemann, London.

MARSHALL V.R., WHITE R.G., TRESIDDER G.C. & BLANDY J.P. (1975) The natural history of renal and ureteric calculi. *Brit. J. Urol.*, **47**, 117.

NORDIN B.E.C. (1973) *Metabolic bone and stone disease*. Churchill Livingstone, Edinburgh.

NORLIN A., LINDELL B., GRANBERG P.O. & LINDVALL N. (1976) Urolithiasis: a study of its frequency. *Scand. J. Urol. Nephrol.*, **10**, 150.

ROBERTSON W.G. & NORDIN B.E.C. (1976) Physico-chemical factors governing stone formation. *Scientific Foundations of Urology*, eds. Williams D.I. and Chisholm G.D., p. 254. Heinemann, London.

WATTS R.W.E. (1976) Cystinuria and cystine stone disease. *Scientific Foundations of Urology*, eds. Williams D.I. and Chisholm G.D., p. 302. Heinemann, London.

WICKHAM J.E.A. (1976) The matrix of renal calculi. *Scientific Foundations of Urology*, eds. Williams D.I. and Chisholm G.D., p. 323. Heinemann, London.

WILLIAMS R.E. (1976) Renal and ureteric calculi. *Urology*, ed. Blandy J.P., p. 291. Blackwell Scientific Publications, Oxford.

Chapter 10
The Kidney–
Neoplasms

AETIOLOGY AND CLASSIFICATION

There are two different types of neoplasm arising in the kidney: those which occur in the renal parenchyma, and those arising from the lining of the collecting system—the calices and pelvis.

TUMOURS OF THE RENAL PARENCHYMA

Two different parenchymal tumours are seen: that which arises in childhood, the embryoma (Wilms' tumour), and that which occurs in adults, the renal cell carcinoma (Grawitz).

1. EMBRYOMA—WILMS' TUMOUR—NEPHROBLASTOMA (fig. 10.1)

This tumour was first described by Rance in 1814, and not by Wilms until 1899, so that there is little point in keeping on using his eponym. They amount to about 10% of all childhood malignancies, about one in every 13,000 live births. There are several family studies showing an association with congenital aniridia, hemihypertrophy of the body, exomphalos and macroglossia, and a few pedigrees have been studied in which multicystic disease and adult renal cell carcinomas occur more often than one would expect.

Pathology

Macroscopic features. The tumour is usually homogeneous, soft and pale, but it may contain cystic areas and have patchy haemorrhages, as may any other rapidly growing tumour. There is no clear line of demarcation between the malignant and the benign part of the kidney, and these tumours are bilateral in approximately one in ten cases, possibly from spread, possibly from independent separate primary growth (how can anyone say?).

Microscopically the embryoma shows a very variable picture: almost every tissue which can arise from mesoderm being found, as if the tumour represented a mesodermal segment gone wild. In the first year of life some of these tumours are virtually benign—the 'mesoblastic nephroma' and have an excellent prognosis.

Spread. Local spread occurs early, invading the perinephric fat and psoas muscle, and occasionally the colon or duodenum. It gets into the renal pelvis rather late, but into the renal vein early, as well as into

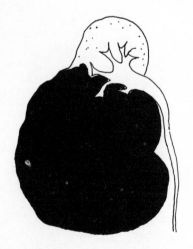

'a large lump in a wasted baby'
Fig. 10.1. Embryoma of kidney (Wilms).

lymphatics. Distant metastases occur both by venous emboli and lymphatic spread. Blood-borne metastases most often occur in the lungs.

CLINICAL FEATURES

'A big lump in a wasted baby' is how to remember the embryoma. The younger the baby, the better the prognosis, so much so that some pathologists have questioned the malignancy of the tumours which occur in neonates, which tend to show atypical histological features, with diffuse mesenchymal proliferation between islands of renal parenchyma. They are sometimes called *mesoblastic nephromas*.

They present with three main features:

a *Abdominal mass*. The mother notices the lump when bathing the baby; there is reason to believe that it can grow very rapidly, and by the time the child is brought to hospital, the lump may be enormous.

b *Haematuria* occurs in about one in three cases: it is seldom obvious, and usually only noticed on testing the urine.

c *Pain*. Sometimes it is obvious that the baby is distressed, but it is curiously seldom a feature.

They may also have certain odd features common to the adult tumour: fever is common, hypertension occurs in a high proportion though its explanation is obscure; and there may be raised levels of erythropoietin.

INVESTIGATIONS

The chief differential diagnosis is between an embryoma and a neuroblastoma: but hydronephrosis and multicystic disease of one kidney need also to be considered. The key investigation is an excretion urogram. Speckled calcification is more common in the neuroblastoma. The embryoma generally shows as a large, soft tissue mass distorting and deforming as well as displacing the kidney: the neuroblastoma tends to shift the kidney bodily downwards, without deforming it.

TREATMENT

The first line of treatment is transabdominal nephrectomy (see page 267). The pedicle of the kidney is ligated first before the mass is mobilized. A wide excision is performed, and the abdomen is not closed until the contralateral kidney has been examined for contralateral disease.

After nephrectomy the child is given a course of radiotherapy, beginning as soon as the wound has begun to heal (e.g. after about a week from operation). This is supplemented by actinomycin D, which appears to potentiate the effect of radiotherapy. The details of the dosage and methods of giving actinomycin are under investigation in MRC-sponsored clinical trials. Similar trials are also under way with respect to vincristine, which appears to be equally effective and has fewer toxic side effects.

RESULTS

Excellent prognosis is obtained in children under one year old: perhaps because many are mesoblastic nephromas, thereafter it gets worse, but thanks to combined surgery, radiotherapy, and chemotherapy, it now approaches 80% in tumours not originally metastasized widely.

ADENOCARCINOMA OF THE KIDNEY—GRAWITZ TUMOUR (fig. 10.2)

Not originally described by Grawitz (who in any case thought it arose from the adrenal), this is a malignant growth arising from renal tubular cells.

It occurs at all ages after childhood, though very rare before puberty, and more common with advancing age. It is more common in men than women.

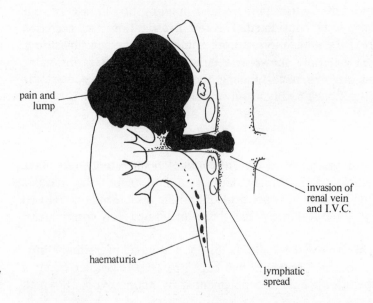

pain and lump

invasion of renal vein and I.V.C.

haematuria

lymphatic spread

Fig. 10.2. Adenocarcinoma of kidney (Grawitz).

Chapter 10/*Kidney: Neoplasms*

Pathology

Macroscopically it cuts with a vivid yellow, blotchy appearance, often with numerous cysts and areas of haemorrhage and necrosis.

Microscopically its chief feature is the clear cell, filled with lipid which gives the growth its yellow hue. Three types are recognized: the most benign of all is the *papillary,* which is histologically identical with the common little benign 'hamartomas' of the kidney, or cortical adenomas, which cause hardly any comment when they are noted at post mortem. By convention if a cortical adenoma is bigger than 3 cm across it is a carcinoma, and there is a good deal of speculation here, as in other similar tumours, as to the concept of a critical mass above which a tumour becomes malignant.

The usual *moderately differentiated tumour* has clear cells in an orderly pattern. There are also exceedingly *anaplastic carcinomas* which spread rapidly and carry a very bad prognosis.

Spread occurs by direct invasion into the perinephric fat and local tissues: it invades the renal pelvis early, and so gives rise to haematuria. Distant spread occurs through massive invasion of the renal vein, in which large blobs of tumour can often be seen waving about in the current of blood.

Curiously, despite early involvement of the renal vein, in recent series it is spread by lymph nodes which seems to carry the most evil prognosis.

CLINICAL FEATURES

1 Haematuria occurs in 80% of cases, and is the main reason why every patient with haematuria is subjected to such a rigorous investigation.

2 Pain is common—a vague, ill-defined discomfort in the loin.

3 A lump may be felt by the examining doctor, or the patient may be aware of a lump—a useful symptom which should never be disregarded lightly.

4 Other unusual features occur in this as in the embryoma of children: some of these seem to reflect an alteration in the immunological defences of the patient, e.g. there is a raised sedimentation rate, an alteration in the albumen/globulin ratio, and the deposition of amyloid in some tissues (which may go away after the tumour has been removed). Fever of unknown origin may bring the patient to hospital into a medical ward, and the tumour in the kidney may only be brought to light in the course of a methodical and painstaking investigation. Sometimes there are strange disturbances of the bone marrow, no doubt due to alterations in the secretion of erythropoietin: as a rule this is shown in an increase in the red cell mass of the body (polycythaemia), but one may find one or all of the white cell population hypertrophied, giving rise to a picture which may be mistaken for a leukaemia.

INVESTIGATIONS AND DIAGNOSIS (fig. 10.3)

The common problem is to find a lump in the kidney shadow in the urogram in the course of a routine examination for haematuria or prostatism. Is it a tumour or a cyst? The pyelogram tends to show distortion and displacement of the calices by tumour, but a smooth lump in a cyst. The nephrogram looks round and empty in a cyst, irregular in tumour. An arteriogram shows abnormal tumour vessels, with escape of contrast into the necrotic parts of the growth in tumour, and if nor-adrenaline has been injected, the vessels of the good part of

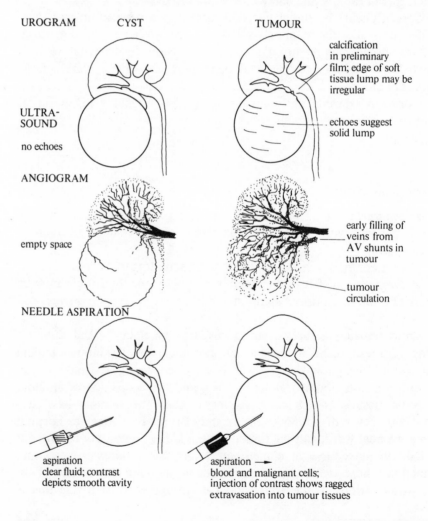

Fig. 10.3. Cyst or tumour in kidney.

Chapter 10/*Kidney: Neoplasms*

the kidney are thrown into spasm, but those going to the tumour do not contract. Ultrasound shows many echoes coming from the debris within the tumour, but no echoes from the fluid inside the cyst. A needle may be passed into either lump: if it is a tumour, aspiration yields blood stained fluid from which malignant cells may be isolated by the Papanicolaou technique; if it is a cyst, clear fluid is produced. (It has been shown that fine-needle aspiration of a tumour carries no increased risk of seeding of growth into the wound or of disseminating metastases.)

TREATMENT

The first line of treatment is transabdominal nephrectomy, removing the kidney, adrenal, and all its surrounding box of Gerota's fascia in one block. There is no evidence that post-operative radiotherapy improves the prognosis, indeed, two controlled studies show it makes it worse. It is possible that pre-operative radiotherapy may improve the outlook, but as yet this belief lacks any substantiation in controlled trials now in progress in London and Rotterdam. If tumour has been left behind by mistake at operation, most surgeons advise post-operative radiotherapy.

When metastases are single, surgical excision should be performed when it is feasible—as in the lung or brain. But localized radiotherapy in some situations may be more appropriate and no less effective. The adenocarcinoma of the kidney is one of those tumours where the prognosis is notoriously unpredictable: cases survive for twenty years before developing a metastasis, and there are a handful of well-documented cases in whom lungs riddled with metastases have become clear after removing the primary, and sometimes after no treatment at all.

Hormonal therapy for adenocarcinoma is still on trial: it is widely believed that progestogens may stave off the development of metastases, or get rid of some which have already formed, but the evidence so far is dubious. Other forms of chemotherapy have, so far, been useless.

TUMOURS OF THE RENAL CALICES AND PELVIS (fig. 10.4)

The aetiology and classification of these tumours are exactly the same as for tumours of the rest of the urothelium, and are fully dealt with in the section on carcinoma of the bladder on page 177. It has recently become clear that in certain parts of the Balkans, where a kind of interstitial nephritis and papillary necrosis is common, and perhaps related to some poison in the drinking water, that there is an increased incidence of carcinoma of the renal pelvis and calices. Similarly, in the analgesic-

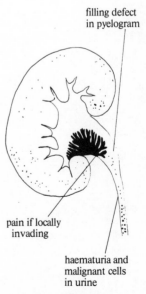

filling defect
in pyelogram

pain if locally
invading

haematuria and
malignant cells
in urine

Fig. 10.4. Salient features of renal papillary transitional cell carcinoma.

addicted population of Huskvarna (Sweden) and Newcastle (Australia) an undue proportion of renal papillary cancer has been found in those already known to have analgesic nephropathy. Most recently, there was a disturbing rumour that coffee had similar effects, fortunately unconfirmed.

Pathology

Macroscopically one finds the lining of the kidney set about with seaweed-like fronded tumours, sometimes becoming more nasty and solid, but rarely ulcerating. Invasion can often be seen as an indurated grey streak tracking up into the renal parenchyma or into the surrounding tissues.

Microscopically these tumours fall into the same classification as urothelial tumours of the bladder: i.e. they may be transitional cell cancers, in which case they are papillary or solid, and well differentiated or anaplastic. Or they may be the products of metaplasia, either forming squamous cell carcinoma (a late sequel of having a stone lodged in the renal pelvis for year upon year), or sometimes an adenocarcinoma secondary to cystitis glandularis.

Spread occurs directly into the surrounding tissues, and early into the rich plexus of lymphatics in the renal sinus; it is impossible to say whether the tumours so often found in association with these cases, further down the ureter or in the bladder itself, are the result of waterborne seeding, or the consequence of the action of a waterborne carcinogen upon the urothelium itself. It is probable that both may occur, and in any case, even after the kidney and ureter on one side have been removed, the patient must be meticulously followed as for any other urothelial cancer.

Diagnosis

The urogram will show filling defects. The urine may show clumps of malignant cells on Papanicolaou staining. In early cases a distinction must be made from a filling defect caused by a lucent uric acid stone, from the cystic defects due to pyelitis cystica, from renal papillary necrosis, and from clots due to other less sinister causes of haematuria.

Treatment

Not only the kidney but the whole of the ureter on that side must be removed right down to and including the entry of the ureter into the bladder. Otherwise recurrence is almost inevitable in the stump of ureter. In many cases the tumour will have spread through the thin lining of the wall of the renal pelvis into surrounding tissues, and post-operative radiotherapy is given. The prognosis, except for patients with very early superficial papillary tumours, is very bad. The follow up necessitates regular cystoscopy and urography to detect other tumours arising *de novo* elsewhere in the urothelium.

OTHER TUMOURS OF THE KIDNEY

Since the kidney is supplied with connective tissue, nerves, and blood vessels, it is subject to sarcomata of every description, but these are all very rare. They have no special features by which they can be recognized until they have been removed in mistake for an adenocarcinoma.

Secondary carcinoma also occurs in the kidney, most commonly from a primary carcinoma of the bronchus. It is usually bilateral, and seldom is any useful purpose served by treating it.

FURTHER READING

General considerations
CLARK P. & ANDERSON K. (1976) Tumours of the kidney and ureter. Chap. 17, *Urology*, ed. Blandy J.P. Blackwell Scientific Publications, Oxford.
DEMING, C. (1970) Tumors of the kidney. *Urology*, ed. Campbell M.F. and Harrison J.H. Saunders, Philadelphia.
EVERSON T.C. (1963) Spontaneous regression of cancer. *Ann. New York Acad. Sci.*, **114**, 721.
HOLLAND J.M. (1973) Cancer of the kidney: natural history and staging. *Cancer*, **32**, 1030.
RICHES SIR E.W. (ed.) (1964) *Tumours of the Kidney and Ureter*. Livingstone, Edinburgh and London.

Nephroblastoma (Wilms)
FAY R., BROSMAN S. & WILLIAMS D.I. (1973) Bilateral nephroblastoma. *J. Urol.*, **110**, 119.
HILTON C. & KEELING J.E. (1974) Neonatal renal tumours. *Brit. J. Urol.*, **46**, 157.
RICKHAM P.P. (1972) Malignant tumours involving the genitourinary system in childhood. Chap. 9, *Problems in Paediatric Urology*, eds. Johnston J.H. and Scholtmeijer R.J. Excerpta Medica, Amsterdam.
LEDLIE E.M., MYNORS L.S., DRAPER G.J. & GORBACH P.D. (1970) Natural history and treatment of Wilms' tumour. *Brit. Med. J.*, **2**, 195.
MOTT M.G. (1975) Nephroblastoma (Wilms' tumour). *Brit. J. Hosp. Med.*, **13**, 161.

Adenocarcinoma (Grawitz)
ALFTHAN O., JUNSELA H., ORAVISTO K.J. & MALMIO K. (1976) Preoperative irradiation in the treatment of renal adenocarcinoma. *Scand. J. Uul. Nephrol.* Supp. **33**, 17.
BLOOM H.J.G. (1973) Adjuvant therapy for adenocarcinoma of the kidney: present position and prospects. *Brit. J. Urol.*, **45**, 237.
FINNEY R. (1973) The value of radiotherapy in the treatment of hypernephroma—a clinical trial. *Brit. J. Urol.*, **45**, 258.
MURPHY G.P. & MOSTOFI F.K. (1970) Histologic assessment and clinical prognosis of renal adenoma. *J. Urol.*, **103**, 31.
MARBERGER M., & GEORGI M. (1975) Balloon occlusion of the renal artery in tumor nephrectomy. *J. Urol.*, **114**, 360.

PEELING W.B., MANTELL B.S. & SHEPHEARD B.G.F. (1969) Post-operative irradiation in the treatment of renal cell carcinoma. *Brit. J. Urol.*, **41**, 23.

PUIGVERT A. (1976) Partial nephrectomy for renal tumours: 21 cases. *Eur. Urol.* **2**, 70.

VAN DER WERF-MESSING B. (1973) Carcinoma of the kidney. *Cancer*, **32**, 1056.

ROBSON C.J., CHURCHILL B.M. & ANDERSON W. (1969) The results of radical nephrectomy for renal carcinoma *J. Urol.* **101**, 297.

Urothelial cancer

ANGERWALL L., BENGTSSON U., ZETTERLUND, C.G. & ZSIGMOND M. (1969) Renal pelvic carcinoma in a Swedish district with abuse of a phenacetin-containing drug. *Brit. J. Urol.*, **41**, 401.

WALLACE D.M. (1976) Carcinoma of the urothelium. Chap. 30. *Urology*, ed. Blandy J.P. Blackwell Scientific Publications, Oxford.

WILLIAMS C.B. & MITCHELL J.P. (1973) Carcinoma of the ureter—a review of 54 cases. *Brit. J. Urol.*, **45**, 377.

INFARCTION (fig. 11.1)

Since the renal arteries are end-arteries, if an embolus occurs, the entire wedge-shaped segment of parenchyma supplied by that artery undergoes necrosis. These infarcts occur in old age and are often found at autopsy as a sequel to the detachment of atheromatous plaques. They may occur in consequence of valvular disease of the heart, when vegetations may separate and get stuck in the renal arterial branches, or they may follow open heart surgery when fragments of blood clot or tissue similarly become dislodged. Local pain, and haematuria from bleeding from the adjacent inflamed areas of the parenchyma at the border of the infarct, are the usual features. The diagnosis may be guessed clinically, or confirmed by the combination of a retrograde pyelogram which shows a normal pelvicalicine pattern and a nephrogram which shows a shrunken renal cortex at the site of the infarct. By the time the infarct has been diagnosed it is too late to save that part of the kidney, and there is seldom any need to meddle with it.

Chapter 11
The Kidney—
Vascular Disorders
and Hypertension

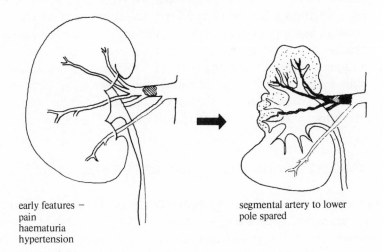

early features –
pain
haematuria
hypertension

segmental artery to lower
pole spared

Fig. 11.1. Infarct of kidney.

VENOUS THROMBOSIS (fig. 11.2)

Occurring *de novo* in dehydrated children, or secondary to some forms of glomerulonephritis, the renal vein or one of its major tributaries may undergo thrombosis. In childhood the clinical features are those of an ill, dehydrated child, who develops a large tender mass in the loin accompanied by haematuria. Urography shows no function on the affected side. Left alone, it may recover, thanks to the rich provision of anastomoses between the renal veins.

In adults there may be severe pain over the kidney, with haematuria

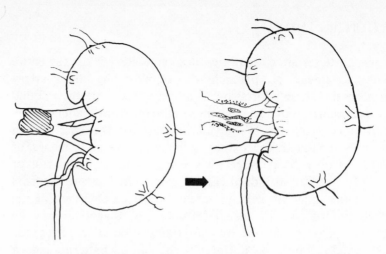

renal vein thrombosis may be followed by recovery thanks to alternative venous drainage – or may lead to atrophy

Fig. 11.2. Venous obstruction.

and proteinuria. If both kidneys are involved, there will be anuria. There may be other evidence of venous thrombosis such as chest pain from small pulmonary emboli. If the condition is borne in mind, the diagnosis can be confirmed by introducing a catheter up the inferior vena cava, and performing a renal phlebogram. Treatment is rapid anticoagulation with heparin in the first instance, but there have been some twenty successful case reports of removal of the clot from the renal vein at open operation, and this may be the safest therapy in bilateral cases.

ANEURYSMS OF THE RENAL ARTERY (fig. 11.3)

A variety of congenital abnormalities may involve the renal artery and its branches. They are brought to light in the course of investigation of hypertension, or polycythaemia, or sometimes of haematuria. Their exact configuration is established by selective angiography, and their treatment depends upon how big they are, and whether there is another healthy kidney present so as to permit nephrectomy of the affected one.

Certain points are worth noting: sometimes a calcified ring in the saccular aneurysm may mimic a calculus. Sometimes these aneurysms have occurred after needle biopsy of the kidney. Sometimes what seems to be an aneurysm turns out to be a very vascular adenocarcinoma of the kidney.

It is not safe to leave them alone once they have been found, though it is often very tempting, because the operation is difficult. Neglected, 83% of renal artery aneurysms rupture, and if they do, the mortality is 90%. In many instances the aneurysmal deformity involves both renal

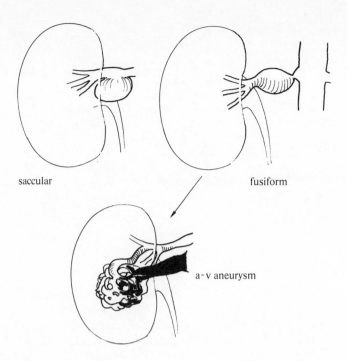

saccular

fusiform

a-v aneurysm

Fig. 11.3. Aneurysms of the renal artery.

artery and veins. The only relevant clinical sign (in addition to hypertension) is a bruit over the loin.

HYPERTENSION

Almost any disorder of the kidney may be complicated by hypertension; this includes pyelonephritic scarring, all forms of glomerulonephritis, tuberculosis, obstructive lesions of any kind, tumours, and polycystic disease. Hypertension may itself lead to damage to the renal parenchyma because fibrinoid necrosis of the walls of arterioles and proliferative endarteritis, may result in ischaemic changes throughout the kidney.

If the renal artery is partially occluded, and the pressure in the afferent arteriole is lowered, juxtaglomerular cells secrete *renin* from their granules. Renin is an enzyme which converts *angiotensinogen* (a protein constructed in the liver) to *angiotensin I*, which in turn is split into the simpler polypeptide *angiotensin II* (fig. 11.4).

Angiotensin II acts directly upon peripheral blood vessels to constrict them, and increase the peripheral vascular resistance. At the same time it stimulates the adrenal cortex to release *aldosterone*. Aldosterone in turn makes the renal tubules conserve sodium by working their pump mechanism harder, exchanging the sodium for potassium.

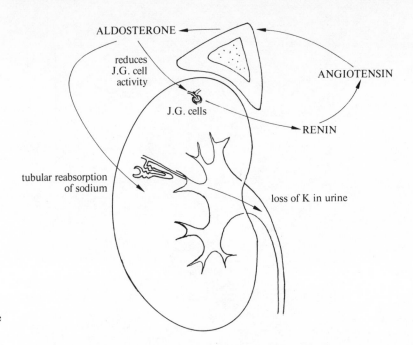

Fig. 11.4. Renin–angiotensin–aldosterone mechanism.

As a result of renin release, there is both a direct effect on peripheral vessels to increase the peripheral resistance, as well as an increase in the extracellular fluid volume, which will be reflected in an increased blood volume.

Precise regulation of the mechanism of renin release is effected by feed-back controls: aldosterone in excess inhibits renin release, and a low plasma sodium promotes it.

If the adrenals are diseased, and aldosterone output is low, there is compensatory increased renin production, and the reverse is seen when the adrenals harbour an aldosterone-secreting tumour (Conn's syndrome).

In chronic hypertension there comes a stage when an increased level of circulating renin can no longer be detected. It is not clear what has taken place: there are endless theories, interminable discussion by the cognoscenti, but nothing for the surgeon to do.

Arterial causes for renal hypertension (fig. 11.5)

1 *Fibromuscular hyperplasia* may affect the main renal arteries, causing an irregular narrowing along the length of either or both arteries and some of their principal branches. The restricted arterial pressure gives rise to renin release and hypertension, which is usually detected in early adult life. Section of the artery shows hypertrophied muscle in some places, with degeneration—amounting to mural aneurysm

Chapter 11/*Vascular Disorders and Hypertension*

1. MAJOR ARTERY AND
   ARTERIAL BRANCHES

fibromuscular hyperplasia

atheroma

2. SMALLER ARTERIES

ARTERIOLAR NEPHROSCLEROSIS

splitting of internal elastic lamina
('onion skinning')

PROLIFERATIVE ENDARTERITIS

thickened muscular wall: onion
skinning of internal elastic lamina

3. AFFERENT ARTERIOLE OF
   GLOMERULUS

FIBRINOID NECROSIS

infiltration of media and intima by
eosinophilic fibrinoid,

necrosis of muscle fibres

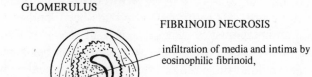

Fig. 11.5. Arterial changes in hypertension.

formation—in others. Angiography gives a characteristic picture. The
treatment is to patch the narrowed renal artery with a vein graft, or to
bypass the diseased segment with a graft taken from the aorta or the
splenic artery.

2   *Atheroma* usually affects the origin of the renal artery at the aorta,
where a thick plaque of atheroma bulges into the lumen and limits blood
flow. If it can be detected sufficiently early, it can be cured by removing

the atheroma, reimplanting the artery, or bypassing the narrow segment with a graft. With careful selection of cases, about half can be cured—at a price of a surgical mortality of about 5%. The selection of cases suitable for surgery demands the most careful collaboration between surgeon and physician, and the nicest exercise not only of investigative skill, but clinical judgement.

3 *Arteriolar nephrosclerosis* may occur as a sequel to prolonged hypertension caused by other conditions, or in diabetics without hypertension. Histologically it is characterized by splitting up of the arteriolar internal elastic lamina by deposits of hyaline material.

4 *Proliferative endarteritis* occurs in malignant hypertension, and is marked by thickening of the muscular walls of the arteries as well as layering of the elastic fibres, resulting in obliteration of the lumen.

5 *Fibrinoid necrosis* is another effect of malignant hypertension which attacks the afferent arteriole of the glomerulus. In addition to infiltration of the media and intima by the characteristic eosinophilic fibrinoid material—which is an altered plasma protein—there are inflammatory cells and necrosis of muscle fibres.

Obviously the surgeon can do nothing about any of the last three arterial lesions in the kidney. Indeed, it is doubtful if more than 5% of hypertensives are capable of being helped by any surgical procedure.

The majority of patients with high blood pressure have, for want of a better term, *essential hypertension*. This is a disease of many, often interrelated causes, and it is important that enthusiasm does not betray the surgeon (who always likes to have his pathology simple, cut, and dried) into unnecessary operations in the hope that his patient has some remediable lesion of the kidney. Equally important is it that the physician should not become completely demoralized and hopeless, and feel that the search for a remediable renal cause for hypertension is a lost cause and that the results are never worth the discomfort and danger of the diagnostic tests. Recently new hope has been kindled by the use of Saralysin, an antagonist of Angiotensin II. It seems as if an infusion of this material will lower the blood pressure if it is being maintained by the Renin–Angiotensin mechanism. Early reports claim that diagnosis by means of this drug can detect renal hypertension even in patients whose renin estimations are normal.

Adrenal tumours

1. PHAEOCHROMOCYTOMA

This is a tumour arising in the adrenal medulla, secreting a group of *catecholamines* of which nor-adrenaline is the most well known and most important. The secretion of the catecholamines occurs when the adrenal is handled, and occurs in episodes, so that there is typically a succession of paroxysms of hypertension. Sometimes the tumours arise not in the adrenal medulla but in other sites. The symptoms are typically attacks of headache, palpitation, faintness, and a sense of terror. One can provoke such an episode by giving the patient various drugs including histamine—a test now abandoned because it is dangerous. Ideally the individual catecholamines are measured in the plasma or the urine, a difficult and specialized assay not generally available. It is more easy to measure the breakdown products of these amines in the urine, notably vanillyl-mandelic acid (VMA). These are measured in 24-hour urine samples. The treatment is to remove the tumour, taking care during the operation to avoid a severe paroxysm of hypertension by blocking the alpha-receptors with phenoxybenzamine and the beta-receptors with propanalol.

2. CONN'S TUMOUR

A tumour of the adrenal cortex may secrete *aldosterone*, leading to overactivity of the sodium pump in the distal tubule, expansion of the blood volume, and hypertension. Since sodium is exchanged in the tubule for potassium, these patients may become seriously short of potassium, and develop muscular weakness and even paralysis. The raised blood volume and sodium inhibits the output of renin, so that while plasma aldosterone levels are high, those for renin are low. So many precautions have to be taken in making and interpreting these tests that the diagnosis of Conn's syndrome calls for the nicest exercise of the physician's skill and acumen. One can reverse the effect of the raised aldosterone levels by giving spironolactone, but this has its own side effects, and in the long run it is probably better to remove the offending gland if there is only one tumour rather than diffuse hyperplasia. The surgical procedure is rather like the exploration of parathyroid tumours: frozen sections are used to check the progress of the work, and to make sure that there is not bilateral diffuse disease.

3. CUSHING'S DISEASE

Here the adrenal glands are secreting too much *cortisol*, and the patient has all the clinical features of steroid overdosage as well as hypertension. There may either be a discrete adrenal adenoma, or diffuse bilateral hyperplasia. The diagnosis is made by confirming the clinical suspicion by detecting an excessive excretion in the urine of 17-hydroxy-corticosteroids, which are the metabolic end products of cortisol. One can distinguish between a tumour and hyperplasia by seeing whether its secretion of cortisol is independent of the pituitary: if

ACTH is given, there is an increased output of cortisol by the hyperplastic glands: conversely if dexamethasone is given, it will suppress the pituitary, and there will be a fall in the 17-hydroxy-corticosteroid output. There are innumerable other and more refined tests sometimes used in practice, which are based on this principle. The treatment for an isolated adenoma (or carcinoma) is to remove it: for hyperplasia, to perform a subtotal or total resection of both adrenals. On the whole it has been found better to remove the glands rather than to try to guess how much to leave behind, and perhaps make the patient go through a second operation a few years later if hyperplasia recurs.

FURTHER READING

DE BAKEY M.E., LEFRAK E.A., GARCIA-RINALDI R.R. & NOON G.P. (1973) Aneurysms of the renal artery: a vascular reconstructive approach. *Arch. Surg.*, **106**, 438.

CHARRON J., BELANGER R., VAUCLAR R., LEGER C. & RAZAVI A. (1975) Renal artery aneurysm. *Urology*, **5**, 1.

FAIR W.R. (1976) Renovascular hypertension—assessment of functional disorders. *Scientific Foundations of Urology*, eds. Williams D.I. and Chisholm G.D., p. 117. Heinemann, London.

GOODWIN T.J. (1974) Renovascular hypertension. *Brit. J. Hosp. Med.* **11**, 625.

JOHNSTON J.H. (1976) Congenital anomalies of the calices, pelvis and ureter. *Urology*, ed. Blandy J.P., p. 521. Blackwell Scientific Publications, Oxford.

LEDINGHAM J.G.G. (1976) Renal disease and hypertension. *Scientific Foundations of Urology*, eds. Williams D.I. and Chisholm G.D., p. 113. Heinemann, London.

MARKS L.S., MAXWELL M.H., SMITH R.B., CAHILL P.J. & KAUFMAN J.J. (1976) Detection of renovascular hypertension: Saralysin test versus Renin determination. *J. Urol.*, **116**, 406.

MESSING E., KESSLER R. & KAVANEY P.B. (1976) Renal arteriovenous fistula. *Urology*, **8**, 101.

O'DEA M.J., MALEK R.S., TUCKER R.M. & FULTON R.E. (1976) Renal vein thrombosis. *J. Urol.*, **116**, 410.

OWEN K. (1976) Renal hypertension. *Urology*, ed. Blandy J.P., p. 375. Blackwell Scientific Publications, Oxford.

PICKERING G. (1974) *Hypertension: causes, consequences & Management*, 2nd edn. Churchill Livingstone, Edinburgh.

TANAGHO E.A. (1976) The ureterovesical junction: anatomy and physiology. *Scientific Foundations of Urology*, eds. Williams D.I. and Chisholm G.D., p. 23. Heinemann, London.

WICKHAM J.E.A. (1976) Diseases of the renal artery, veins, and lymphatics. *Urology*, ed. Blandy J.P., p. 348. Blackwell Scientific Publications, Oxford.

WILLIAMS D.I. (ed.) (1974) *Urology in Childhood*. Handbuch der Urologie XV Supplement. Springer Verlag, Berlin.

ACUTE RENAL FAILURE

The kidneys may fail as a result of a wide range of insults, but the final common pathway for most of these appears to be a gross degree of hypotension accompanied by vasoconstriction or blockage of renal capillaries. Table 12.1 lists some of the conditions which give rise to acute renal failure.

Pathology (fig. 12.1)

The kidney in acute renal failure is typically large, pale and oedematous: the medulla is typically congested and the cortex pale and ischaemic. Microscopically one may find nothing wrong at all, or there may be patches of necrosis involving all or part of the tubules, which appear to be choked with cellular debris, an appearance formerly thought to mean that they were blocked. In fact, it seems as if it is the falling-off in the glomerular filtration which allows the tubules to get silted up with the debris.

This histological picture seems to require not only a period of hypotension but also a coexisting and inappropriate vasoconstriction. If hypovolaemic shock can be overcome by early and adequate transfusion of blood and plasma, and if inappropriate vasoconstriction can be prevented by giving (if necessary) an alpha-blocker such as phenoxybenzamine, then acute renal failure can be largely prevented, at least after trauma.

Table 12.1. Causes of acute renal failure

1 *Poor renal perfusion*
   blood loss
   burns
   diarrhoea/vomiting
   bacteraemic shock
   coronary thrombosis
   ischaemia in transplanted kidney

2 *Renal tubular poisons*
   mercury
   phenol
   carbon tetrachloride
   glycol
   Clostridium welchii toxin

3 *Tubular blockage*
   myoglobin (in severe crush injury)
   porphyrins
   bilirubin
   haemoglobin (in mismatched transfusion)
   sulphonamide crystals
   hyperuricaemia

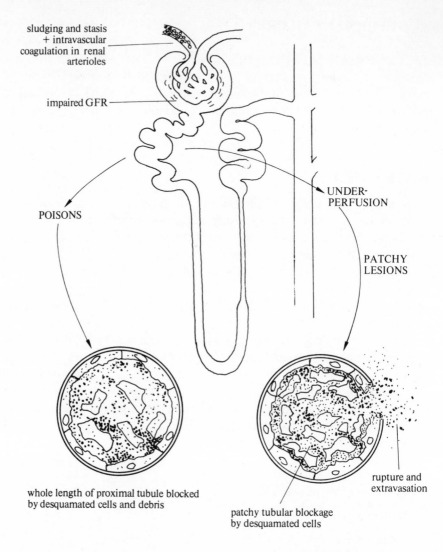

sludging and stasis + intravascular coagulation in renal arterioles

impaired GFR

POISONS

UNDER-PERFUSION

PATCHY LESIONS

whole length of proximal tubule blocked by desquamated cells and debris

patchy tubular blockage by desquamated cells

rupture and extravasation

Fig. 12.1. Acute renal failure.

POISONS   UNDER-PERFUSION

Accompanying the vasoconstriction is an opening up of arteriovenous anastomoses which shunt the blood away from the cortex of the kidney. If the cause of the acute renal failure is allowed to continue unchecked, and this shunting continues, then the renal cortex may become infarcted and never recover. The condition is called 'renal cortical necrosis', and probably represents an extreme stage in the deterioration of the kidney rather than a separate pathological process.

Clinical features

In addition to the features of the causative illness, such as severe traumatic shock, bacteraemia, or a septic abortion, there are certain features common to most cases of acute renal failure. First comes a *prodromal* phase: there is a continuance of some glomerular filtration, before the tubules become blocked by sludge. This gradually falls off—but it is a most useful feature, for it may help to distinguish acute tubular necrosis from accidental surgical trauma to the ureters. If the ureters have been blocked, then the anuria is of abrupt onset. In acute tubular necrosis, the anuria comes on more gradually.

After the prodromal phase comes the period of *anuria* or *oliguria*. Even here there is a wide range of variation in the clinical picture: many patients have a normal volume of urine, though it is qualitatively far from normal, being virtually unprocessed proximal tubular fluid.

After the phase of oliguria or anuria comes the phase of *recovery*. Phagocytosis has cleared the blocked tubules, and glomerular filtration has begun again. Urine begins to trickle down the collecting ducts. But at first it is urine of very low specific gravity and osmolarity, as if hardly acted upon at all by the tubules. During this phase, because the distal tubule is unable to conserve water or salt, the patient may lose a vast quantity of fluid, and it may take considerable effort and many litres of intravenous fluid to keep up with the salt and water loss. This is the *diuretic* phase. It will last as long as it takes the tubules to clear themselves, and to regenerate their cells.

The amount of recovery is variable, and after a very severe episode of acute tubular necrosis, recovery is seldom complete: one can usually detect some impairment of tubular function and of glomerular filtration even many years later.

Treatment

If only the patient can be kept alive, he should recover, unless the initial damage has been so severe as to lead to cortical necrosis. So the principles of treatment are to sustain life during the 3 to 6 weeks which may be necessary before the kidney recovers, the blocked tubules become clear, and their cells regenerate.

During this phase of anuria, the patient is in danger of being given so much water as to drown him, and so much food as to poison him with nitrogenous breakdown products.

He only needs as much water as he is sweating and respiring, and for most patients this is barely a litre per day.

He needs about 1000 calories a day, to minimize the catabolism of his own protein for energy requirements. But there is little point in giving more.

In many cases the disorder—e.g. trauma or sepsis—which caused the initial renal shutdown is likely to dictate what has to be done, for the immense breakdown of protein which occurs in these clinical circumstances may impose a huge load of nitrogenous waste on the body. In such a patient the blood urea may mount by 100 mgm/100 ml every day, and one cannot afford to wait and hope that the kidneys will recover in time. Along with this breakdown of intracellular protein comes a release of intracellular potassium which cannot be eliminated so long as the glomerular filtrate is not being got rid of. Hyperkalaemia may call for the emergency administration of glucose and insulin, or an ion-exchange resin, which will bring down the level of extracellular potassium to safe limits. But in such a hypercatabolic patient the only safe course is to dialyse the patient. With increasing experience the lesson has been learned that it is better to dialyse early and often rather than late and little. The patient can be allowed a more liberal diet, can take more fluid by mouth, and seems to be able to resist infection better if the blood urea is kept below 100 mgm/100 ml by regular dialysis.

The method by which the dialysis is performed may be either intraperitoneal, or haemodialysis using an artificial kidney. Each has its merits and its drawbacks. Peritoneal dialysis may be difficult and may run the risk of introducing infection in the presence of existing peritonitis or a recent abdominal operation (though this is not a complete contraindication). Haemodialysis has the advantage of being able to bring down the urea more rapidly, and ultrafilter off an excess of water more quickly, but has the disadvantage of requiring a machine, a trained team to run it, and careful attention to heparinization if the patient is not to develop haemorrhagic complications, which, after recent severe trauma, can be a major hazard.

CHRONIC RENAL FAILURE

Whatever the cause of the renal disease, if it goes on long enough, the patient enters upon the last phase, when his remaining nephrons cannot keep him dialysed.

If the rate of deterioration is slow, the next step is to restrict his dietary protein. When the glomerular filtration rate has fallen to about 20 ml/min, reducing the protein in the diet from 120 gm/24 hours to 40 gm/24 hours may be enough to bring the urea down from about 200 to about 70—a very useful reduction. By further restricting the protein input to about 20 gm per day, the patient can be maintained in reasonable health with a clearance as low as 5 ml/minute. By means of such a dietary regime—which is irksome in the extreme to the patient—a year or two may be bought before the decision has to be reached whether or not to take the patient on for long term treatment.

This is not the place for a discussion of the many aspects, both social and medical, which have to be weighed in the balance before this decision can be arrived at.

Complications of chronic renal failure

Thanks to the success with which it has been possible to treat patients year after year by intermittent dialysis and diet, a new batch of disease entities has emerged, with which one ought to be at least acquainted, even though their expert management rests, fortunately, with the nephrological physicians.

Pigmentation of the skin, accompanied by *itching*, is a feature of patients on chronic dialysis and is probably due to the deposition of urinary pigment in the skin. It clears after successful transplantation.

Anaemia is inevitable in renal failure, since the kidney no longer manufactures sufficient erythropoietin and the bone marrow works inefficiently. Transfused blood is quickly lost, and there is in fact little point in trying to keep the haemoglobin level above 5 gm/100 ml, since it soon falls again, and repeated transfusions tend to sensitize the patient to transplant antigens on the accompanying white cells.

Neuropathy occurs in some patients more than in others. It appears to be due to loss of myelin from peripheral nerves, resulting in weakness and sensory loss. Paraesthesiae, especially in the feet which 'burn' may be distressing.

Pericarditis resulting from uraemia is accompanied by evidence of tamponade and a rub. It is seldom seen when the patient is being adequately dialysed and the blood urea is kept low.

Bone changes are a common and important cause of pain and disability in chronic renal failure patients. There are three separate processes, all of which may be going on at the same time to a varying extent. The understanding of the clinical picture is not made any easier by the tiresome terminology which is sometimes used to confuse the issue by dog-Latin gobbledygook (fig. 12.2).

1 In renal failure less calcium is absorbed by the gut, because it seems to be in some way insensitive to vitamin D. Because of this, when new bone is formed, only osteoid is laid down, but not properly calcified, and so it bends under stress causing deformity and sometimes pathological fractures. This is called *rickets* when it happens in children, *osteomalacia* in adults.

2 In renal failure the level of phosphate in the blood is high, and that of calcium correspondingly low: to this low calcium level, the parathyroid responds by putting out more parathormone, causing the osteoclasts to work harder at leaching calcium out of the bones. Hence there may be an element of *osteitis fibrosa cystica*, as in classical primary hyperparathyroidism.

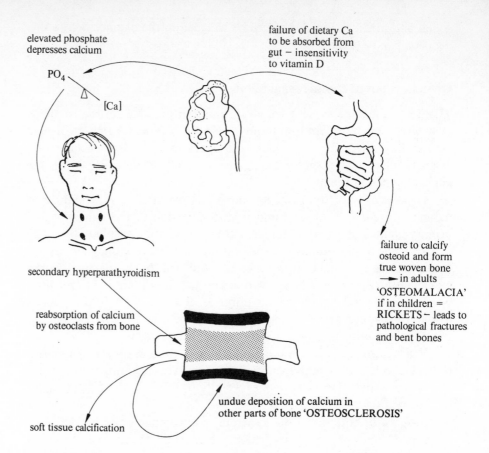

elevated phosphate
depresses calcium

failure of dietary Ca
to be absorbed from
gut – insensitivity
to vitamin D

PO$_4$

[Ca]

failure to calcify
osteoid and form
true woven bone
— in adults
'OSTEOMALACIA'
if in children =
RICKETS – leads to
pathological fractures
and bent bones

secondary hyperparathyroidism

reabsorption of calcium
by osteoclasts from bone

soft tissue calcification

undue deposition of calcium in
other parts of bone 'OSTEOSCLEROSIS'

Fig. 12.2 Bone changes in renal failure.

3   But, when the phosphate is raised in renal failure, and the calcium is
lowered, this is because the calcium is precipitated as calcium
phosphate somewhere. This may be in soft tissues, giving rise to
heterotopic ossification and calcification of tendons, arteries, and other
tissues, or it may be in bone—giving the paradox that in the same bone
there may be an excess deposition of calcium salts at one end, and
reabsorption of bone in the middle. This entire crazy maladjustment is
called *osteodystrophy*, whose classical feature is the banded appearance
of the *osteosclerotic* vertebrae—the 'rugger-jersey spine'.

DIALYSIS AND TRANSPLANTATION

In many contemporary centres where the treatment of terminal renal
failure is undertaken, patients are accepted for treatment with the
understanding that, to begin with, arrangements will be made for them
to look after themselves at home. This means that a kidney machine will
be installed in the patient's home, and that the patient's husband, wife,

or parent will undertake to look after the patient during the two or three nights in the week when dialysis is performed.

The hospital therefore runs a training ward, in which patients accepted on to the programme are made fit and instructed in the technique of home dialysis. During this training period arrangements are made for the house to have the necessary modifications carried out to the electricity or water supply, and the dialysis machine is installed.

Once the patient has been accepted, and once he or she has been trained in home dialysis, the patient's name is placed on a standby list for a renal transplant.

If a correctly matched kidney is provided from a cadaver, the patient is offered the chance of a transplant. Many patients will eagerly avail themselves of the chance of escaping the twilight life which is part of regular intermittent dialysis. Others opt for going on as they are, and one hopes that for several years to come, this choice will remain open to them.

It is futile to enter any argument as to which is best: there is no doubt that a well functioning transplant offers the patient a return to normal life, at the expense of a small daily dose of steroids and azathioprine. On the other hand at the end of a year only about 70% of cadaver grafts are still surviving, and there is a 10 to 15% chance that the patient will have died as a result, direct or indirect, of the transplant operation or its aftermath. Compared with this, the chance of living (leaving aside the quality of life) is substantially better on intermittent dialysis. Once more, each case must be most carefully evaluated on its merits, and transplantation or dialysis is not a simple decision about which there is room for polemics, but a choice which the physician and surgeon should offer to the patient only after taking every circumstance into consideration.

Dialysis

Although the principles of intermittent haemodialysis or peritoneal dialysis can be understood very easily, the art and craft of dialysing a patient is one which can only be learned by practical instruction, and no useful purpose is served by the medical student attempting to memorize any of the details of the procedure.

HAEMODIALYSIS

The design of haemodialysis machines has undergone constant improvement over the past 15 years, and is still changing. Nevertheless the principle is simple. The machine in most common use in Britain today is the Kiil flat plate dialyser (fig. 12.3). Blood from the patient,

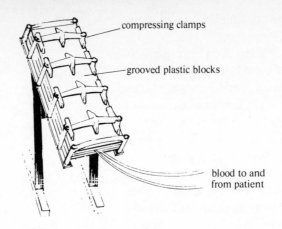

compressing clamps

grooved plastic blocks

blood to and
from patient

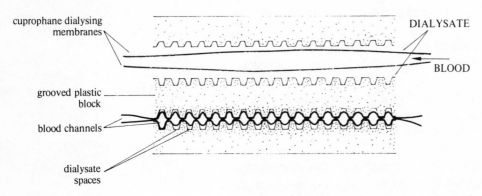

cuprophane dialysing
membranes

DIALYSATE

BLOOD

grooved plastic
block

blood channels

dialysate
spaces

Fig. 12.3. Kiil artificial kidney.

treated with heparin to stop it coagulating, is allowed to flow under the patient's arterial pressure, along tiny grooves in a plastic plate, which is covered by a very thin semi-permeable cuprophane membrane. On the other side of the membrane there circulates the dialysate fluid—which is for practical purposes physiological saline modified according to the needs of the patient. Thus, if it is necessary to remove water from the overloaded patient the dialysate is made more hypertonic by the addition of glucose. If the patient is hyperkalaemic, potassium is omitted from the fluid; if short of calcium, calcium can be added to the fluid, and so on. Urea, creatinine and phosphates, being absent from the dialysate, diffuse out into the fluid and are removed from the blood.

By modifying the design of the machine, it is possible to increase the pressure within the blood compartment, and so force water out, rather like the glomerulus itself, a process called *ultrafiltration*.

Access to the bloodstream is often provided by inserting a Scribner shunt (fig. 12.4) into the radial artery and cephalic vein of the forearm, or some other suitable pair of vessels. The Scribner shunt has a U-piece which can be disconnected and attached to the dialysis circuit. The material of which the shunt is made is one which does not react with the

Chapter 12/*Renal Failure*

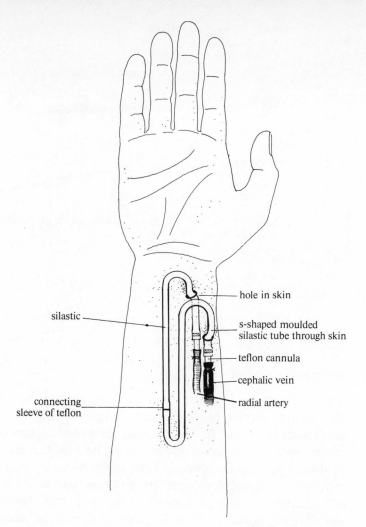

silastic

hole in skin

s-shaped moulded
silastic tube through skin

teflon cannula

cephalic vein

radial artery

connecting
sleeve of teflon

Fig. 12.4. Scribner shunt.

blood, and so does not give rise to clotting. The flexible piece is made of Silastic; the inserts into vein and artery of Teflon. But where the firm Teflon tubes are tied into the artery and vein they rub, leading to spasm and thrombosis, and 'shunt troubles' cause a good deal of minor practical emergency surgery in every dialysis unit, as well as a good deal of distress.

Equally good access is provided by forming an arteriovenous anastomosis between the radial artery and a cephalic vein in the forearm, the Cimino fistula. In consequence the patient develops 'varicose' veins of enormous size, into which he is trained to insert large bore needles to remove and restore the blood when the time comes for dialysis (fig. 12.5).

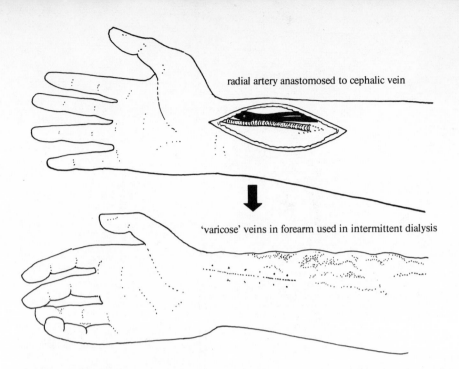

radial artery anastomosed to cephalic vein

'varicose' veins in forearm used in intermittent dialysis

Fig. 12.5. Cimino–Breschia fistula.

PERITONEAL DIALYSIS (fig. 12.6)

A plastic catheter is inserted into the peritoneal cavity through a small stab wound. Into the catheter is run a known volume of the dialysate; it is left there for about 20 minutes, and allowed to siphon out again. The semipermeable membrane made use of here is the peritoneum itself. Peritoneal dialysis is cheap, and can easily be set up and supervised by relatively untrained personnel. Its disadvantages are the obvious ones that peritonitis may follow in time, and that the cannula may inadvertently injure bowel or large blood vessels. In practice peritoneal dialysis has the disadvantage that it is a slow process compared with haemodialysis, and may not be rapid enough in patients who are breaking down masses of protein in consequence of trauma or sepsis.

Transplantation

The operation of renal transplantation is easy. Technically the steps have now been worked out in many centres, and are virtually standardized. The kidney is obtained from a cadaver (or from a living donor) and is removed together with a length of ureter, renal artery and vein. The surgeon removing the kidney must take great care not to damage the rather delicate vessels running in the triangle of fat between the renal vein and the ureter, since the blood supply to the ureter depends upon them.

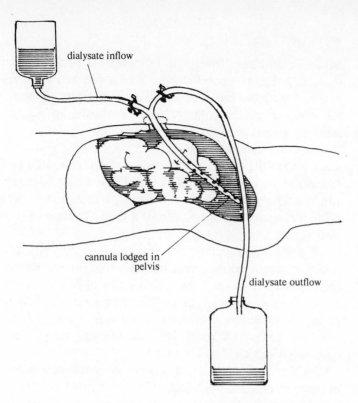

dialysate inflow

cannula lodged in
pelvis

dialysate outflow

Fig. 12.6. Peritoneal dialysis.

An incision is made in one or other iliac fossa. The internal iliac artery is ligated just where it divides, its proximal end is occluded by a bulldog clamp, and it is cut and washed out with heparin solution. A window is carefully cut out of the side of the external iliac vein. The renal artery of the donor kidney is anastomosed to the internal iliac artery of the recipient, and the donor vein to the external iliac vein. The clamps are then removed and blood allowed once more to course through the kidney.

The ureter is then anastomosed to the bladder taking care to provide it with a non-refluxing tunnel. The wound is closed with appropriate drainage. The new kidney can now be easily felt sitting in the iliac fossa, where it is easily palpated, biopsied, and assessed from time to time.

The technical work of renal transplantation is the most easy part of the whole procedure. Since the donor kidney usually comes from a patient who is not an identical twin, the recipient begins to mount an immunological defence process against the foreign material as soon as the graft enters his body. The real difficulty with transplantation is the difficulty of overcoming this immunological hurdle.

When an unrelated transplant (allograft) is performed for the first time, there is a latent period during which the anastomoses heal and the kidney functions. But after an interval of 10 to 14 days lymphocytes in the regional nodes enlarge, as if provoked to anger, become pink-staining (with pyronin) and divide. Others are provoked into the manufacture of immunoglobulin. Pink-staining cells now appear in the graft, and at the same time a coating of immunoglobulin is deposited on the intima of the vessels of the graft, to which platelets stick, and on which a thrombus soon forms, leading within a short while to occlusion of the vessels, and infarction of the graft. The whole process is called a 'first set reaction'.

If a second graft from the first donor is put into the same recipient, rejection again takes place, but this time at an accelerated pace: the more rapid 'second set' reaction is different in that, among other things, more leucocytes play a part. The second set reaction signifies that the patient has become sensitized to antigens on the first graft, specific to the first donor. (A graft from a different donor is handled in the relatively sluggish 'first set' manner.)

Neither a first set nor a second set reaction is seen when a graft is exchanged between identical twins, or when tissue is moved from one site in the body to another. The transplantation antigens are evidently inherited, and studies in inbred strains of animals suggested that it was probable that only one group of antigens, and that elaborated by genes on only one pair of chromosomes, was responsible for the 'strong' rejection reaction which would cause a graft to die.

Although no large numbers of 'inbred strains' of humans were available for similar transplantation studies to be carried out, it was not long before sufficient numbers of live donor transplants had been performed between members of families for it to be apparent that—so long as both siblings had the same chromosomes, the transplants would have a survival of the order of 90%, whereas if they had neither in common, the survival was reduced to about 40%—despite chemotherapeutic immunosuppression. In sibling donors it was possible to detect the chromosomes carrying these strong transplantation antigens by certain 'marker genes', manufacturing antigens to which it was possible to identify antibodies by well-tried laboratory methods—by serological methods (the serologically defined or SD antigens) or by watching the behaviour of the lymphocytes from donor and recipient when cultured together (lymphocyte detected or LD antigens).

The strong histocompatibility antigens in man were called the Human Lymphocyte Antigens (A) or HLA for short. Soon there was no question but that HLA identity signified a good result in sibling transplants, and HLA incompatibility a bad one. But it was an entirely different matter to apply the results of family studies to the question of cadaveric transplants, for the transplant antigens from a stranger's chromosomes would doubtless keep company with a whole group of antigenic material capable of eliciting rejection.

The only way to see if HLA applied in unrelated cadaveric transplants was to do a large number of transplants, making sure that there were a sufficient number of HLA identical ones to allow comparison to be made with transplants in which the HLA antigens were different.

Unfortunately the chance of finding a perfect HLA match in a crowd of strangers is less than one in 5,000—an impossibly large pool to find even in one country, let alone one hospital. So followed the first of the great international transplant-sharing schemes. Essentially what happened was that when a kidney became available from a cadaver, the tissue typing was carried out on the donor's lymphocytes (obtained from blood or a lymph node). The resulting information was telephoned to a central register, on which were kept the HLA details of all the patients awaiting a kidney transplant. The kidney was then despatched to the hospital where the patient was waiting.

This enormous international experiment was only made possible by the finding that a kidney would keep fresh if it were removed from the cadaver soon after death, and if it were then cooled and stored in a thermos flask at 4°C. Such stored kidneys functioned even after 18 hours of 'cold ischaemia'.

A development of this storage method has been to make a machine which slowly trickles ice-cold oxygenated diluted plasma through the kidney. Such machines have now been developed in several countries, based on the same principles. They have one useful advantage over transport and storage on ice: if the circulation through the kidney becomes clogged up after a few hours, it suggests that there has been irreversible tissue damage to the kidney, and the organ should be discarded. So the Belzer and Gambro storage machines allow the donor kidney to be evaluated for damage it may have sustained during the period of hypotension or anoxia which immediately preceded death of the donor.

Thanks to the pooling of results from many hospitals, it is now clear that transplants between donors and recipients who share all four HLA antigens in common have a 2-year survival which is double that of transplants between donors and recipients in whom none of the antigens are identical.

SHORTAGE OF DONORS

There remains one outstanding obstacle to the development of renal transplantation in our day, namely the difficulty of obtaining cadaver kidneys. Despite publicity on the topic, the real hurdle has always been the reluctance of doctors and nurses to consider the question of transplantation. The next generation will, we hope, be less muddled in their thinking. In Britain today it is necessary (and, the writer believes) civilized and polite, to obtain the permission of the next of kin of the patient who has just died before removing the kidneys for transplantation. Despite the obvious difficulties and embarrassments surrounding the interview with the distressed and bereaved parents or husband or wife, it is seldom indeed that one meets with a refusal. Most sensible folk, when asked, are only too glad to think that some part of their beloved is continuing to live and be useful to someone else.

SELECTION OF DONORS

If a living relative, with a satisfactory HLA match, insists on giving his or her child or sibling a kidney, it is no part of the surgeon's duty to play the Deity and refuse to perform the operation. But never should the least pressure be applied in any case.

Any cadaver is suitable as a source of donor kidneys unless there has been a carcinoma anywhere at any previous time, or recent sepsis, or severe hypertension. Because so many of the kidneys from the very aged have so much atheroma in the main renal vessels, it is seldom feasible to use a kidney from a donor who is more than 70 years old: age is otherwise no barrier.

IMMUNOSUPPRESSION

The combination of azathioprine (Imuran) and steroids was the turning point in transplantation. Thanks to these two drugs it is possible to achieve a 45% 2-year success even in badly mismatched kidneys. The dosage and the side effects of these drugs are closely watched for the first 6 weeks after transplantation, and it would be a futile task to attempt to memorize their details.

1 Bone marrow depression. This toxic effect of azathioprine is dose-related in most patients, and all that is necessary is for the drug to be stopped, or its dose lowered for a few days. For this reason in the early days after transplantation a daily full blood count is performed.

2 Peptic ulceration. During the period of uraemia, when the patient is on intermittent dialysis, there is an increased incidence of peptic ulceration, perhaps related to the increased level of circulating gastrin, and perhaps to other factors as yet unknown. (Forty per cent of gastrin is normally destroyed by the kidney.) Steroids tend to induce multiple peptic ulcers, mainly in the duodenum and upper small bowel. If, in the period of anuria after transplantation, to the high level of gastrin is added the additional insult of steroid overdosage, it is small wonder that peptic ulceration tends to appear. Haematemesis and perforation are an important and lethal post-operative complication after transplantation.

3 *Renal artery thrombosis* seldom occurs nowadays, since the technique of renal artery anastomosis is standardized. Narrowing may however occur at the anastomosis, and the restricted blood flow may, occasionally, be responsible for hypertension in the early post transplant period.

4 *Rejection* occurs at any stage after transplantation. It ought only to occur after 10 to 14 days, if the laws of the 'first set' reaction were followed in clinical practice. But some patients have previously been sensitized by antigens on the white cells of the blood they have previously been transfused with, and rejection may take place even 'on the table', though it is fortunately very rare.

The clinical diagnosis of rejection calls for the utmost judgement and skill: the pathological process is the laying down of immunoglobulin on the intima of the vessels of the graft, upon which platelets and then fibrin are deposited. The partly ischaemic kidney becomes swollen, and the local tissues react by becoming painful and tender. Blood flow in the graft is diminished. The creatinine clearance falls off, and the volume of urine diminishes.

The differential diagnosis is from obstruction to the main artery (which can be diagnosed only by an arteriogram) or to the ureter, or infection in and around the kidney. Biopsy of the kidney may show telltale infiltration of the graft by lymphocytes, and deposition of immunoglobulin upon the smaller vessels may be shown with immunofluorescent stains. But in practice the interpretation of these tests often takes too long, and the decision whether or not to treat for rejection has to be made without delay.

The treatment of rejection episodes consists of giving as large a dose of steroids as the patient can tolerate, together with as much azathioprine as his marrow can stand. In some centres local radiotherapy is also given to the graft, since this has been shown in some animal studies to be of benefit.

SECOND AND THIRD TRANSPLANTS

In the end it seems likely that most transplants will ultimately fail, and be rejected. There is no reason why these patients should not have a second or a third or even a fourth transplant, if a sufficient number of kidneys can be found. While they are waiting, they are returned to dialysis, preferably at home. And for this reason there is much to be said for a policy which ensures that the patient has been trained for home dialysis, so that when the transplant fails, all does not seem to have been lost.

FURTHER READING

Acute renal failure
Acute renal failure (Editorial) (1973) *Lancet*, July 21, **2**, 134.
BRIGGS J.D., KENNEDY A.C., YOUNG L.N., LUKE R.G. & GRAY M. (1967) Renal function after acute tubular necrosis. *Brit. med. J.* **2**, 513.
GALLAGHER L. & POLAK A. (1967) The management of acute renal failure. *Brit. J. Hosp. Med.*, **1**, 286.
Prognosis of acute renal failure (Editorial). (1973) *Brit. med. J.* May 26, **2**, 435.
SHARPSTONE P. (1970) Acute renal failure. *Brit. med. J.*, **2**, 158.

Chronic renal failure
EVANS, D.B. (1976) Acute and chronic renal failure. Chap. 18, *Urology*, ed. Blandy J.P. Blackwell Scientific Publications, Oxford.

Peritoneal dialysis
RAE A.I. & PENDRAY M. (1973) Advantages of peritoneal dialysis in chronic renal failure. *J. Amer. med. Ass.*, **225**, 937.
LANKISCH P.G., TONNIS H.J., FERNANDEZ-REDO E., GIRNDT J., KRAMER P., QUELLHORST E. & SCHELER F. (1973) Use of Tenckhoff catheter for peritoneal dialysis in terminal renal failure. *Brit. med. J.*, **4**, 712.
LEDINGHAM J. (1970) Peritoneal dialysis. *Brit. J. Hosp. Med.*, **4**, 85.

Haemodialysis
BELL P.R.F. & CALMAN K.C. (1974) Surgical aspects of haemodialysis. Churchill, Livingstone, Edinburgh.
BRESCIA M.J., CIMINO J.E., APPEL K. & HURWICH B.J. (1966) Chronic haemodialysis using venepuncture and a surgically created arteriovenous fistula. *New Eng. J. Med.*, **275**, 1089.
GORDON P.M. (1973) Home dialysis. *Brit. J. Hosp. Med.*, **9**, 629.
LUMLEY J.S.P., CATTELL W.R. & BAKER L.R.I. (1973) Access to the circulation for regular haemodialysis. *Lancet*, **1**, 510.
ROBINSON B.H.B. (1971) Intermittent dialysis in the home. *Brit. Med. Bull.*, **27**, 173.

Disease of bone in renal failure
COCHRAN M. (1970) Bone disease in renal failure. *Brit. J. Hosp. Med.*, **3**, 451.
STANBURY S.W. (1967) Bony complications of renal diseases. *Renal Disease* 2nd edn, p. 696, ed. Black D.A.K. Blackwell Scientific Publications, Oxford.
TATLER G.L.V., BAILLOD R.A., VARGHESE Z., YOUNG W.B., FARROW S., WILLS M.R. & MOREHEAD J.F. (1973) Evolution of bone disease over 10 years in 135 patients with terminal renal failure. *Brit. Med. J.*, **2**, 315.

Transplantation
CALNE R.Y. (1971) *Clinical Organ Transplantation*. Blackwell Scientific Publications, Oxford.
CALNE R.Y. (1976) Renal Transplantation. Chap. 19, *Urology*, ed. Blandy J.P. Blackwell Scientific Publications, Oxford.

CALNE R.Y. (1973) *Immunological Aspects of Transplantation Surgery*. Medical and Technical Pub. Co., Lancaster.

FESTENSTEIN H. (1976) Tissue typing and logistics of renal transplantation. Chap. 20, *Urology*, ed. Blandy J.P. Blackwell Scientific Publications, Oxford.

ROBERTS C.I. (1972) Transplantation immunity. *Brit. J. Hosp. Med.*, **8,** 695.

Chapter 13
Pelvis and Ureter–
Structure

SURGICAL RELATIONS (fig. 13.1)

On each side the ureter lies *posteriorly* in relation to the psoas muscle, crossing the iliohypogastric and ilioinguinal nerves. It is sheathed in a slippery envelope of connective tissue which permits free movement from side to side and up and down, so that one can watch the ureter (at operation) writhing up and down like a sleepy snake.

Medially the right ureter is related to the inferior vena cava, the duodenum, and the colon. On the left, the relations are similar—e.g. the aorta, the duodenojejunal flexure, and the descending colon (fig. 13.2).

It is the *anterior* relations of the ureter which are most important to remember: above, the renal artery and vein lie in front of the upper part of the renal pelvis. The segmental artery to the lower pole of the kidney crosses over the pelvis, and may lie in front of the pelviureteric junction. Half way down, the ureter is crossed over in front by the gonadal vessels, ovarian in the female, testicular in the male. Now the ureter passes anterior to the bifurcation of the common iliac artery, an infallible guide at operation, and then passes behind the first main division of the internal iliac artery—the superior vesical pedicle—from which springs off the so-called obliterated umbilical artery (which always bleeds when it is cut) and the uterine artery in women.

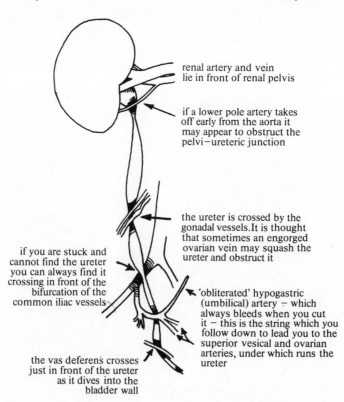

renal artery and vein lie in front of renal pelvis

if a lower pole artery takes off early from the aorta it may appear to obstruct the pelvi–ureteric junction

the ureter is crossed by the gonadal vessels. It is thought that sometimes an engorged ovarian vein may squash the ureter and obstruct it

if you are stuck and cannot find the ureter you can always find it crossing in front of the bifurcation of the common iliac vessels

'obliterated' hypogastric (umbilical) artery – which always bleeds when you cut it – this is the string which you follow down to lead you to the superior vesical and ovarian arteries, under which runs the ureter

the vas deferens crosses just in front of the ureter as it dives into the bladder wall

Fig. 13.1. Surgical relations of the ureter.

Lastly the vas deferens crosses the ureter just before it tunnels through the bladder muscle to reach its lumen.

In women the ureter has an important surgical relationship with the 'cardinal ligament' of the uterus, a tough band of fibromuscular tissue which holds up the cervix like the guy rope of a tent. The ureter passes through the middle of this ligament, and so if the uterus descends, as in prolapse, it may drag the ureter down with it. Since this ligament is situated just at the upper corner of the vaginal fornix, next to the cervix, it offers a method of reaching a stone in a ureter *per vaginam*—a surgical route favoured in the earlier days of surgery when any laparotomy was likely to be fatal (fig. 13.3).

Because the ureter lies so close to the side of the cervix of the uterus it is easily damaged during a difficult dissection at hysterectomy. If damaged, the ureter may be *cut* (when it will leak, usually into the vagina) or it may be *tied* (when the kidney and ureter on that side will become obstructed).

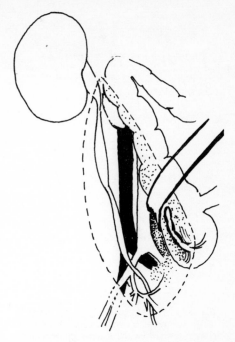

Fig. 13.2. Medial relations of the ureter are the colon and the duodenum and the inferior vena cava. Posteriorly it lies on the psoas, and crosses the ilio-inguinal, ilio-hypogastric nerves. The surgical approach to the ureter by drawing the colon over medially: note how the retrocaecal position of the appendix makes it lie on top of the ureter: many a ureter has been damaged during appendicectomy, and it is easy to mistake pain in the appendix for pain in the ureter.

BLOOD SUPPLY (fig. 13.4)

Along the front of the ureter runs a conspicuous artery and vein, mainly deriving from the renal vessels, but reinforced at intervals from lumbar vessels and the superior vesical pedicle nearer the bladder. Thanks to this longitudinal arrangement of its blood supply it is possible to preserve a fairly long length of viable ureter during transplantation.

NERVE SUPPLY (fig. 13.5)

Sensory fibres emerge from the ureter in a segmental pattern. Its upper

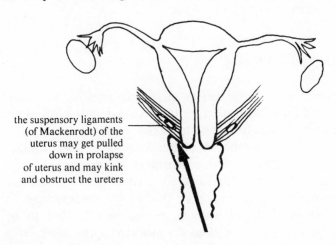

the suspensory ligaments (of Mackenrodt) of the uterus may get pulled down in prolapse of uterus and may kink and obstruct the ureters

Fig. 13.3. Note close relationship of ureter to cervix, and fornix of vagina. This makes it easily damaged during hysterectomy; when it leaks after injury, it leaks into the vagina as a ureterovaginal fistula. In the old days stones in the lower inch of the ureter were sometimes removed through the fornix where they could be felt and cut down upon.

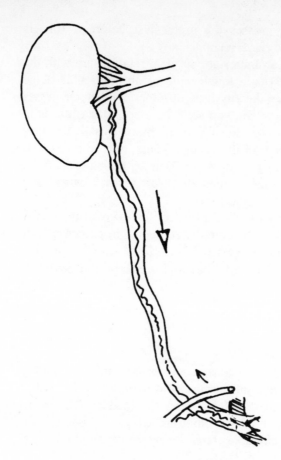

Fig. 13.4. The blood supply of the ureter is lucky for renal transplantation, because it comes down from the arteries of the kidney and renal pelvis in longitudinal ureteric vessels. Trivial additional blood supply is derived from branches of the artery of the vas deferens and the arteries of the bladder wall.

In removing a donor kidney for a transplant one must take care not to damage the little branches of the renal artery in the sinus of the kidney.

part is supplied from T 10, hence pain is referred to the umbilical region: lower down pain in the ureter is felt at progressively lower intervals until finally where it goes into the bladder pain may be referred to groin, vulva, or penis.

PERISTALSIS IN THE URETER

The ureter is constructed of long helices of smooth muscle, interlaced with one another, and the whole muscular tube is lined with a thin layer of urothelium on a very thin submucosal layer (fig. 13.6).

Each muscle bundle is composed of hundreds of smaller smooth muscle cells, each one fitted by microscopical interlocking jig-saw fittings into its neighbour: these jig-saws are termed nexuses, and are found in other muscular systems such as that of the myocardium. It seems as if they allow electrical activity in one muscle fibre to be transmitted directly to the next, and so do away with the need for a

Chapter 13/*Pelvis and Ureter: Structure*

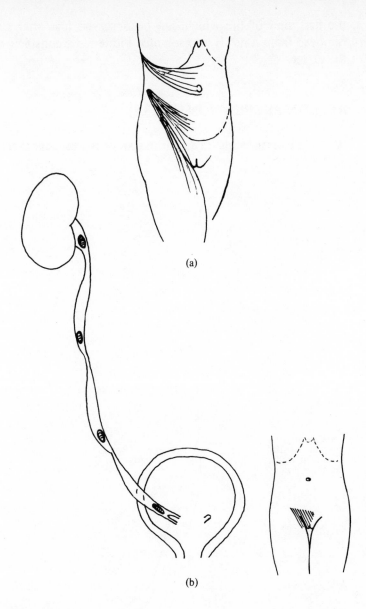

(a)

(b)

Fig. 13.5. Nerve supply of the ureter. It gets segmental nerve supply: hence pain arising from a stone in the upper part is felt in the loin, radiating towards the umbilicus. (a) As the stone works down the ureter so the pain gets lower and lower, radiating to groin, testicle and thigh. (b) As the stone works through the wall of the bladder pain is felt as 'cystitis' or referred to penis or vulva.

nervous network or for ganglia. In fact electron microscopy of the ureter fails to show any ganglia at all, and the slow writhing motion of the ureter is now thought to be purely a muscular conduction, determined by distension of the upper part (i.e. calix or renal pelvis) and perhaps governed to some extent by a 'pacemaker' situated in the renal pelvis (fig. 13.7).

This is fortunate for transplantation, because it means that the completely denervated ureter will work perfectly well. Indeed, almost the first sign of life which can be observed just after the clamps are removed from a newly transplanted kidney is a conspicuous writhing of the ureter.

REFLUX-PREVENTION (fig. 13.8)

Where the ureter slips through the wall of the bladder there is an oblique

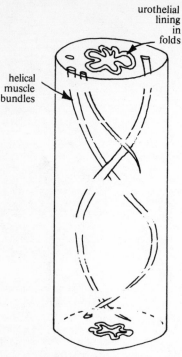

urothelial
lining
in
folds

helical
muscle
bundles

Fig. 13.6. Ureter is lined with urothelium like bladder and renal pelvis. At rest, it seems all folded up in longitudinal folds, which fill out on being distended.

Its muscle fibres appear to be longitudinal and transverse in cross section: in fact they form a series of helices of varying obliquity, and are grouped together like the strands of a Chinese fingerstall.

Fig. 13.7. Ureteric peristalsis seems to be determined by a pacemaker in the renal pelvis, whose timing is governed by the volume of urine put out by the kidney, and the distension of the renal pelvis. There are no ganglia in the wall of the ureter. One smooth muscle fibre forms a very intimate connection with the next by means of a jigsaw puzzle arrangement. Hence the electrical activity of one smooth muscle fibre is communicated to the next. This communication works both ways, so peristalsis can go upwards as well as downwards.

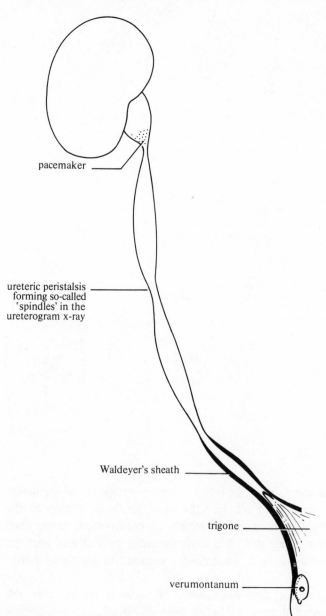

pacemaker

ureteric peristalsis
forming so-called
'spindles' in the
ureterogram x-ray

Waldeyer's sheath

trigone

verumontanum

Chapter 13/*Pelvis and Ureter: Structure*

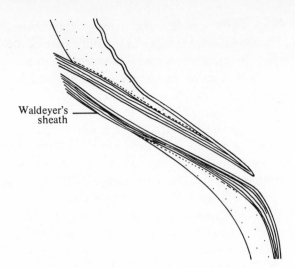

Waldeyer's sheath

Fig. 13.8. Where the ureter passes through the wall of the bladder there is very beautiful valvular arrangement first described by Leonardo da Vinci. Lubricated areolar tissue allows the ureter to move in and out in a sleeve (described by Waldeyer) which is tethered at its lower end to the urethra near the verumontanum in the male. Note the thick 'backing' to the valve made by the wall of the bladder, and the thin delicate flap of the valve itself where it issues into the bladder. As the bladder contracts, this valve shuts, so that urine is not forced up the ureter to the kidney. Many children are born with incompetent valves and so get vesico-ureteric reflux of urine, which may injure the kidney, and perpetuate urinary infection.

tunnel, forming a flap-valve. If the pressure increases in the bladder the valve is shut, so that urine does not run up the ureter each time the patient voids. The actual structure of the valve is more complicated than this: it is provided with a lubricated areolar sheath allowing it to slide up and down, and there is a firm attachment of the lower part of the ureter to the trigonal muscle.

EFFECT OF DILATATION (fig. 13.9)

Thanks to persistent peristalsis, or to obstruction, the wall of the ureter may become dilated. When this occurs the tube cannot contract completely, i.e. its walls do not meet. If this happens, then peristalsis cannot form the bolus of urine into a compartment, and squeeze it down to the bladder. It merely allows the urine to run up and down. Under these circumstances the ureter is converted into an open hose-pipe, and the only force pushing the urine into the bladder is the glomerular filtration pressure.

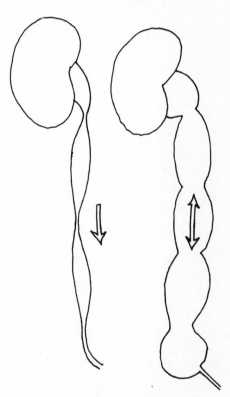

Fig. 13.9. To be effective, peristalsis needs the walls of the ureter to come together to form closed compartments in which a bolus of urine is carried down to the bladder.

When the ureter is dilated as the result of obstruction or congenital deficiency in the muscle fibres, the walls do not occlude the lumen, a bolus cannot be formed, and urine merely washes up and down.

FURTHER READING

GOODWIN F.G. (1976) Urinary obstruction and renal function. *Urology*, ed. Blandy J.P., p. 554. Blackwell Scientific Publications, Oxford.

NOTLEY R.G. (1976) Anatomy and physiology of the ureter. *Urology*, ed. Blandy J.P., p. 568. Blackwell Scientific Publications, Oxford.

ORMOND J.K. (1975) A classification of retroperitoneal fibrosis. *Urol. Survey*, **25**, 53.

TANAGHO E.A. (1976) The ureterovesical junction: anatomy and physiology. *Scientific Foundations of Urology*, eds. Williams D.I. and Chisholm G.D., p. 23. Heinemann, London.

WEISS R.M. (1976) Initiation and organisation of ureteral peristalsis. *Urol. Survey*, **26**, 2.

WHITAKER R.H. (1976) Pathophysiology of ureteric obstruction. *Scientific Foundations of Urology*, eds. Williams D.I. and Chisholm G.D., p. 18. Heinemann, London.

Chapter 14
Pelvis and Ureter–Congenital Anomalies

The ureter develops as an important branch from the mesonephric (Wolffian) duct leading to the only part of the row of nephrons which is used in the adult human—the metanephros.

This ureteric bud branches as it nears the metanephros into, at first, two main branches, one supplying the upper group of nephrons, the other the lower part.

With the continued growth of the hind part of the foetus, the relative position of the kidneys seem to rise up into the abdomen and loin. At the same time the bladder grows upwards and outwards taking in the lower end of the Wolffian (mesonephric) ducts together with their budding ureters. If these bud off separately, from the region of the elbow bend of the mesonephric duct, because the bladder rises upwards and outwards, so it comes about that the ureteric bud from the upper half-kidney comes to enter the trigone below and medial to the bud belonging to the lower half-kidney (fig. 14.1).

PROBLEMS ASSOCIATED WITH DUPLEX URETER

Ureterocele (fig. 14.2)

Where the ureter enters the bladder, it may have a very small orifice, and the mucosa just behind it becomes distended like a little balloon. This deformity may occur with a single ureter, or with a duplex pair of ureteric orifices, in which case it affects the ureter of the upper moiety, the medial ureter, the one which enters the trigone nearest the internal meatus.

Ureterocele may cause no trouble at all: it may cause some

Fig. 14.1. Development of the ureter.

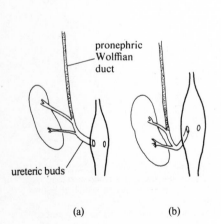

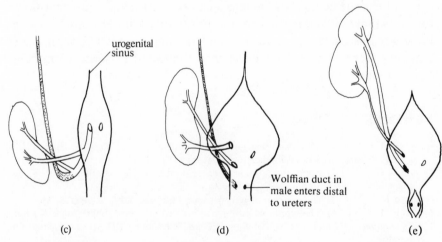

(a)   (b)   (c)   (d)   (e)

as the urogenital sinus elongates, it loops up the Wolffian duct and ureters which now cross each other

lateral expansion of the trigone incorporates the ends of the ureters

the kidneys now move upwards

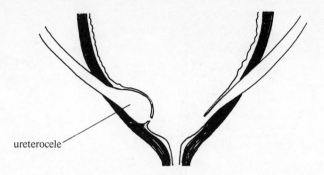

ureterocele

Fig. 14.2. Ureterocele.

obstruction, and sometimes a calculus forms within its little balloon. Its radiographic appearance is quite characteristic and has been likened to the head of a cobra (fig. 14.3). If it is slit up cystoscopically, there may be insufficient flap valve to prevent reflux, and the ureter may then have to be reimplanted. In children the ureterocele may really be gigantic, and actually be extruded from the bladder as the child tries to pass urine, appearing at the vulva as a peculiar cyst. Ureteroceles may occur in ureters opening in ectopic positions.

Ectopic ureter

Where the Wolffian ducts debouch into the cloaca is just where the urorectal septum falls down like a shutter to demarcate the bladder from the rectum. Just lateral and behind the entry of the Wolffian ducts are the paramesonephric ducts, which, it will be remembered, were special additional tubes formed by the mesonephros which become taken over in the female to form the uterus, and Fallopian tubes, and the upper part of the vagina. These paramesonephric (Müllerian) ducts lie close to the Wolffian ducts, and, while the Wolffian ducts are spreading out to form the trigone, and the Müllerian ducts are expanding to form the upper end of the vagina, it is hardly surprising that occasionally the upper part of the vagina may take up the lower end of the

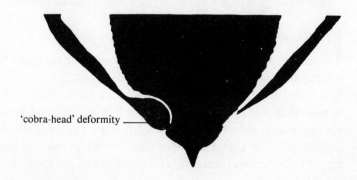

'cobra-head' deformity

Fig. 14.3. Radiographic appearance of ureterocele.

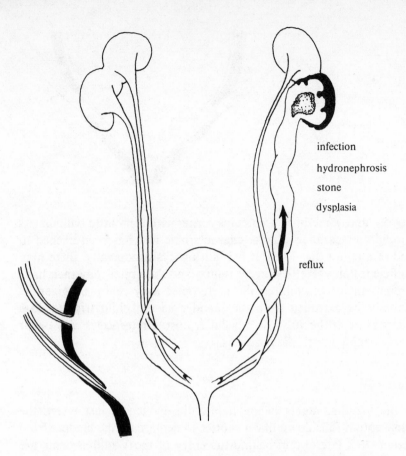

infection

hydronephrosis

stone

dysplasia

reflux

Fig. 14.4. Duplex kidneys and reflux.

Wolffian tissue, or the most medial of a pair of duplex ureters finds itself opening in the vagina rather than the bladder. Ectopic ureters cause persistent wetting by day and by night, and always drain the upper half-kidney. They may be associated with a ureterocele.

In little boys, thanks to the fact that the ureters arise as diverticula of the Wolffian mesonephric duct, and this duct is borrowed in the male to serve as the gonadal duct and turns into the vas deferens and seminal vesicles, it is not surprising that occasionally a ureter is found to drain into a seminal vesicle or the lower end of the vas.

Reflux (fig. 14.4)

The most medial of the two duplex ureteric orifices follows a long course through the wall of the bladder, but the most lateral opening, which drains the lower half-kidney, may have such a short intramural course that there is ineffectual flap-valve action, and reflux takes place. Occasionally unfortunate babies are born with a 'full-house' of duplex pathology—i.e. they have ureteroceles with ectopic ureters draining the upper half-kidneys, and reflux taking place to the lower half-kidneys.

Abnormal dilatation may occur at any part in the collecting system of the urinary tract.

Chapter 15
Pelvis and Ureter—Hydronephrosis

TUBULES

In congenital medullary sponge kidney there are congenital dilatations of the collecting tubules (fig. 15.1) in the renal papilla (see page 46). Calculi and infection tend to lurk in these dilated tubules. The condition may be unilateral or bilateral, and affect all or only part of a kidney. It presents as episodes of ureteric colic or infection. The radiographic picture is characteristic: the kidney is enlarged, and streaks, like little necklaces of minute calculi outline each of the dilated tubules. Urography shows these streaks to be filled with contrast. It may be associated with hemihypertrophy of the body.

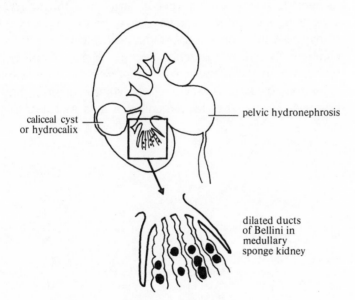

caliceal cyst or hydrocalix

pelvic hydronephrosis

dilated ducts of Bellini in medullary sponge kidney

Fig. 15.1. Dilatation of tubules and calices.

CALICES

Congenital dilatation of a calix (caliceal diverticulum or cyst) occurs for no good reason. One postulate is a dyssynergy of the muscle at the neck of the calix, as if putting the thing into Greek makes it easier to understand. In other cases a similar narrowing of the neck of the calix occurs as a result of inflammation and scarring, sometimes from tuberculosis. Occasionally the narrowing of the neck of the calix, affecting the main upper pole calix, seems to be related to its proximity to the main upper renal segmental artery, and a plastic operation may correct the trouble.

Clinically such patients present with a stone or infection or both, or the deformity is noticed in a routine urogram done for some other reason.

The only important differential diagnosis is from tuberculosis. The treatment is to uncap the cyst, and divide the affected calix in the renal sinus, if it is causing trouble. Many of them can be safely left alone.

RENAL PELVIS (fig. 15.2)

Dilatation of the renal pelvis may be the result of a stone impacted at the junction of pelvis and ureter, a tumour, or a post-traumatic scar, but far and away the most common and most important cause of hydronephrosis is due to the collection of collagen fibres in the wall of the ureter, just where the pelvis turns into the ureter. Why collagen collects here is still not known: it may be the result of inflammation, or it may be some congenital anomaly (it is certainly seen in very young children). Whatever the aetiology, once a ring of stiff collagen has been laid down in the ureteric wall, it prevents it from expanding, and in conditions of diuresis when a large volume of urine has to be pumped down the ureter, the ring of collagen acts like a collar, and prevents

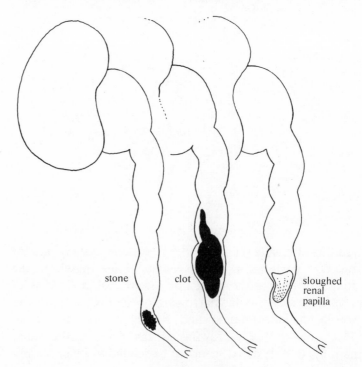

stone   clot   sloughed renal papilla

Fig. 15.2. Causes of obstruction within the lumen of the ureter.

expansion to the necessary calibre. The pressure rises in the pelvis proximal to the pelviureteric junction, hypertrophy takes place, the pelvis expands and dilates, and eventually the kidney begins to undergo progressive atrophy (fig. 15.3).

In a large proportion of cases, the expansion of the pelvis causes it to bulge forward between the main leash of renal vessels and the artery going to the lower pole. In time it begins to look as though the lower polar artery is actually causing the obstruction—and indeed it may be making it worse, if not actually causing it in the first place. Hence the tradition of the 'PUJ' obstruction caused by an 'aberrant lower pole artery'.

Clinically patients with the PUJ obstruction present with episodes of pain, coming on after drinking large volumes of fluid, and associated with unusual feelings including indigestion—perhaps from the proximity of the duodenum or colon. Many patients get relief from the pain by lying in odd positions, bending forward over the bed, or lying on the side, and it is easy to form the impression that the patient is mad. Later on, when the kidney pelvis has become converted into a fibrotic and more or less inert bag, there is less pain, and the condition may go unnoticed for years until infection takes place in the residual urine, or until for some reason a lump is found on abdominal palpation, or an excretion urogram is performed because of haematuria, trauma, or the investigation of recurrent urinary infection.

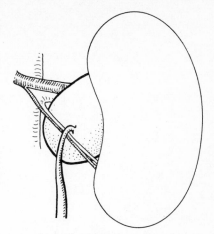

Seen from behind the lower polar vessels appear to be causing the PUJ obstruction

Fig. 15.3 Pelvi-ureteric junction obstruction.

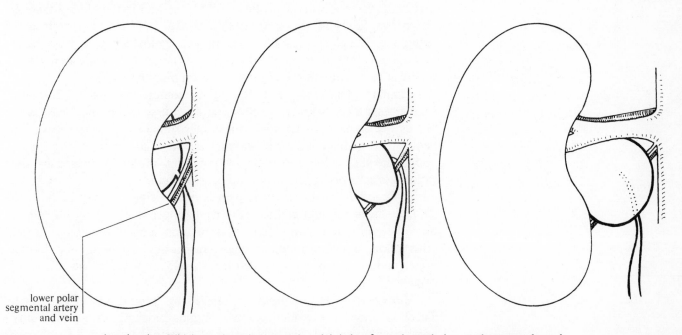

lower polar segmental artery and vein

Anterior view. With increasing enlargement the pelvis bulges forward over the lower pole segmental vessels

There are many operations to correct the trouble: in Britain the procedure most usually performed is the pyeloplasty of Anderson and Hynes (see page 273). Provided this is done before the renal parenchyma is utterly destroyed, the results are excellent.

Stones, hypertension and haematuria are common complications of hydronephrosis.

OTHER CAUSES OF HYDRONEPHROSIS

Causes within the lumen of the ureter and pelvis

1. STONE

Ureteric calculus is the most common cause of dilatation of the ureter and kidney. If under 0.5 cm diameter the stone is likely to pass without any need for surgical interference. If larger than this, it is probably going to need an operation.

Aetiology. The stones form in the kidney (see page 91). They become detached and are carried down the ureter. They are more common in men than in women, occur at any age, but usually in middle age, and they are more common in hot climates where the urine become concentrated from water loss in the sweat.

Pathology. Behind the stone there is oedema of the mucosa of the ureter, the ureteric wall is swollen and dilated, and in the kidney there is distension, followed by extravasation (leakage) of urine permitting a continuance of glomerular filtration, though against a higher pressure. If there is infection, tremendous damage is done to the renal parenchyma by the intravasation of the organisms accompanying the urine.

Clinical features. Ureteric colic comes on with dramatic suddenness: there is severe pain, radiating at first to the umbilicus, later on, as the stone courses down the ureter, felt in the groin, vulva, or penis. The pain comes in waves, and is accompanied by gross abdominal distension and often by vomiting, probably caused by the exudate of retroperitoneal urine and oedema fluid.

Differential diagnosis. If the pain is on the right, it may be hard to distinguish the clinical picture from acute appendicitis. If on the left, it may be mistaken for acute diverticulitis or even small bowel obstruction. When in doubt, an emergency urogram will show a dilated ureter ending at the site of obstruction, and may show the offending calculus.

Management. Pain should be relieved by large doses of pethidine. There is very little evidence that ganglion-blocking drugs offer any additional advantage. The urine must be examined to see if it is infected or not: if it is infected (i.e. if the gram stain teems with organisms and there are masses of pus cells) then a far more active line of treatment is called for, and one will almost certainly want to get the stone out without much delay. But in the absence of infection, it is safe to wait and see, being confident in the knowledge that small calculi generally pass on their own.

Indications for surgery. A stone bigger than 0.5 cm diameter; one that has got stuck in the ureter for several months, and does not budge; one associated with persistent hydronephrosis and hydroureter; or the complication of infection—all these circumstances call for surgical intervention.

If the stone is anywhere in the ureter except the lowermost two or three centimetres, it is removed by open operation (*ureterolithotomy* see page 288). In the lowermost part of the ureter, it can be got out occasionally by passing a *basket* up the ureter which catches (fig. 15.4) the stone and removes it cystoscopically. Used for any but small stones in the lower reaches of the ureter the basket is a most dangerous weapon. Sometimes the stone gets held up at the opening of the ureter

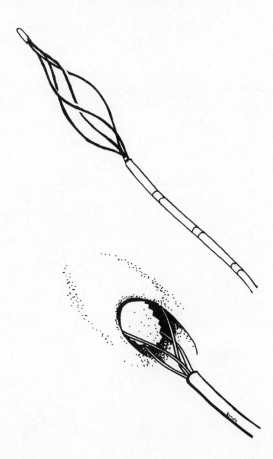

Fig. 15.4. Dormia's basket.

itself, and can be seen down the cystoscope like a rabbit looking out of its hole. It is then easy to enlarge the hole with a diathermy or scissors and release the trapped calculus.

2. BLOOD CLOT

Clot may obstruct the ureter, from any cause of haematuria.

3. DETACHED RENAL PAPILLA

In countries where analgesic abuse is common, dead papillae stuck in the ureter are a common surgical emergency. They can usually be removed with the Dormia basket.

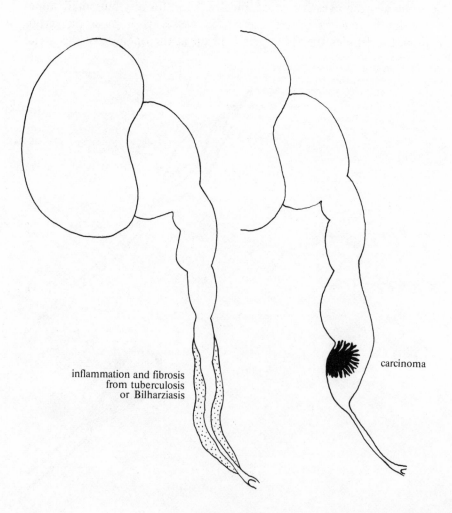

inflammation and fibrosis
from tuberculosis
or Bilharziasis

carcinoma

Fig. 15.5. Causes of obstruction arising in the wall of the ureter.

Chapter 15/*Pelvis and Ureter: Hydronephrosis*

Causes within the wall of the ureter (fig. 15.5)

1. INFLAMMATION

Oedema and fibrosis cause obstruction in tuberculosis and schistosomiasis. Fibrosis may follow radiotherapy for cancer in the cervix or bladder.

2. CARCINOMA

If carcinoma occurs in the urothelium of the ureter it may occlude its lumen like a cherry on a stalk, or invade its muscular wall, making it rigid, narrow, and stiff.

Carcinoma in adjacent organs e.g. the cervix of the uterus or the colon may infiltrate the wall of the ureter. So may retroperitoneal spread from a distant primary such as a carcinoma of breast or lung.

Causes outside the wall of the ureter (fig. 15.6)

1. COMPRESSION BY BLOOD VESSELS

There is a rare congenital anomaly in which the ureter passes behind the inferior vena cava. Proximal to the vena cava the ureter and kidney are enormously dilated by the time the diagnosis is made. In pregnancy, dilatation of the ovarian veins on the right side may compress the ureter, though it is by no means certain how often this takes place, or whether there are other, more important causes for the ureteric dilatation seen in pregnancy.

2. PREGNANCY

Although pathologists have strained for years to conceive of something other than the baby which squashes the ureter, and have invoked vascular and hormonal causes for the hydroureter of pregnancy, it seems somewhat more likely that ureteric compression is caused by that rather large and obvious swelling—the pregnant uterus. However, the question is still open.

3. COMPRESSION BY EXTRAURETERIC TUMOURS

Unless a tumour actually invades the wall of the ureter it hardly ever causes obstruction, and benign tumours may cause gross deviation of the line of the ureter without producing any dilatation above it.

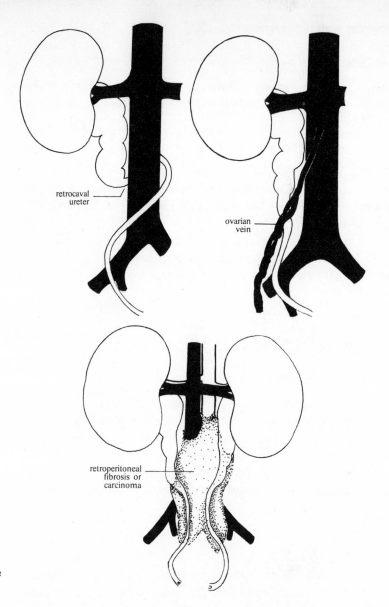

Fig. 15.6. Causes of obstruction outside ureter.

4. IDIOPATHIC RETROPERITONEAL FIBROSIS

Fibrous tissue is laid down in the retroperitoneal connective tissue, which infiltrates and compresses the ureter and cava and sometimes the aorta. Nobody knows why it gets there: in some cases it seems to be associated with the ingestion of methysergide, and more recently, with analgesic abuse. It may be associated with mediastinal fibrosis, nodules in the ear-lobes, and Dupuytren's contracture of the palms of the hands. If caught early, it may respond to steroids: more established and mature fibrous tissue has to be dissected off the ureter which is then wrapped in omentum.

Vesicoureteric reflux (fig. 15.7)

Reflux may be due to a congenital abnormality in the construction of the intramural part of the ureter, and as described above, is often associated with duplex ureter, when it affects the more laterally placed ureter which drains the lower half-kidney.

Or reflux may be caused by oedema around the ureteric orifice, and so can occur as a transient event in association with urinary infection. Similarly, reflux can follow operations upon the lower end of the ureter such as transurethral resection of a bladder cancer, or diathermy of a papilloma, or indeed any pathological process which is followed by scarring of that part of the wall of the bladder. Hence it is seen after

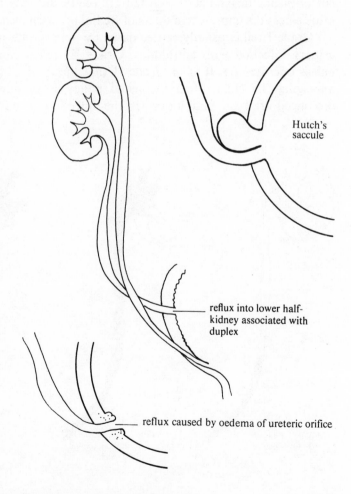

Hutch's saccule

reflux into lower half-kidney associated with duplex

reflux caused by oedema of ureteric orifice

Fig. 15.7. Some causes of reflux.

tuberculosis has been treated, and in interstitial and other forms of chronic bladder inflammation.

If peristalsis in the ureter is effective, then reflux is probably not going to matter very much, since the ureter will keep the bladder urine away from the kidney. If the urine is sterile, it does not damage the kidney. Even if it is infected, it can only get into the parenchyma when the renal papillae are misshaped so as not to act like valves—a condition only present in some papillae in some children.

DIAGNOSIS

Reflux is diagnosed by a micturating cystogram, in which special films are taken as the child is voiding. Reflux is classified into three grades: in Grade I the lower end of the ureter is barely filled, and the contrast does not reach the renal pelvis. In Grade II the contrast reaches the kidney, but does not distend it. In Grade III reflux distends the kidney and urine enters the unprotected ducts of Bellini of misshapen papillae.

Grade I reflux usually settles down by appropriate treatment of the urinary infection with antibiotics. Grade III reflux rarely gets better, unless operated on. It is in Grade II that the main difficulty arises in managing the child. Here the usual policy is to allow the child a prolonged trial on antibiotics. If the infection is controlled, and if

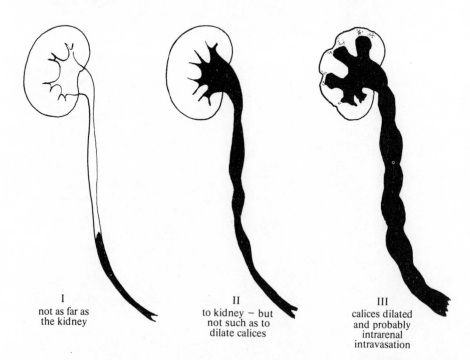

I
not as far as
the kidney

II
to kidney – but
not such as to
dilate calices

III
calices dilated
and probably
intrarenal
intravasation

Fig. 15.8. Grades of reflux.

Chapter 15/*Pelvis and Ureter: Hydronephrosis*

successive urograms show that the kidney is growing properly, and not forming scars, then nothing need be done. But if infection repeatedly relapses, or if the urograms show failure of the parenchyma to grow, or the development of cortical scars, then the ureters should be reimplanted.

REIMPLANTATION OF THE URETERS

Several techniques are in use (see page 290). In expert hands there is little to choose between them. Given an experienced surgeon and a well tried technique, reflux is prevented in about 90% of ureters reimplanted, infection is cured in about 80%, and there is a 2 to 3% incidence of sloughing or stricture of the reimplanted ureter necessitating nephrectomy. When the ureter is grossly enlarged, it may be necessary to 'tailor' it to size over a catheter.

FURTHER READING

Butler M.R., Devine H.F. & O'Flynn J.D. (1973) Medullary Sponge Kidney: review of the literature and presentation of 33 cases. *J. Irish Med. Ass.*, **66**, 5.

Derrick F.C., Rosenblum R. & Frensilli F.J. (1973) Right ovarian vein syndrome: six year critique. *Urology*, **1**, 383.

Glenn J.F. & Anderson E.E. (1973) Complications of ureteral reimplantation. *Urol. Survey*, **23**, 243.

Golding P.L., Singh M. & Worthington B. (1972) Bilateral ureteric obstruction caused by benign pelvic lipomatosis. *Brit. J. Surg.*, **59**, 69.

Hendren W.H. (1974) Reoperation for the failed ureteral reimplantation. *J. Urol.*, **111**, 403.

Johnston J.H. (1976) Congenital anomalies of the Calices, Pelvis and Ureter. *Urology*, ed. Blandy J.P., p. 521. Blackwell Scientific Publications, Oxford.

Johnston J.H. & Goodwin W.E. (1975) *Reviews in Paediatric Urology*. Excerpta Medica, Amsterdam.

Lewis C.T., Molland E.A., Marshall V.R., Tresidder G.C. & Blandy J.P. (1975) Analgesic abuse, ureteric obstruction and retroperitoneal fibrosis. *Brit. Med. J.*, **2**, 76.

Notley R.G. (1976) Anatomy and physiology of the ureter. *Urology*, ed. Blandy J.P., p. 568. Blackwell Scientific Publications, Oxford.

Notley R.G. & Beaugié J.M. (1973) The long term follow-up of Anderson Hynes pyeloplasty for hydronephrosis, *Brit. J. Urol.*, **45**, 464.

Ormond J.K. (1975) A classification of retroperitoneal fibrosis. *Urol. Survey*, **25**, 53.

Ransley P.G. (1976) The renal papilla and intrarenal reflux. *Scientific Foundations of Urology*, eds. Williams D.I. and Chisholm G.D., p. 79. Heinemann, London.

Scott J.E.S. (1972) A critical appraisal of the management of ureteric reflux. *Problems in Paediatric Urology*, eds. Johnston J.H. and Scholtmeijer R.J., p. 271. Excerpta Medica, Amsterdam.

Williams D.I. & Mininberg D.T. (1968) Hydrocalycosis: report of three cases in children. *Brit. J. Urol.*, **40**, 541.

Williams D.I. (1974) Vesicoureteric reflux. *Encyclopaedia of Urology XV*, Supplement, p. 111. Springer.

Williams D.J. (1974) Ectopic ureter. *Encyclopaedia of Urology XV*, Supplement, p. 137. Springer.

Chapter 16
The Bladder— Surgical Anatomy

SURGICAL RELATIONS OF THE BLADDER

Superiorly the bladder is covered by peritoneum, and is overlain by various loops of small bowel, the transverse colon, the sigmoid, and the omentum. A long tail of urachus joins the dome of the bladder to the umbilicus, and represents the foetal allantois.

Anteriorly the bladder when empty is tucked behind the symphysis pubis, but when full rises up behind the lower part of the rectus abdominis muscles. In this state it is a close relation of the gap between the lateral edge of the rectus sheath and the curved conjoined tendon, through which emerge direct and and indirect inguinal herniae, so the bladder can be injured at herniorrhaphy, or a diverticulum of the bladder can bulge out as part of the medial wall of a hernial sac.

Posteriorly the bladder is separated from the rectum in the male by the two layers of peritoneum, here stuck together to form Denonvilliers' fascia. In the female the bladder lies in front of the uterus, cervix, and vagina.

Below the bladder in the male sits the prostate, encircling the urethra like a doughnut, and below this lies the 'pelvic diaphragm' i.e. the levator ani muscle sandwiched between two tough layers of fascia.

Fig. 16.1. Surgical relations of the bladder.

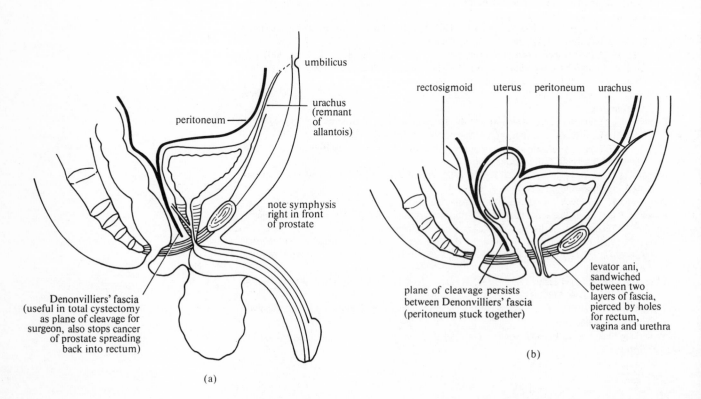

(a)

(b)

BLOOD SUPPLY (fig. 16.2)

The bladder has a very rich blood supply, derived from three pedicles on either side. The main one is the superior vesical artery, the first big branch of the internal iliac artery. This crosses just in front of the ureter, and has always to be cut when carrying out surgical operations on the side of the bladder or the ureter.

There are two other less well-defined groups of vessels entering the side of the bladder further down towards the levator ani diaphragm.

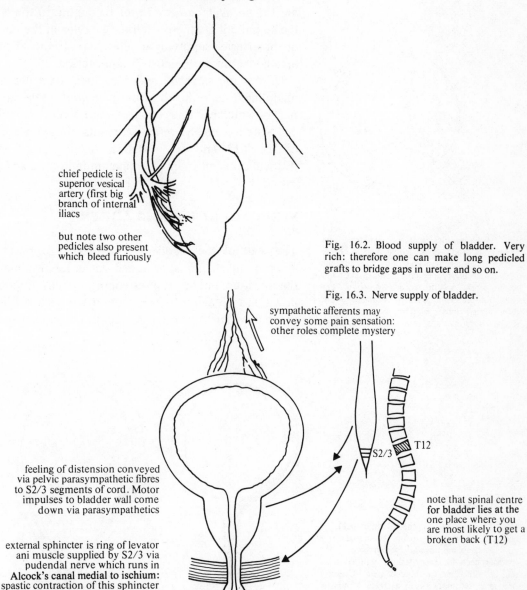

chief pedicle is superior vesical artery (first big branch of internal iliacs

but note two other pedicles also present which bleed furiously

Fig. 16.2. Blood supply of bladder. Very rich: therefore one can make long pedicled grafts to bridge gaps in ureter and so on.

Fig. 16.3. Nerve supply of bladder.

sympathetic afferents may convey some pain sensation: other roles complete mystery

S2/3   T12

note that spinal centre for bladder lies at the one place where you are most likely to get a broken back (T12)

feeling of distension conveyed via pelvic parasympathetic fibres to S2/3 segments of cord. Motor impulses to bladder wall come down via parasympathetics

external sphincter is ring of levator ani muscle supplied by S2/3 via pudendal nerve which runs in Alcock's canal medial to ischium: spastic contraction of this sphincter will stop the bladder from emptying

INNERVATION (fig. 16.3)

Although there is a thick band of *sympathetic* fibres passing to, or from, the bladder, which courses down in front of the bifurcation of the aorta, and was once entitled the 'presacral nerve', nobody quite knows what these fibres are supposed to be doing. Probably they carry pain sensation up from the bladder, and possibly they are important in ejaculation. No doubt in time more will be found out about them.

The most important nerves of the bladder (as far as we know today) are the *parasympathetic* fibres belonging to the S2 and S3 segments of the spinal cord, which reach the bladder in the connective tissue sheaths of the arteries supplying it. These serve both afferent and efferent reflex arcs concerned with detrusor contraction.

From the same S2 and 3 segments are derived the *somatic motor* medullated nerve fibres of the *pudendal nerve*, going to the levator ani, part of which encircles the urethra and acts as an external sphincter.

Note that the S2 and 3 segments of the cord are situated at the level of the T12 and L1 vertebral disc—just where vertebral fracture-dislocation is most apt to happen in industrial and mining accidents.

STRUCTURE OF THE BLADDER

The wall of the bladder is formed by a basket-work of interlacing smooth muscle fibres, arranged not in longitudinal or circular coats like the intestine, but as an intertwining system of loops, many of which dip down and up again to curl around the neck of the bladder, and to give the impression of a collar of smooth muscle at the bladder neck.

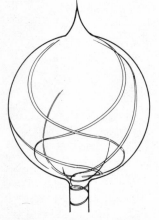

Fig. 16.4. Muscle wall of bladder. The detrusor is made up of helical muscle fibres, not an inner circular and outer longitudinal layer as formerly depicted. This makes (1) lattice work, so in hypertrophy you get trabeculation and a coarse network, (2) some fibres loop round bladder neck to form 'internal sphincter', (3) others encircle urethra.

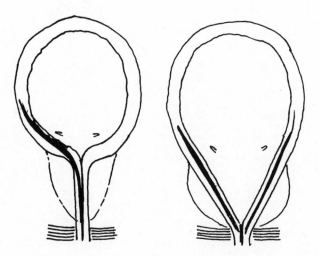

Fig. 16.5. Effect on the bladder neck of contraction of the detrusor. As the detrusor contracts, some fibres, which cross the bladder neck like bow-strings, will contract and so pull open the bladder neck. Concept of an automatically separate 'internal sphincter' is not so simple as we once thought.

Chapter 16/*Bladder: Surgical Anatomy*

Some of these helical fibres continue down the urethra and are attached to the connective tissue of the urethral wall in the region of the verumontanum, while others are continued down amongst the other muscle fibres of the wall of the urethra itself.

The result of this beautiful and unique construction is that when the detrusor contracts, it also opens the internal meatus.

Lining the wall of the bladder is the urothelium. This is about two cells thick when the bladder is fully distended but, when empty, wrinkles up, so that it seems as if the cells are five to seven layers thick and piled on top of each other. Electron microscope studies however show that this is not the case, but that each cell retains its attachment by a long thin stalk to the basement membrane.

Beneath the urothelium is a plexus of arteries and veins, but remarkably few lymphatics (except in disease).

FURTHER READING

AWAD S.A. & DOWNIE J.W. (1976) Relative contributions of smooth and striated muscles to the canine urethral pressure profile. *Brit. J. Urol.*, **48**, 347.

DONKER P.J., DROES J.T.P.M. & VAN ULDEN B.M. (1976) Anatomy of the musculature and invervation of the bladder and urethra. *Scientific Foundations of Urology*, eds. Williams D.I. and Chisholm G.D., p. 39. Heinemann, London.

GOSLING J.A. & DIXON J.S. (1975) The structure and innervation of smooth muscle in the wall of the bladder neck and proximal urethra. *Brit. J. Urol.*, **47**, 549.

SMITH J.C. (1976) The function of the bladder. *Urology*, ed. Blandy J.P., p. 672. Blackwell Scientific Publications, Oxford.

TANAGHO E.A. (1976) The ureterovesical junction: anatomy and physiology. *Scientific Foundations of Urology*, eds. Williams D.I. and Chisholm G.D., p. 23. Heinemann, London.

ZINNER N.R., RITTER R.C. & STERLING A.M. (1976) The mechanism of micturition. *Scientific Foundations of Urology*, eds. Williams D.I. and Chisholm G.D., p. 51. Heinemann, London.

Chapter 17
The Bladder—
Congenital
Abnormalities

EMBRYOLOGY (fig. 17.1)

The bladder is formed from two parts: its dome and the long tail of urachus which leads up to the umbilicus are formed from the primitive hind-gut or cloaca. Draining into this cavity are the two mesonephric ducts and their lowermost branches, the ureters. Parallel and lateral to the mesonephric (Wolffian) ducts are the paramesonephric (Müllerian) ducts. Separating the bladder from the rectum is the curtain of urorectal septum, which carried with it the paramesonephric ducts which are going to turn into the vagina, uterus, and Fallopian tubes of the female. The urethra and trigone are formed by the expansion and flattening-out of the lower ends of the Wolffian ducts.

CONGENITAL ABNORMALITIES

1. Agenesis

A very rare anomaly in which the cloaca does not develop. Ureteric obstruction usually coexists.

2. Duplication

Sometimes the bladder is split in half by a median septum, in other cases the septum is more or less incomplete. In rare instances there is a horizontal septum giving the bladder an hour-glass appearance.

3. Patent urachus

Sometimes the urachus remains open, and urine leaks after the umbilical cord has sloughed off. It may be associated with a congenital obstruction at the neck of the bladder. Sometimes a cyst remains half way along the urachus, which gets infected in later life and forms an abscess, which may discharge at the umbilicus.

4. Extrophy (fig. 17.2)

The basic abnormality occurs at the 5 mm embryo stage and is caused by the growth of an abnormally large cloacal membrane, which extends over and up to the lower abdominal wall, keeping its lateral walls from migrating inwards, as they normally would to close the defect. The cloacal membrane normally dissolves in the region of the perineum in order to open up the rectum vagina and urethra: but in extrophy, when it dissolves, it leaves the whole infraumbilical triangle raw. The gap may

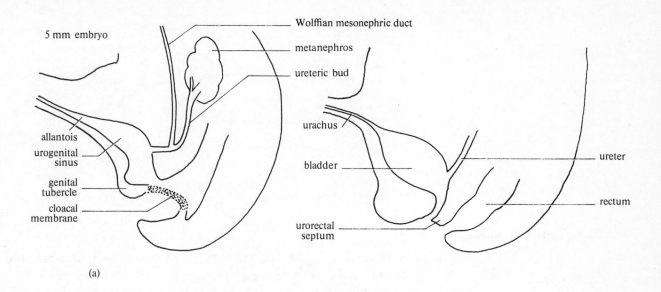

5 mm embryo

Wolffian mesonephric duct

metanephros

ureteric bud

allantois

urogenital sinus

genital tubercle

cloacal membrane

urachus

bladder

urorectal septum

ureter

rectum

(a)

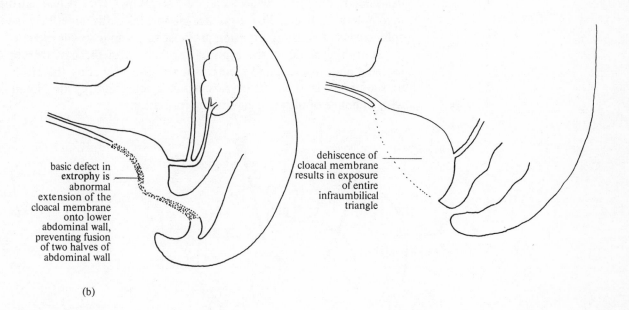

basic defect in **extrophy** is abnormal extension of the cloacal membrane onto lower abdominal wall, preventing fusion of two halves of abdominal wall

dehiscence of cloacal membrane results in exposure of entire infraumbilical triangle

(b)

Chapter 17/*Bladder: Congenital Abnormalities*   161

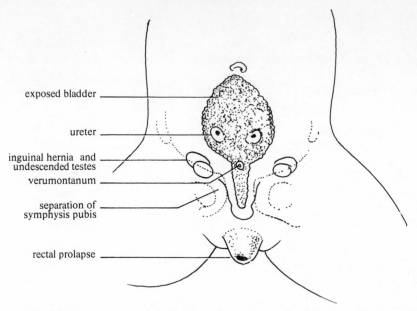

exposed bladder

ureter

inguinal hernia and
undescended testes

verumontanum

separation of
symphysis pubis

rectal prolapse

Fig. 17.2. The syndrome of extrophy.

be of varying degree, and extrophy may range from a mere defect in the dorsum of the penis, to complete extrophy of the entire cloaca.

The common problem is vesical extrophy: here the abdominal wall below the umbilicus is wanting in skin and muscle, and the bladder lies exposed on the surface. The penis is represented by a curved flat stump with a narrow strip of epithelium on its dorsum. Neither testis is descended into the wide, shallow scrotum. The pelvic girdle is incomplete in front. The anus lies abnormally far anteriorly and its sphincter is often lax, permitting prolapse to complicate the picture.

If nothing is done, the exposed urothelium of the bladder becomes irritated and infected, and metaplasia sets in, converting the urothelium to squamous epithelium, or to cystitis cystica and cystis glandularis, with a chance of ultimate carcinoma formation.

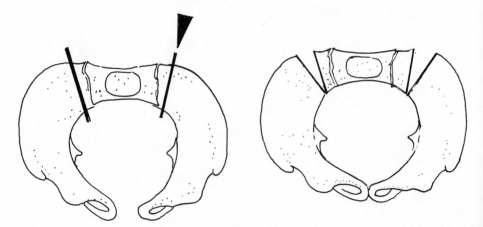

Fig. 17.3. Iliac osteotomy allows pelvis to be closed together to assist in closure of extrophied bladder.

Chapter 17/*Bladder: Congenital Abnormalities*

a   In the first stage, the bladder is reconstructed: the edge of the bladder is dissected from the abdominal wall, and rolled up to form a hollow ball. The abdominal wall is closed, with the assistance of division of the iliac bones on either side of the sacroiliac joint, so that the bony pelvis can be closed up too (fig. 17.3).

b   If the child is fortunate, she may become continent of urine. Boys may grow up to be able to ejaculate and to father children, but in most cases it is not possible to preserve urinary continence, and a urinary diversion is necessary, either into the sigmoid or by an ileal conduit (see page 289).

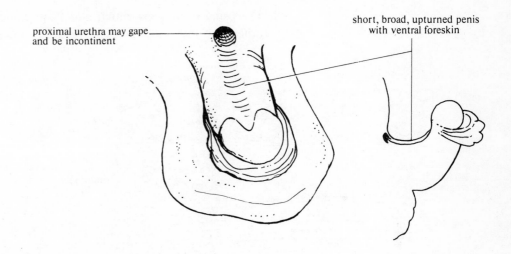

proximal urethra may gape and be incontinent

short, broad, upturned penis with ventral foreskin

5. Epispadias (fig. 17.4)

This also varies in severity, and may be limited to the glans penis or continue down to its base. Staged reconstruction of the defect is performed, if necessary including plication of the bladder neck in the hope of restoring continence.

FURTHER READING

JOHNSTON J.H. (1976) Congenital abnormalities of the bladder and urethra. *Urology*, ed. Blandy J.P., p. 619. Blackwell Scientific Publications, Oxford.

JOHNSTON J.H. & KULATILAKE A.E. (1973) Posterior urethral valves: results and sequelae. *Problems in Paediatric Urology*, eds. Johnston J.H. and Scholtmeijer R.J., p. 161. Excerpta Medica, Amsterdam.

WHITAKER R.H. (1973) The ureter in posterior urethral valves. *Brit. J. Urol.*, **45**, 395.

WILLIAMS D.I. (1974) Epispadias and Extrophy. *Encyclopaedia of Urology XV*, Supplement p. 266. Springer

WILLIAMS D.I. (1975) Epispadias. *Proc. Roy. Soc. Med.*, **68**, 399.

Chapter 18
The Bladder—
Inflammation

CYSTITIS

'Cystitis' is an extremely common condition. In one survey of the healthy mothers and wives accompanying their husbands or children to doctors' surgeries it was found that on being questioned, 70% admitted to having had 'cystitis' at some time or other. Of women who come to the doctor complaining of painful and frequent micturition, only half of them are found to have urinary infection. Others have urinary infection without any symptoms. Not every stinging urethra is infected, and not every infection causes stinging.

Pathology

The usual organisms which infect the bladder are *Escherichia coli* and other normal inhabitants of the intestine. In ill, debilitated,

Fig. 18.1. Changes in chronic cystitis.

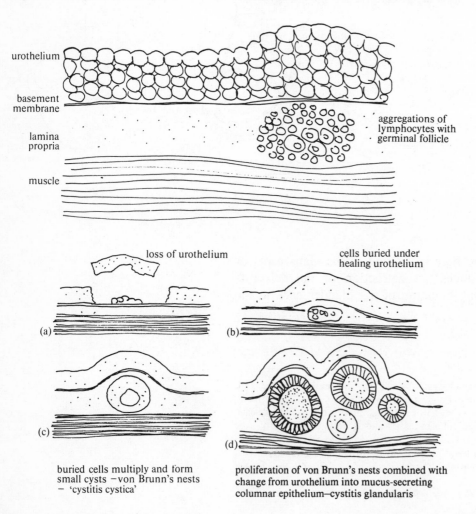

urothelium

basement membrane

lamina propria

muscle

aggregations of lymphocytes with germinal follicle

loss of urothelium

cells buried under healing urothelium

(a)

(b)

(c)

(d)

buried cells multiply and form small cysts —von Brunn's nests — 'cystitis cystica'

proliferation of von Brunn's nests combined with change from urothelium into mucus-secreting columnar epithelium—cystitis glandularis

immunosuppressed patients, other more exotic organisms are found in the bladder: and in patients given broad-spectrum antibiotics, the strains of *E. coli*, *Proteus* and *Pseudomonas* which occur in the stools, on the perineum, and in the urine, may be derived from resistant strains occurring in the hospital environment.

Tuberculosis causes chronic inflammation with granulomata of the wall of the bladder; so also in Africa, and to an increasing extent in the near and middle East, *Schistosoma haematobium, mansoni,* and *japonicum* cause granulomata in the wall of the bladder.

Chemical causes of cystitis which are currently recognized include cyclophosphamide, given to patients with lymphoma, and mandelic acid, given to patients for infection. There may well be others as yet unrecognized.

Acute cystitis

Macroscopically (i.e. at cystoscopy) the bladder looks red, and oedematous, and is sometimes ulcerated. Histologically there is oedema and leucocyte infiltration.

Chronic cystitis

A. NON SPECIFIC FORMS

Macroscopically the bladder may be oedematous, strands of mucus may obscure the view, and the epithelium may be irregular, with small nodules resembling tubercles. Biopsy shows these to be aggregations of lymphocytes, and there is a spectrum of change from mere collections of lymphocytes, to large nodules with follicles and germinal centres.

As the bladder loses its urothelium, and regenerates it over the denuded area, islands of urothelium may become buried under the new covering. The buried islands grow, and form small cysts. At first these are lined by transitional epithelium (*cystitis cystica*, or *Von Brunn's nests*), but with the passage of time they undergo metaplasia and form true mucus. Aggregations of these cysts now appear as if they were columnar celled glands of the bowel, and the condition is recognized as *cystitis glandularis*.

In certain chronic infections with *E. coli* curious yellow plaques may be seen on the mucosa at cystoscopy, and histological section reveals the changes of *malakoplakia*, which is a variant on the theme of chronic inflammation in which little round calcified bodies—named after Michaelis and Guttman—can be identified. This condition can form quite large masses which bleed, and are easily mistaken for a tumour.

B. SPECIFIC FORMS

Tuberculosis causes characteristic small caseating tubercles under the mucosa in which giant cells and epithelioid cells can be recognized, and in which, occasionally, acid-fast bacilli can be detected with the Ziehl–Neelsen stain.

The eggs of the worm *S. haematobium* (fig. 18.2) (and occasionally *S. mansoni*) secrete enzymes which digest the wall of the bladder, and the egg is extruded into the urine. The live egg excites a considerable acute inflammatory reaction, so that around each egg there is oedema and leucocyte infiltration. The dead eggs gradually become calcified, and excite a foreign body reaction, so that histological section reveals fibrosis and foreign body giant cells. As time goes by the mixture of live and dead eggs causes such intense local inflammatory change that the mucosa of the bladder becomes heaped up into 'polypi': at first these are entirely innocent, but later on their overlying mucosa undergoes squamous metaplasia, and in amongst the inflammatory polypi the patient develops a squamous cancer.

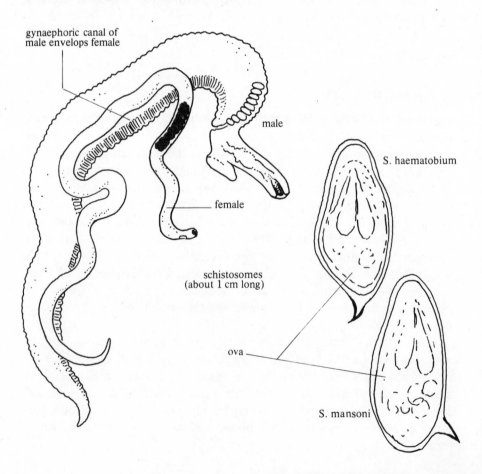

Figs. 18.2. Schistosoma.

Chapter 18/*Bladder: Inflammation*

The worms which lay the eggs which cause the mischief are nematodes, and they dwell in the portal and pelvic veins (fig. 18.3). The male has the nasty habit of completely enveloping the female within a groove on his abdominal wall—hence the name *schisto-soma*. When the eggs are liberated in the patient's urine, and he passes his water into an African or Egyptian river, the egg, on contact with fresh water, dissolves, liberating a tiny free-swimming intermediate form, the *miracidium*, which swims off to find the intermediate host, which in Africa is the fresh-water snail *Bulinus globosus*. Boring into the snail, the miracidia make for the snail's liver, where they grow and form cysts full of *cercariae*. These leave the snail in thousands. They are tiny hair-like creatures a millimetre or so in length. A single snail can shed a thousand in an hour.

Fig. 18.3. Bilharzia life cycle.

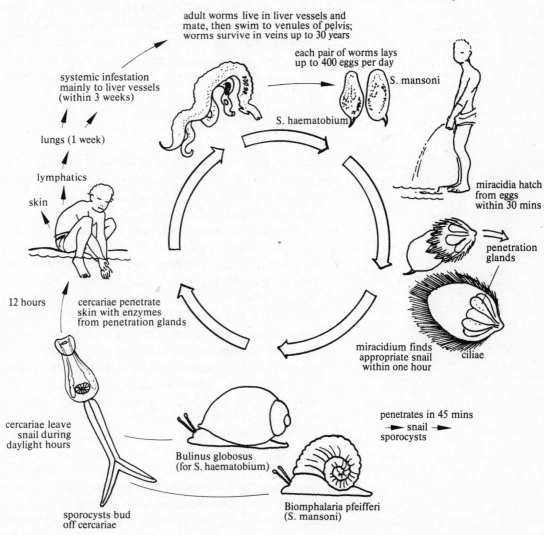

adult worms live in liver vessels and mate, then swim to venules of pelvis; worms survive in veins up to 30 years

each pair of worms lays up to 400 eggs per day

S. mansoni

S. haematobium

systemic infestation mainly to liver vessels (within 3 weeks)

lungs (1 week)

lymphatics

skin

miracidia hatch from eggs within 30 mins

penetration glands

12 hours

cercariae penetrate skin with enzymes from penetration glands

ciliae

miracidium finds appropriate snail within one hour

penetrates in 45 mins
→ snail →
snail sporocysts

cercariae leave snail during daylight hours

Bulinus globosus (for S. haematobium)

Biomphalaria pfeifferi (S. mansoni)

sporocysts bud off cercariae

Visiting the river to fish, to wash her clothes, or just to have a chat, the unwary victim steps into the water. Within 30 seconds her skin is penetrated by a few score cercariae. They travel in the dermal lymphatics until they get into the systemic venous system, and are then disseminated all over the body. No tissue is immune but in practice most of the cercariae fail to survive, except those which get a lodgement in the portal and pelvic veins. The survivors mature into adult worms. African children repeatedly infested with wave after wave of cercariae may grow so many worms that the portal vein is occluded, and they then develop splenomegaly and oesophageal varices. Others, less severely infested, develop the complications of having these worms in their pelvic veins and viscera. In the intestine the eggs give rise to polypi and inflammatory changes. In the bladder they cause chronic cystitis.

As a cause of morbidity, and as a cause of haematuria, schistosomiasis is beyond question the single most important disease affecting the urinary tract. It lays special claim also to being the most unpleasant, since death from inoperable cancer of the bladder, today the fate of so many Egyptians and Africans, is arguably the most dreadful of all ways of dying.

Clinical features

It is not possible to distinguish between the clinical features of infection confined to the bladder and those involving the upper tract as well, so the discussion of the investigation and management of urinary tract infection applies to that of cystitis.

In schistosomiasis, the most important investigations are to search the urine for the eggs of the worm, which are usually easy to find, and are present in large numbers. In doubtful cases one may take a biopsy of the lining of the bladder, but it is more simple to take a snip from the rectal mucosa and examine the fresh preparation squashed between a slide and a coverslip, which readily reveals the ova under the lower power of the microscope. Treatment of schistosomiasis involves giving antimony compounds which are notoriously toxic to skeletal and myocardial muscle, and must be given with great care.

Prevention of schistosomiasis is an almost insoluble problem. Every spadeful of earth dug from even a dried up river bed in those parts of Africa where the disease is common is found to contain hundreds of the infected snails. It is not feasible to prevent villagers from urinating in the streams, or the womenfolk from washing their clothes there, since there is no other source of water. Extensive irrigation schemes, while they cause deserts to blossom, also spread the scourge of schistosomiasis, and the attractive artificial lakes formed behind grandiose new dams, which look so well suited to fishermen and water-skiers, teem with

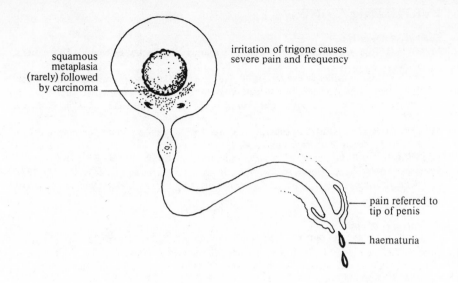

squamous
metaplasia
(rarely) followed
by carcinoma

irritation of trigone causes
severe pain and frequency

pain referred to
tip of penis

haematuria

Fig. 18.4. Clinical features of vesical calculus.

deadly cercariae. Search for a protective vaccine still seems a long way from achieving its objective.

STONE IN THE BLADDER

One uncommon cause of chronic infection and irritation of the bladder is a vesical calculus, which in Europe today is virtually confined to elderly men who have outflow obstruction. No doubt a small ureteric calculus is the origin of most of these stones, and they cannot get out of the bladder because there is outflow obstruction due to an enlarged prostate or tight bladder neck. As time goes by they grow, and their rate of growth is accelerated when infection ensues, as it almost inevitably does.

Complicating stones there may be metaplasia of the urothelium, and squamous-cell carcinoma.

The diagnosis is made by the typical pain referred to the tip of the penis which is worse when the patient walks about and is better when he is lying down at night.

The treatment is to crush and evacuate the calculus with a lithotrite, an instrument which cracks the stone into tiny fragments which can then be evacuated through special cannulae (see page 262). If there is some excuse to perform an open operation—e.g. to deal with coexisting prostatic obstruction or a carcinoma of the bladder, then the stone should be removed at the same time. It may also be necessary to open the bladder to remove the stone if the surgeon does not possess, or does not know how to use a lithotrite.

FURTHER READING

General considerations

MARSH F. (1976) Cystitis. Chap. 28, *Urology*, ed. Blandy J.P. Blackwell Scientific Publications, Oxford.

MARSH F.P., BANERJEE R. & PANCHAMIA P. (1974) The relationship between urinary infection, cystoscopic appearance and pathology of the bladder in man: I. Lymphocytes in the lamina propria; II. Squamous change in the bladder epithelium. *J. Clin. Path.*, **27**, 297.

MEHROHTRA R.M.L. (1953) An experimental study of the vesical circulation during distension and in cystitis. *J. Path. Anat.*, **66**, 79.

PUGH R.C.B. (1967) Pathology of urinary tract infection. *Hospital Medicine*, **1**, 1001.

SHAH M.S., NABONG R., ROGIN A., ZARIF A., JAVADPOUR N., SASSON H. & BUSH I.M. (1973) Sequestration of the total bladder mucosa caused by Clostridial infection. *J. Urol.*, **110**, 54.

Special types of cystitis

CHAMPION R.H. & ACKLES R.C. (1966) Eosinophilic cystitis. *J. Urol.*, **96**, 729.

GINGELL J.C. & BURN J.I. (1970) Cystitis glandularis. *Brit. J. Urol.*, **42**, 446.

GOLDSTEIN A.G., D'ESCRIVEN J.C. & ALLES S.D. (1968) Haemorrhagic radiation cystitis. *Brit. J. Urol.*, **40**, 475.

JOHNSTON F.R. (1957) Some proliferative and metaplastic lesions in transitional epithelium. *Brit. J. Urol.*, **29**, 112.

LETCHER H.G. & MATHESON N.M. (1935) Encrustation of the bladder as a result of alkaline cystitis. *Brit. J. Surg.*, **23**, 716.

MARSH F.P., VINCE F.D., POLLOCK D.J. & BLANDY J.P. (1971) Cyclophosphamide necrosis of bladder causing calcification, contracture and reflux: treated by colocystoplasty. *Brit. J. Urol.*, **43**, 324.

Hunner's ulcer

HUNNER G.L. (1915) A rare type of bladder ulcer in women: report of cases. *Boston Med. Surg. J.*, **172**, 660.

BADENOCH A.W. (1971) Chronic interstitial cystitis. *Brit. J. Urol.*, **43**, 718.

Schistosomiasis (Bilharzia)

ADAMS A.R.D. and MAEGRAITH B.G. (1971) *Clinical Tropical Diseases*, 5th edn, ed. Maegraith B.G. Blackwell Scientific Publications, Oxford.

BELL D.R. (1974) Bilharzia (schistosomiasis). *Brit. J. Hosp. Med.* **11**, 29.

SINGH M. (1976) Tropical parasitic infections of the urinary tract. Chap. 13, *Urology*, ed. Blandy J.P. Blackwell Scientific Publications, Oxford.

DIMMETTE E., SPROAT H.F. & SAYEGH E.S. (1956) The classification of carcinoma of the bladder associated with schistosomiasis and metaplasia. *J. Urol.*, **75**, 680.

EL-BOUKANY M.N., GHONEIM M.A. & MANSOUR M.A. (1972) Carcinoma of the bilharzial bladder in Egypt. *Brit. J. Urol.*, **44**, 561.

Calculus in the bladder

BIGELOW H.J. (1876) On lithotrity by a single operation. *Boston Med. Surg. J.*, **98**, 259 and 291.

BLANDY J.P. (1976) Stones and foreign bodies in the bladder. Chap. 29, *Urology*, ed. Blandy J.P. Blackwell Scientific Publications, Oxford.

ELLIS, HAROLD (1969) *A History of Bladder Stone*. Blackwell Scientific Publications, Oxford.

AETIOLOGY

In 1894 Rehn noted that workers in the aniline dyestuff industry making fuchsin were developing more than their fair share of bladder cancer. It turned out that it was not aniline which was responsible, but an intermediary product, *2-naphthylamine* which was metabolized into a carcinogen and excreted in the urine. Later another group of compounds of similar benzene-ring structure were indicted: these included *1-naphthylamine* and *benzidine* (fig. 19.1).

Industries in which these compounds were used include the chemical industry, dyeing, rubber moulding and rubber cable covering, pitch and gas works, and the optical industry where pitch was used to hold the lenses during the grinding process. Other industries with an unduly high proportion of bladder cancers, even though the offending carcinogen remains to be traced, are hairdressing, nursing, and leather work.

It is likely that smoking and analgesic abuse is a cause of urothelial cancer. The incidence of the disease increases with every year in Europe.

Today men outnumber women as victims of this disease 4:1, perhaps because of the smoking habits of a generation ago.

Some industrial cancers are a notifiable industrial hazard in Britain, and you should notify the case as being 'prescribed disease number 39' on the medical certificate you issue to the patient.

PATHOLOGY

Macroscopic features

Bladder tumours may be single or multiple, and they may appear at cystoscopy as either papillary (cauliflower) growths, solid ones, or ulcers (fig. 19.2).

Histologically they are classified as follows (fig. 19.3):

1 *Transitional cell tumours* (*urothelial cancer*): these may be either *solid* or *papillary* according to their microscopic architecture, and *well-differentiated* or *anaplastic* according to their degree of cellular dedifferentiation.

Chapter 19
The Bladder—
Urothelial
Neoplasms

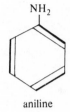

aniline

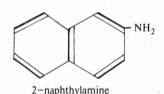

2—naphthylamine

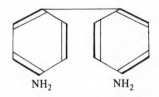

4, 4—diaminodiphenyl (benzidine)

Fig. 19.1. Structural formulae of some carcinogens.

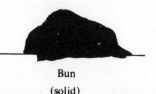

Cauliflower
(papillary)

Bun
(solid)

Ulcer

Fig. 19.2. Macroscopic features of bladder cancer.

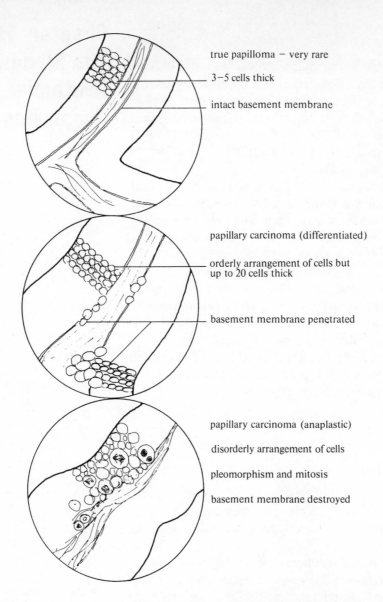

true papilloma – very rare

3–5 cells thick

intact basement membrane

papillary carcinoma (differentiated)

orderly arrangement of cells but
up to 20 cells thick

basement membrane penetrated

papillary carcinoma (anaplastic)

disorderly arrangement of cells

pleomorphism and mitosis

basement membrane destroyed

Fig. 19.3. Variants of 'papilloma'.

2 *Squamous cell carcinoma* arises from metaplasia of the urothelium to a squamous form, generally in consequence of prolonged irritation e.g. inside a diverticulum of the bladder, after prolonged contact with a stone, or as a result of repeated infestation with schistosoma ova.

3 *Adenocarcinoma.* This only occurs in relation to the urachus, at the dome of the bladder, and is very rare, or in the trigone in consequence of prolonged irritation causing the urothelium to develop cystitis cystica and ultimately cystitis glandularis.

Bladder tumours spread locally, and through the wall of the bladder. They tend not to get into lymphatics early perhaps because these are

Chapter 19/*Bladder: Urothelial Neoplasms*

rather sparse in the superficial layers of the wall of the bladder. However lymphatics are plentiful deeper in the bladder muscle, and once the tumour has begun to invade the muscle deeply, spread into lymphatics is swift.

CLINICAL AND PATHOLOGICAL STAGING OF BLADDER TUMOURS

Two systems are used in parallel: the first is the surgeon's guess as to the depth of the tumour: this is supplemented by whatever pathological information the biopsy he has been able to take can provide him with. One must remember two sources of error: first, the surgeon's guess as to the depth of invasion of the tumour is based upon whether or not he can feel induration—a very subjective sign—on bimanual examination under anaesthesia. Secondly the pathologist can only report on the tissue he is given, and it may be difficult or impossible for the surgeon to take a biopsy from the worst part of the tumour, or take it so deeply that the pathologist can say whether deep muscle is invaded or not (fig. 19.4).

There is an imaginary half-way line in the wall of the bladder dividing T2 and T3. It was claimed that in a large series of cases all treated by total cystectomy there was a very sharp dividing line in prognosis according to whether or not the tumour had got past this imaginary line. Unfortunately in practice in a bulky invasive tumour it

Fig. 19.4. Stages in carcinoma of the bladder. Note that the 'T' stage is the *surgeon's guess* as to the extent of invasion of the tumour, based upon his assessment at cystoscopy, and the evidence given to him by the pathologist based on the small bit obtained by biopsy. The 'P' stage is what the *pathologist finds*, but is often based upon incomplete evidence—i.e. biopsy less than full thickness of bladder wall.

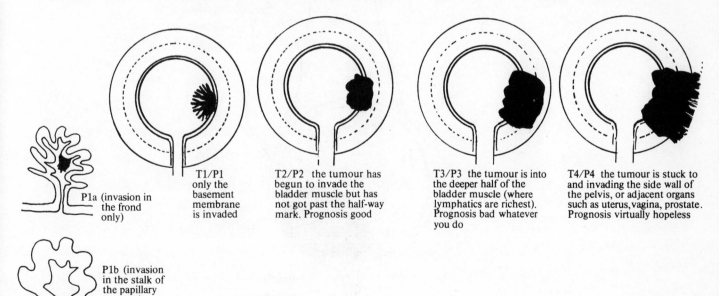

P1a (invasion in the frond only)

P1b (invasion in the stalk of the papillary tumour)

T1/P1 only the basement membrane is invaded

T2/P2 the tumour has begun to invade the bladder muscle but has not got past the half-way mark. Prognosis good

T3/P3 the tumour is into the deeper half of the bladder muscle (where lymphatics are richest). Prognosis bad whatever you do

T4/P4 the tumour is stuck to and invading the side wall of the pelvis, or adjacent organs such as uterus, vagina, prostate. Prognosis virtually hopeless

is quite impossible even with the total cystectomy specimen to draw such a line, and too much reliance should never be attached to clinical or pathological staging.

CLINICAL FEATURES (fig. 19.5)

Patients usually complain of haematuria. This is present in 80% of bladder cancer patients, and is the cardinal reason why every patient with haematuria must be cystoscoped sooner or later. But one must remember that the other 20% do not notice haematuria. They may have other symptoms. First are those who have frequency of urination and

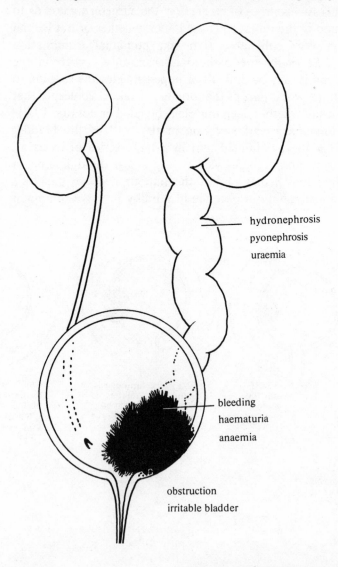

hydronephrosis
pyonephrosis
uraemia

bleeding
haematuria
anaemia

obstruction
irritable bladder

Fig. 19.5 Clinical features of bladder carcinoma

Chapter 19/*Bladder: Urothelial Neoplasms*

pain on voiding. It is very easy to jump to the conclusion that these patients merely have cystitis, and need a bottle of antibiotic tablets. Their urine may show pyuria, but if it is sterile this ought to ring a warning bell. Since bladder cancer is a disease of elderly men, and since elderly men nearly always have some degree of enlargement of the prostate it is important not to accept the prostate as the cause of the symptoms.

Others present with true urinary infection, developing perhaps on the breaking down surface of the carcinoma. It should be a rule that every new incident of urinary infection taking place in an elderly man should be regarded as a sign of underlying bladder cancer until proved otherwise.

Physical signs are very seldom helpful. Occasionally one will encounter an advanced case where there is a large fixed indurated mass to be felt either suprapubically, or on rectal examination, but this is the exception. Diagnosis therefore depends on intelligent investigation of the subject at risk.

INVESTIGATIONS

1. URINE

Sterile pyuria, or a positive Papanicolaou stain in the urinary deposit should call for confirmatory cystoscopy.

2. EXCRETION UROGRAPHY

The bladder cancer may show a filling defect in the bladder, or it may have grown into the wall of the ureter and be causing obstruction to the upper tract.

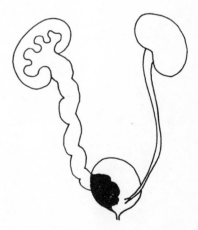

3. CYSTOSCOPY AND BIOPSY UNDER ANAESTHESIA

Note that it is no good attempting to make the diagnosis without a general anaesthetic, since it is important to have the patient deeply asleep and relaxed if the examination is to be worthwhile. At cystoscopy the surgeon discovers how many tumours there are, where they are situated in the bladder, and what they look like. Solid and ulcerated tumours are nearly always those which have begun to invade deeply (fig. 19.6).

A biopsy must be taken (it is no good sending bits of dead tumour washed off the surface of the growth and hoping that the pathologist can

Fig. 19.6. Every patient who has had haematuria requires a cystoscopy and an IVP. To do less (in the absence of albuminuria and other evidence of glomerular disease) is negligent.

The IVP may show (1) dilatation of one or other ureter: this always signifies invasion of the wall of the ureter by tumour. (2) A filling defect in the bladder films.

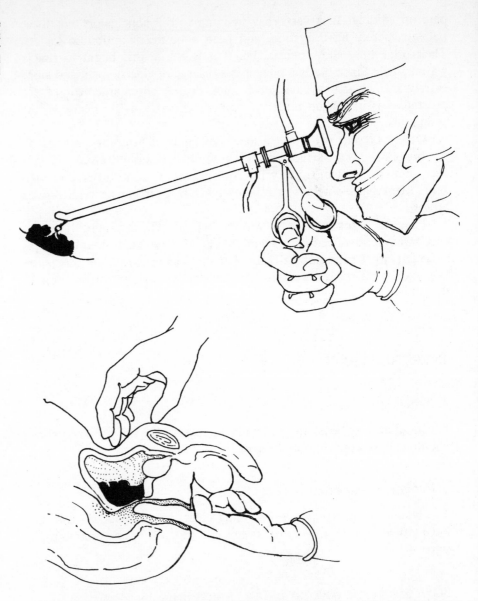

Fig. 19.7. Cystoscopy for tumour must be done under a deep general anaesthetic, at which a biopsy is taken from the tumour (for histological grading) and a bimanual palpation is made to determine the clinical stage of infiltration of the tumour.

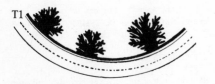

Fig. 19.8. T1 tumours—no invasion of the muscle.

make something out of the debris). The biopsy is taken either with the resectoscope loop or special sharp cup forceps.

Bimanual palpation is then carried out under deep relaxation in order to try to estimate the depth to which the carcinoma has invaded (fig. 19.7).

TREATMENT

T1 superficial tumours (fig. 19.8)

When they are small, and there are not too many of them, after taking a

Chapter 19/*Bladder: Urothelial Neoplasms*

biopsy, they are destroyed by coagulation with a cystoscopic electrode, or resected with the diathermy loop.

When there are so many of them that this is not feasible, the bladder may be treated by instillation of thiotepa or epodyl, locally acting antimitotic agents, which may result in reduction in the numbers of small tumours, and sometimes in complete clearance of the bladder.

With bulky fronded tumours the bladder may be treated by the Helmstein distension method, using an inflated rubber balloon which causes pressure necrosis of the projecting growths.

If all these measures fail, it may be necessary to perform a total cystectomy.

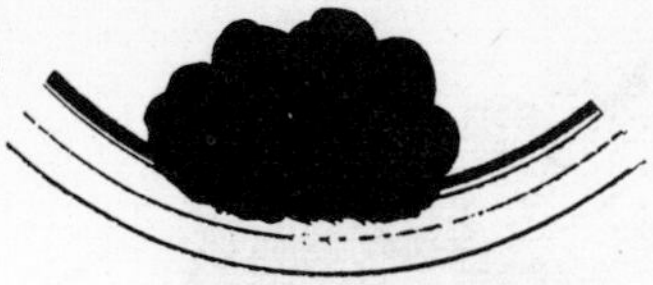

Fig. 19.9. T2 tumours—invasion of the superficial half of the bladder muscle.

T2 tumours, invading superficial muscle (fig. 19.9)

If reasonably small these are best treated by transurethral diathermy resection carrying the excision down to deep muscle. If they are too big for this method to be safe, the bladder may be opened and the tumour removed with a diathermy loop, and the seared base implanted with radioactive gold grains to destroy any tumour which has escaped the diathermy destruction. In tumours favourably placed at the vault of the bladder the same end can be achieved by a wide partial cystectomy.

T3 tumours, invading deeply into muscle (fig. 19.10)

Nobody knows how best to treat these tumours. At present most urological surgeons attempt some combination of total cystectomy and irradiation, but it is not known what dose of radiotherapy is best, or whether to take the bladder out before, during, or after the radiation has been given. Unfortunately carcinoma of the bladder so often occurs in elderly patients, where the mortality and morbidity of total cystectomy is very high, that the attempt at a curative form of treatment is all too likely to result in death of the patient. Currently the author prefers to administer a radical course of radiotherapy, and follow this, if he must, by salvage cystectomy if the tumour does not go away, or if it comes back and causes symptoms.

T4 tumours—inoperable (fig. 19.11)

All one can attempt here is to make the patient comfortable. Radiotherapy may get rid of the local tumour and all its distressing symptoms for several years, and should be tried first. But in time it may

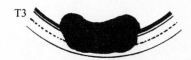

Fig. 19.10. T3 tumours—indurated and deeply invasive but thought to be removable by surgery.

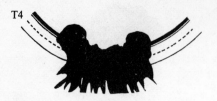

Fig. 19.11. T4 tumours—where there is fixation to the pelvis or to surrounding viscera.

be necessary to consider urinary diversion as a form of palliation. Bleeding and pain may be controlled by Helmstein's distension therapy or by local hyperthermia.

FURTHER READING

ATANASSOR H. & DONOVSKI L. (1975) Characteristics of the tumours of the urinary tract in patients with Endemic Nephropathy. *Eur. Urol.*, **1**, 26.

ENGLAND H.R., RIGBY C., SHEPHEARD B.G.F., TRESIDDER G.C. & BLANDY J.P. (1973) Evaluation of Helmstein's distension method for carcinoma of the bladder. *Brit. J. Urol.*, **45**, 593.

O'FLYNN J.D., SMITH J.M. & HANSON J.S. (1975) Transurethral resection for the assessment and treatment of vesical neoplasms: a review of 840 consecutive cases. *Eur. Urol.*, **1**, 38.

PUGH R.C.B. (1976) Histopathology. *Scientific Foundations of Urology*, eds. Williams D.I. and Chisholm G.D., p. 291. Heinemann, London.

KIPLING M.D. (1976) Occupational considerations in carcinoma of the urogenital tract. *Brit. J. Hosp. Med.*, **15**, 465.

RATHERT P., MELCHIOR H. & LUTZEYER W. (1975) Phenacetin: a carcinogen for the urinary tract? *J. Urol.*, **113**, 653.

REECE R.W. & KOONTZ W.W. Leukaplakia of the urinary tract: a review. *J. Urol.*, **114**, 165.

RIDDLE P.R., CHISHOLM G.D., TROTT P.A. & PUGH R.C.B. (1975) Flat carcinoma-in-situ of the bladder. *Brit. J. Urol.*, **47**, 829.

WALLACE D.M. (1976) Carcinoma of the urothelium. *Urology*, ed. Blandy J.P., p. 774. Blackwell Scientific Publications, Oxford.

WALLACE D.M. (1976) General principles of tumour staging. *Scientific Foundations of Urology*, eds. Williams D.I. and Chisholm G.D., p. 199. Heinemann, London.

Chapter 19/*Bladder: Urothelial Neoplasms*

The basic anatomical arrangement of the bladder consists of a muscular bag, the detrusor, with a pipe leading from it, the urethra, which is surrounded by the levator ani ring which constitutes the external sphincter. Arrangement of the helical muscle fibres around the internal meatus amounts to an 'internal sphincter' or 'bladder neck'.

Chapter 20
The Bladder–
Neuropathy

NORMAL MICTURITION

When the bladder is full, parasympathetic afferent fibres signal a state of distension to the reflex centre for the bladder situated at S2/3 in the spinal cord, which lies at the level of the T12/L1 intervertebral disc (Fig. 20.1)

In babyhood (as in the newborn puppy), the reflex arc is sparked off: there is an emission of parasympathetic impulses towards the detrusor muscle, and at the same time there is inhibition of the tone of the external sphincter.

As the detrusor contracts, the fibres of its muscle which are joined on to the urethra in the region of the verumontanum act to pull open the bladder neck. The external sphincter relaxes, and the detrusor muscle continues to contract until the bladder is completely empty.

As the baby (or the puppy) is house-trained, inhibition from higher centres prevents the S2/3 reflex arc from working. At first this cortical inhibition is active during the waking hours, and the baby is dry in the day time, i.e. empties his bladder when it is convenient. Later this inhibition is carried over into sleep.

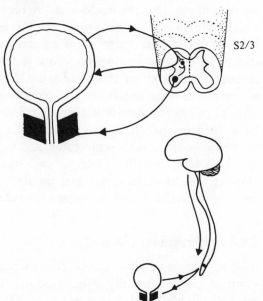

S2/3

Fig. 20.1. The bladder and the spinal reflex centre for micturition at S2/3.

In anxiety or under extreme emotional stress, the cortical inhibition may alter, and the bladder reflex becomes either less inhibited, or facilitated. There are some Jacksonian epileptic fits which begin by an aura associated with the whole business of going to the lavatory, undressing, and making water, and, as everyone knows, the sensory component of a full bladder is represented at the highest cortical levels.

INVESTIGATION OF THE NEUROGENIC BLADDER

In addition to a complete physical and neurological examination, and an excretion urogram and microbiological examination of the urine, the cystometrogram is a helpful diagnostic investigation.

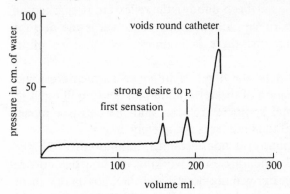

Fig. 20.2. Investigation of the neurogenic bladder. 1. Cystometrogram.

The normal cystometrogram (fig. 20.2) is obtained by passing a fine sterile catheter into the bladder of the recumbent patient. While sterile water is run in at a constant rate, the pressure in the bladder is measured by a recording manometer. Most normal patients will show only a very trivial rise in pressure (measured above the symphysis pubis) until the bladder contains about 150 ml of urine. At this stage the patient may be aware of the 'first sensation' to void (which should be recorded) and often at this filling there is a slight increase in pressure, probably caused by a detrusor contraction aborted at once by cortical inhibition. Later the filling becomes less comfortable, and the patient expresses a stronger desire to void. Finally, when he can stand it no longer, the bladder empties around the catheter and the detrusor contraction registers an increase in pressure until the catheter is expelled.

Cystourethrography (fig. 20.3)

This performed by filling the bladder through a similar fine catheter with contrast medium (usually sodium iodide), and then asking the patient to void as the bladder is examined with Xrays and image intensifier. (In

Chapter 20/*Bladder: Neuropathy*

ideal circumstances the cystometrogram and cystogram can be combined on a simultaneous recording—a method which requires very elaborate equipment.)

The normal cystourethrogram will show the bladder neck at rest, and during micturition, relaxation of the external sphincter, detrusor contraction, widening of the internal sphincter, emptying of the bladder contents, and finally the drop of urine left between the sphincters is milked back up into the bladder.

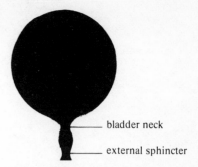

bladder neck

external sphincter

Fig. 20.3. Investigation of the neurogenic bladder. 2. Cysto-urethrography.

ENURESIS

The most simple form of 'neurogenic' disturbance of the bladder which gives rise to symptoms is enuresis. Daytime cerebral inhibition of the sacral reflex occurs in most babies at around 18 months, but sleeping inhibition does not develop until much later, and many children still wet the bed even at the age of 7 who are perfectly normal. Here, as in other aspects of human activity, there is a broad spectrum of normality. One should therefore hesitate before regarding bed-wetting before the age of 5 or 6 as being in any way abnormal behaviour, nuisance to the parents though it may be.

Certain things may make the bladder reflex more powerful: e.g. if there is abnormal afferent stimulation because the mucosa of the bladder is more sensitive in consequence of infection and oedema. Hence it is useful to make sure that the enuretic child does not have a urinary infection or threadworms and treat them if found. Very few enuretics have anything physically wrong with their urinary tract, but what has gone wrong seems to have been a failure of daytime cortical inhibition to carry over into sleeping inhibition of the sacral reflex to empty the bladder when it is full.

Since the critical time for the establishment of this reflex habit is around the age of 4 to 6 years, and since any severe emotional disturbance can bring on other bad habits in the child such as nail biting, it is prudent to enquire sensibly into the possibility of family emotional disturbances which could have prevented the establishment of nocturnal control over the bladder's reflex arc; and in a few cases, this is rewarding, and it may help matters for the parents and child to talk the whole matter out with a child psychiatrist.

It is important never to be stampeded by an over-anxious mother into a series of investigations and treatments for what is not in fact an abnormal situation at all. However after the age of 7 something needs to be done.

Having excluded urinary infection, threadworms and overt emotional problems in the family, the first thing to do is to explain to the child and his mother what has gone wrong, and how you propose to put it right.

Your aim is to establish such a strong daytime conditioned reflex inhibition that it will carry over into sleep. To do this your method is to make the child think throughout the day about his bladder: he must drink so much water that almost all the time he wants to go to the lavatory. He should be encouraged to pass water when it suits him, not his bladder. Let him go every hour, or every two hours, or between every lesson in school: the timing is less important than that there should be regularity about the process.

Let him have a diary, and put a tick in the dates when the bed is dry in the morning. A small reward from his mother never does any harm, but punishment is probably unnecessary, since the poor child is usually sufficiently miserable and ashamed already.

The next line of treatment is to lighten the child's sleep. It is fashionable today to administer amitryptiline in order to prevent the child sleeping too deeply. It certainly works, but so also does a cup of tea or coffee. (The dose may have to be adjusted.) The latter are a good deal more safe than amitryptiline and serve the same purpose.

It will help if the parents lift the child before the adults retire to bed, and make sure he is properly awake, and has emptied his bladder.

As a last resort, one may use the buzzer: two metal foil sheets, separated by a cotton sheet, are placed over the waterproof sheet in the child's bed, and covered with a second cotton sheet. The top foil sheet is perforated with numerous holes. When the bed is soaked with urine, contact is established and the electric alarm goes off. (When testing the device, make sure urine is used, not tap water, which has insufficient electrolytes to make the circuit complete.)

The object of the buzzer is to wake the child up. No useful purpose is accomplished if all the buzzer does is to wake his mother, who gets wearily out of bed to change the wet bedclothes, while the child sleeps deeply on. For the first few weeks it may be necessary for the mother to wake up, and in turn wake the child, but before long a pattern is established: at first the child wakes just after he has emptied his bladder. A few days or weeks later he wakes just when the first few drips of urine have escaped. Before long he wakes when the bladder is full, and before it has emptied.

One should be very wary of investigating children with enuresis. There is seldom anything wrong with them, and a combination of urography, cystometrography, and micturating urography will make them feel sure that there is, even if nothing else has done. Nevertheless the older child deserves a thorough examination, as do all adults, lest one misses a more serious underlying lesion which ought to be treated. One should be careful not to miss an ectopic ureter in a girl, even though she says she has been dry in the day time, and even though the wetness seems only to come on after the onset of her menstrual periods.

One should be even more careful not to start investigating without good thought, the child who having once been dry, starts to wet the bed again. This is often a manifestation of some serious underlying emotional problem which hospital investigation may magnify, and which ought to be treated by a psychiatrist interested in children.

PATTERNS OF NEUROGENIC ILLNESS OF THE BLADDER

1. The denervated bladder (fig. 20.4)

If the parasympathetic pathways to and from the bladder have been destroyed, as they may be in the course of a radical operation for uterine or rectal cancer, when the side walls of the pelvis have been dissected clean, then there is neither an afferent nor an efferent limb from the detrusor. Filling continues without any sensation until the bladder holds a huge volume. In theory it ought to burst, but this seldom occurs. Since there is nothing to cause the external sphincter to relax, nothing to inhibit its tonic muscle contraction, it remains closed, but not so tightly as to prevent some urine escaping from the distended bladder on coughing or straining. The cystometrogram is flat: the cystogram shows no relaxation of the external sphincter, and the internal sphincter remains half open, since its detrusor does not contract to pull it open.

If the diagnosis suggests no hope that the injured pelvic parasympathetics can ever recover, then one must try to make the best of what is left. It is sometimes possible by transurethral section of the internal and external sphincters to leave the patient with a bladder sufficiently well balanced that increasing the abdominal pressure by straining will cause the bladder to empty, and yet enough tone remains in the external sphincter to keep the patient dry.

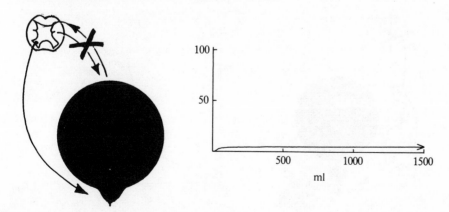

Fig. 20.4. The denervated bladder resulting from injury to the parasympathetic pathways.

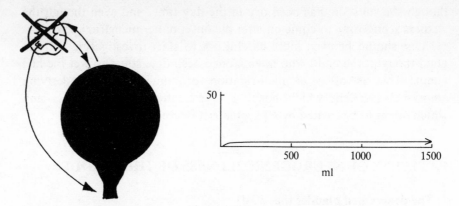

Fig. 20.5. The destruction of the spinal reflex centre for the bladder will result in the same situation as will injury of the parasympathetic pathways.

2. Destruction of the spinal reflex centre S2/3 (fig. 20.5)

The usual cause of this lesion is a fracture at the thoracolumbar junction which compresses the last few segments of the cord in the conus medullaris. (This is a common site for back injuries occurring in sports or industrial accidents.)

The cystometrogram is flat, as in the previous type of lesion: the external sphincter is usually flaccid, but otherwise the cystogram looks similar. There is retention with overflow, and abdominal straining may more or less empty the bladder. In treatment one can seldom hope to keep the patient continent, and one's efforts are spent on making sure that the bladder empties completely to get rid of any residual urine which might invite infection. It may be necessary to cut tissue away from the bladder neck and the external sphincter before the bladder empties completely.

3. The reflex bladder (fig. 20.6)

If the higher pathways to and from the cortex are interrupted by a lesion higher up the spinal cord, and the spinal sacral segments together with

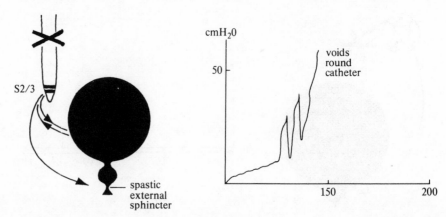

Fig. 20.6. Cortical inhibition cut off by an upper motor neurone lesion.

Chapter 20/*Bladder: Neuropathy*

their innervation are preserved, one may expect reflex emptying of the bladder. Such a situation is seen after gun-shot injuries and cervical spine lesions, and after operations for angiomata and other tumours of the spinal cord. Other causes include multiple sclerosis, whiplash injuries and transverse myelitis.

The cystometrogram shows a jumpy bladder which wants to contract when only 100 ml or less are filling it, and there is nothing to inhibit the contractions. Indeed, some of the contractions appear to continue without obvious cause, and the wall of the bladder becomes enormously hypertrophied.

The cystogram shows a very trabeculated thick-walled bladder, often with many sacculations and diverticula. Because there is poor coordination of the reflex, intact though the spinal cord segment may be, there is seldom correct inhibition of the tone of the external sphincter, which remains spastic and tightly closed. The detrusor contractions, forceful as they are, do not completely empty the bladder, so that there is always residual urine and usually some infection. Cystography may show an increased bulk of tissue at the bladder neck, in addition to a tightly closed external sphincter.

In practice though one may occasionally succeed in getting the bladder to empty by a combination of judicious weakening of both external and internal sphincters, and careful training, few of these bladders ever work safely and effectively, and the patient is better with the spincters completely severed, and the system converted into a urinary conduit. Even then there may be so much residual urine within the sacculated bladder that the patient ends up with a urinary diversion. In many instances in clinical practice there is a mixed picture because the lesion is not clear cut and there is a degree of sensation, some cortical inhibition, and some element of external sphincter spasticity. Here one must go carefully, by stages, aiming to get the right balance between the contractility of the detrusor and the power of the sphincters to retain the urine.

THE NEUROGENIC BLADDER IN THE FEMALE

From what has been said it will be clear that there are rather few instances in which it is possible to restore satisfactory function to a neurogenic bladder even in the male, when one can at least provide the penis with a satisfactory and waterproof urinal by which to keep the patient dry. But in women this is virtually impossible, and for practical purposes they are better off with a urinary diversion, using an ileal conduit.

THE DANGERS OF THE NEUROGENIC BLADDER

The chief danger is of infection, following upon the residual urine. If the patient does not die of the effects of upper tract infection, renal scarring, and renal failure, he is likely to perish from amyloid disease of the renal parenchyma. Therefore in all cases one must not go on trying for too long to get the normal anatomy working properly: there comes a time when one must cut one's losses, and settle for a urinary diversion. Remember that every attack of upper tract infection in a paraplegic is likely to lead to the loss of more precious nephrons.

MANAGEMENT OF THE BLADDER IN INJURY TO THE SPINAL CORD

First aid

Until you know whether the patient has sustained a stable or an unstable fracture of the spine, the spine should not be moved. Hence transport from the accident to the hospital should be performed without disturbing the position of the patient.

On arrival in the casualty department the first concern of the orthopaedic team will be to determine whether the fracture is stable or not. If it is stable (i.e. will come to no harm by turning the patient) then he is transferred to the ward, where arrangements are made for him to be turned regularly, to avoid the development of bedsores.

If the injury is unstable (as judged by the type of fracture shown on the radiograph) an emergency operation to decompress the spinal cord and fix the fragments will be carried out. It should be noted that this type of injury is very uncommon. Do not meddle with the bladder at this stage: there is no urgency about catheterization.

Later on—i.e. up to 24 hours after admission—when the patient's shock has been treated and a decision has been made as to the definitive management of the fracture of the spine, then the bladder should be catheterized.

Under strict asepsis (preferably in the theatre or a special side room) a 6 Ch. Gibbon catheter is passed, and attached to the penis with adhesive strapping. The urine is led to a sterile receiver containing antiseptic. There is no need to change the catheter for a week, and when it is changed strict asepsis should be observed.

After the first three weeks (depending on the severity of the injury) a bruised or oedematous spinal cord may be showing signs of recovery of reflex action below the injury. Now you should look for evidence that the S2/3 segments are intact: elicit the bulbocavernosus reflex, i.e. tweak the end of the penis and feel the bulbospongiosus muscle: if it contracts, the segments are intact. If the reflex is intact, then there is some hope of a return of reflex activity to the bladder.

When the patient is mobilized and up and about in his wheel-chair, you may, after 3 to 6 weeks, start to see whether he can empty his bladder. Remove the Gibbon (at the time it is usual to change it) and see if, when the bladder is full, he can get it to empty reflexly by 'bumping' up and down in his wheel-chair, or by pinching the skin of the thigh. If he can, then carry out a pyelogram in the next few days to see whether there is a significant residual urine. If no residual, well and good. If there is residual—i.e. he is not able to empty the bladder by his reflex activity, then do a cysto-urethrogram, to see if the hold-up is in the bladder neck or the external sphincter, and cut either or both by the appropriate transurethral manoeuvre of bladder neck incision or external sphincterotomy.

If there is no reflex activity, i.e. the spinal centre for S2/3 is destroyed (or the cauda equina nerve roots at this level are destroyed) then the main thing is to make sure that the paralysed floppy bladder can be emptied. Here emptying will have to be by abdominal compression and straining. Control is not to be expected, and the best one can hope for is that the patient will avoid having to have a diversion. You need to measure his residual urine and again cut either the bladder neck, or the external sphincter, if they are preventing him from expressing his urine completely. A urinal is applied to the penis (fig. 20.7).

In women, unless perfect control and reflex activity returns (a rare event) it is better to cut your losses and carry out a diversion. If the patient is paraplegic, she will be unable to get to the WC anyway in time to avoid being wet even if she has a reflex bladder, so a diversion is probably going to be necessary. So far there is no known device or gadget which can keep a woman dry if she cannot control her bladder.

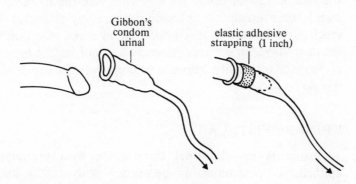

Gibbon's condom urinal

elastic adhesive strapping (1 inch)

Fig. 20.7. The application of a urinal to the penis.

STRESS AND URGE INCONTINENCE

A very common problem is posed by the patient who leaks urine when she laughs or coughs: this is 'stress' incontinence, and is caused by want of resistance at the outflow of the bladder. Normally the urine is kept inside the bladder by the combination of the tone of the external and internal sphincters, and the squeeze of intra-abdominal pressure on the short part of the urethra above the pelvic diaphragm. In women who have had several children, and whose pelvic floor has become weakened, this short length of the urethra no longer lies above the pelvic floor, and is no longer held tight automatically when the intra-abdominal pressure is increased. The diagnosis is made by showing that leakage no longer occurs when the tissues on either side of the urethra are lifted up by fingers introduced into the vagina (Bonney's or Marshall's test): it can be confirmed by measurements of outflow resistance and by stress cystography. The remedy is to lift up the bladder and urethra by one of the many 'repair' procedures which are now available: if there is a large cystocele a vaginal repair is tried first, otherwise a retropubic technique is used, as described by Marshall, Marchetti and Krantz.

It is important to distinguish this stress incontinence from the leakage which occurs when the patient has such a violent urge to void that she cannot reach the lavatory in time. Sometimes this 'urge' incontinence is brought on by coughing or by stress, and the diagnosis is by no means as simple as it sounds. There are many causes of 'urge' incontinence: sometimes it seems to be due to something irritating the detrusor, of which the most simple examples are bacterial cystitis or a calculus in the bladder. Sometimes it is the manifestation of an incomplete upper motor neurone lesion and, as time goes by, the whole tragic pattern of multiple sclerosis unfolds itself. Nowadays the diagnosis is made with some precision thanks to the use of urodynamic measurements of detrusor contraction, pressure profiles of the outflow of the bladder, and the simultaneous observation of the cystogram on the image intensifier, the pressures recorded in the bladder and rectum, and the rate of flow of urine. As a general rule the irritable bladder which causes 'urge' incontinence cannot be cured by measures which correct a mechanical fault, and it is important to make sure that a woman who seems to have 'stress' incontinence does not in fact have a hidden form of detrusor instability before subjecting her to a repair operation which will do no good.

URINARY FISTULAE

A fistula is an abnormal track lined with granulation tissue or epithelium, communicating between a body cavity and the skin, or another body cavity. In the urinary tract fistulae are common and important.

Transient leakage of urine after an operation on the urinary tract is almost inevitable, and of little consequence, provided the wound has been efficiently drained. If a leak persists, it means one of five things:

1 There is persisting obstruction distal to the site of operation: e.g. a stricture or a stone further down the ureter.

2 The track has become lined with epithelium.

3 A foreign body or calculus lies in the track.

4 There is a chronic inflammatory granuloma, e.g. tuberculosis or malakoplakia, deep in the wound.

5 There is carcinoma in the track.

Renal fistulae

Persistent post-operative fistulae occur when there is a residual calculus, tumour, or carcinoma, or when there is uncorrected obstruction further down the ureter. After nephrectomy persistent leakage of pus from a sinus rather than a fistula may be seen when a non-absorbable suture has been used to ligate the renal vessels, in tuberculosis, or when an undrained abscess has led to the formation of innumerable sinus tracts ramifying in the psoas muscle. Fistulae into the colon occur with xanthogranuloma around a stone, or when a carcinoma of the colon works its way into the renal pelvis.

Ureteric fistulae

Congenital ectopic ureteric orifices have been mentioned elsewhere, and occur in association with duplex kidneys and ureteroceles. One should always suspect their existence when a girl is seen who is constantly wet, day and night. Accidental or wartime injuries of the ureter are followed by fistulae, but more often the ureter is injured in the course of a difficult operation in the pelvis. Either the ureter is caught up in the ligature placed on the ovarian artery, or is accidentally involved in the suture used to close the pelvic peritoneum. In either event there is at first some degree of obstruction to the ureter, and later, as the offending ligature cuts through, urine comes away per vaginam. The excretion urogram shows which ureter has been injured because it is slightly obstructed. Nowadays the sooner they are explored and dealt with the better: the ureter is anastomosed to the bladder, if necessary making use of a Boari flap to bridge the gap, or the ureter may be anastomosed to its uninjured fellow on the other side—uretero-ureterostomy.

Vesical fistulae

Persistence of the urachus is responsible for a rare kind of congenital urinary fistula at the umbilicus, and is only seen when there is associated outflow obstruction. When fistulae persist after operations on the bladder, there is always persistent uncorrected outflow obstruction, and it is very seldom that one needs to excise the fistula itself once the obstruction has been corrected. Occasionally carcinoma of the bladder presents in the old cystostomy wound to cause a distressing and dreadful malignant fistula—one good reason for avoiding any open operations for cancer of the bladder whenever possible.

Vesico-vaginal fistulae are usually caused by accidental injury to the trigone at a difficult hysterectomy, when the gynaecologist enters the bladder when trying to dissect it off the cervix. These are small fistulae and can be closed per vaginam or through an abdominal approach, the two layers of bladder and vaginal wall being dissected away from each other, closed, and kept separate with a plug of omentum. Far more difficult are the fistulae which occur as a result of neglected and protracted labour in under-developed countries lacking obstetric services. The baby is forced against the symphysis pubis of the contracted pelvis, and pressure necrosis leads to loss of the trigone, part of the urethra, the cervix and the upper part of the vagina. When the slough finally separates and the damage is healed, the ureters are seen to open into a kind of cloaca formed of the vagina and bladder. It may be necessary to make a new bladder out of an ileocaecal segment (caecocystoplasty) to restore some semblance of normal anatomy, but in many cases the only possible remedy is to divert the urine into the colon or an ileal conduit.

Vesico-uterine fistula is a rare complication of operations or neoplasm in the uterus. The menses flow into the bladder causing periodic haematuria.

Vesico-colic fistulae caused either by diverticulitis of the sigmoid colon, which leads to a pericolic abscess which then secondarily ruptures into the bladder, or are due to direct invasion of the wall of the bladder by a carcinoma of the sigmoid. In either event the patient has severe cystitis, with mixed faecal organisms and vegetable fibres in his urine, and passes gas when he voids—the symptom of *pneumaturia*. On cystoscopy one can sometimes see the hole distinctly, but more often it is obscured by a papillary mass of oedema which the inexperienced surgeon may mistake for a bladder carcinoma. A barium enema usually shows whether the disorder in the bowel is a carcinoma or merely diverticulitis. The remedy is to resect the offending segment of diseased sigmoid and protect the end-to-end anastomosis of the bowel with a temporary colostomy.

Vesico-intestinal fistulae occur as a result of Crohn's disease in the ileum. Note how rarely a carcinoma of the bladder works its way into the bowel.

Prostato-rectal fistula

This usually follows an operation on the prostate for carcinoma, in which no plane of cleavage exists between benign adenoma and capsule, and a hole is made into the rectum. It is more common in the perineal approach to prostatectomy still practised in some North American centres. It can also occur in consequence of unskilled transurethral resection. The best way to close such a fistula is Parks' method, which first removes the mucosa from the lining of the rectum down to the anus, and then brings the mobilized sigmoid down through the sleeve of rectal muscle, sewing it to the frill of mucosa inside the anus. This maintains continence and plugs the hole into the prostatic urethra. Prostato-rectal fistula is also a rare complication of tuberculosis of the prostate.

Urethral fistulae

Pent-up behind a urethral stricture, infected urine bursts through the wall of the urethra to form a periurethral abscess, and then the abscess bursts onto the skin, usually through more than one opening, to form the 'watering-can' perineum, which is made up of a labyrinth of fistulae. In long-standing cases these are associated with squamous cell carcinoma.

FURTHER READING

ALEXANDER S. (1976) Electronic stimulation of the urinary bladder and urinary sphincter. *Scientific Foundations of Urology*, eds. Williams D.I. and Chisholm G.D., p. 107. Heinemann, London.

CALDWELL K.P.S. (ed.) (1975) *Urinary Incontinence*. Sector Publishing, London.

EDWARDS L.E. (1976) Incontinence of Urine. *Urology*, ed. Blandy J.P., p. 687. Blackwell Scientific Publications, Oxford.

EDWARDS L.E. (1976) The pharmacology of the bladder and its sphincter. *Scientific Foundations of Urology*, eds. Williams D.I. and Chisholm G.D., p. 75. Heinemann, London.

GIBBON N.O.K. (1976) The bladder in disorders of the nervous system. *Urology*, ed. Blandy J.P., p. 807. Blackwell Scientific Publications, Oxford.

GIBBON N.O.K. (1976) The pathology of incontinence and principles of treatment. *Scientific Foundations of Urology*, eds. Williams D.I. and Chisholm G.D., p. 95. Heinemann, London.

HOLDEN S., HICKS C.C. O'BRIEN D.P., STONE H.H., WALKER J.A. & WALTON K.N. (1976) Gunshot wounds of the ureter: a 15 year review of 63 consecutive cases. *J. Urol.*, **116**, 562.

THOMAS D.G. (1976) The urinary tract following spinal cord injury. *Scientific Foundations of Urology*, eds. Williams D.I. and Chisholm G.D., p. 59. Heinemann, London.

WHITESIDE C.G. & TURNER WARWICK, R.T. (1976) Urodynamic studies: the unstable bladder. *Scientific Foundation of Urology*, eds. Williams D.I. and Chisholm G.D., p. 84. Heinemann, London.

WILLINGTON F.L. (ed.) (1976) *Incontinence in the elderly*. Academic Press, London.

Chapter 21
The Prostate Gland
Surgical Anatomy

SURGICAL ANATOMY

Surgical relations (fig. 21.1)

The normal prostate gland lies like a doughnut around the urethra as it emerges from the male bladder. It is behind the symphysis pubis, to which it is attached by a tough fascia containing huge veins. On either side the pubis and ischium curve around it. Behind lies the rectum, separated by the fascia of Denonvilliers (two layers of peritoneum stuck together). In the groove between prostate and bladder behind, lie the seminal vesicles and the ampullae of the vasa deferentia.

The normal prostate (fig. 21.2) is made up of two elements, acini, and smooth muscle fibres. Most of the smooth muscle fibres are longitudinal, and are really detrusor muscle fibres running down from the wall of the bladder to be attached to the urethra in the region of the external sphincter. Each acinus secretes a prostatic secretion, of unknown function—the entire volume of prostatic fluid in man is perhaps 0.5 ml, and is probably secreted with the semen during ejaculation. These acini empty, thanks to a sleeve of smooth muscle surrounding each one, disposed radially between outer capsule and urethra, whose contraction tends to empty the secretion like emptying a syringe.

The prostate is pierced obliquely from behind forwards by the common ejaculatory ducts, which emerge just on either side of the verumontanum. A tiny pit in the very middle of the verumontanum

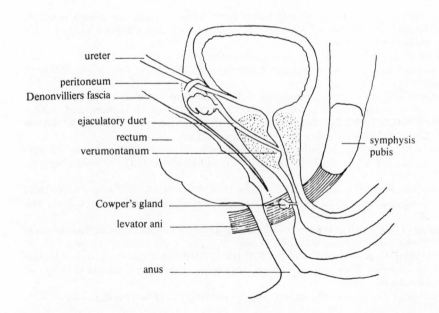

Fig. 21.1. Surgical relations of the prostate.

Chapter 21/*Prostate Gland*

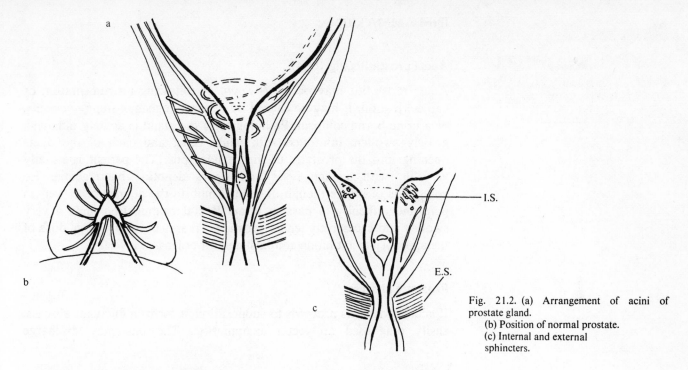

Fig. 21.2. (a) Arrangement of acini of prostate gland.
(b) Position of normal prostate.
(c) Internal and external sphincters.

marks the vestige of the Müllerian (paramesonephric) ducts—glorified with the name *utriculus masculinus*.

The *'internal sphincter'*—i.e. the apparent circular ring of smooth muscle at the neck of the bladder, which is in fact made up of loops of detrusor fibres slinging round the bladder neck, is inextricably mixed up with the acinar tissue of the prostate gland.

Below the prostate lies the *external sphincter*, and the verumontanum is always situated about 1 cm or more above it (fig. 21.3).

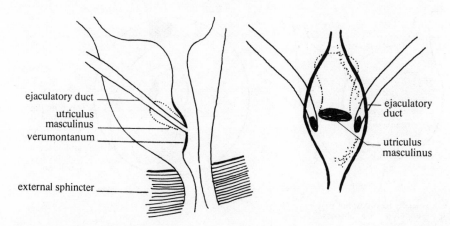

Fig. 21.3. The verumontanum.

INFLAMMATION

Acute prostatitis (fig. 21.4)

Acute prostatitis may occur *de novo*, or following instrumentation or catheterization. It may be caused by a haematogenous *staphylococcus*, or a urine-borne coliform. Pathologically the gland is acutely inflamed, grossly swollen, infiltrated with white cells, and each of the ducts opening into the prostatic urethra exudes pus. The patient is usually very ill, with a high fever and rigors denoting bacteraemia. He complains of severe though ill-defined pain in the perineum, as well as pain and difficulty in passing urine. Rectal examination finds a very swollen and excessively tender prostate. Treatment is by a large dose of the appropriate antibiotic administered for at least two weeks.

Prostatic abscess

If acute prostatitis proceeds to suppuration, it forms a fluctuant abscess, easily diagnosed on rectal examination. The pus may discharge

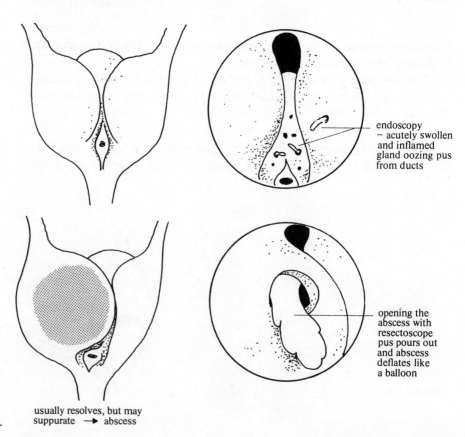

endoscopy
– acutely swollen and inflamed gland oozing pus from ducts

opening the abscess with resectoscope pus pours out and abscess deflates like a balloon

usually resolves, but may suppurate → abscess

Fig. 21.4. Acute inflammation in the prostate.

spontaneously per urethram, or (less commonly) into the rectum. On endoscopy the bulging prostatic urethra may be ruptured by the beak of the cystoscope, or unroofed by taking a slice out of it with a resectoscope loop. Pus pours out, the balloon collapses and the patient gets better.

Chronic prostatitis

This is a condition which is very difficult to diagnose objectively. A good many men who have vague perineal pain, no fever, sterile urine, some difficulty and discomfort on voiding (and often a guilty conscience) get this diagnostic label attached to them. Vigorous prostatic massage may expel pus in the tissue fluid which can be produced, and occasionally organisms may be cultured therefrom. Chronic infection may be an important sequel of incompletely treated gonorrhoea, and may linger long after non-specific urethritis has been treated. For these conditions appropriate treatment will make the patient better. But for the majority of patients the least done the better. Some of these men have an unresolved psychosexual problem at the root of their pains. Histological evidence of infection, i.e. white cell infiltration of the gland, should not be taken as indicating prostatitis, since it is detected in virtually all prostatic tissue removed from elderly men with nodular hyperplasia. 'Chronic prostatitis', if you have excluded gonorrhoea and non-specific urethritis, is a diagnosis to be avoided. Do not fall into the trap of starting the patient off on a protracted course of 'prostatic massage' without asking yourself whether you can think of any other inflammation in the body which you would treat by deliberately squeezing it.

BENIGN ENLARGEMENT OF THE PROSTATE

Aetiology

Virtually every man over the age of 40 has some degree of benign nodular hyperplasia of the prostate, but only one in ten will get obstruction from it. The size of the nodular enlargement has nothing to do with the degree of obstruction, for some of the smallest prostates are accompanied by some of the worst outflow obstruction, and many huge glands are unaccompanied by any obstruction at all. The type of nodular hyperplasia varies from race to race: Anglo-Saxons seem to get rather big bulky glands, Africans and Chinese rather small fibrous ones. But no race of mankind is immune from outflow obstruction.

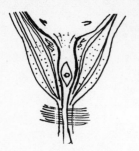

Fig. 21.5. The normal prostate.

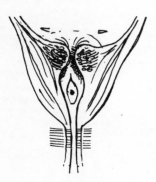

Fig. 21.6. Bladder neck hypertrophy.

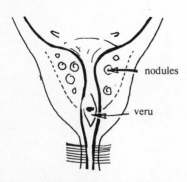

Fig. 21.7. Prostate at 40 years of age.

Pathology

There seem to be two zones in the prostate, an inner one which may be a target for oestrogens, since it enlarges for a week or two in the newborn boy, under the influence, it is thought, of maternal oestrogens, and an outer zone, which may be androgen-influenced. In the normal young male one can see no histological or anatomical difference between the two zones. The prostate of a 20-year-old is made of acini, interlaced with detrusor muscle fibres running from bladder to just below verumontanum. Note position of veru half way down prostatic urethra (fig. 21.5).

It is possible to get pure hypertrophy of the muscular tissue at the neck of the bladder. It may be that this is secondary to some other underlying, possibly neurogenic condition. It occurs in younger men, sometimes in boys, and may cause considerable outflow obstruction (fig. 21.6).

At the age of 40 or thereabouts, nodular hyperplasia commences as tiny collagenous whorls interspersed here and there amongst the glandular acini (fig. 21.7). As the years go by, the benign nodular hyperplasia progresses, and takes one of two forms. In some men, the gland becomes stiff, gnarled, and fibrous, and there is an alteration in its consistency, even though the gland is not much enlarged (fig. 21.8). Others form large bulky 'adenomas' like fibroids in the uterus, which compress the longitudinal muscle fibres of the prostate towards the periphery as a 'capsule' (fig. 21.9). As these nodular 'adenomas' grow larger, they bulge inwards, compress the prostatic urethra from side to side into a sagittal cleft, and may bulge upwards through the ring of muscle at the neck of the bladder, which moulds them into the form of a rounded 'lobe'. Surgeons by tradition talk of this as the 'middle lobe' of the prostate, and the lateral bulges as 'lateral lobes'. They are however not real anatomical entities, but the distorted forms which anatomical limitations have forced the adenomas to adopt (fig. 21.10).

As the adenomas become larger they displace the surgical capsule outwards and downwards, and the verumontanum is pushed nearer and nearer towards the external sphincter. It should be noted that the verumontanum is still proximal to the sphincter, but only just: hence the risk of incontinence if the verumontanum is injured.

The pathological consequences of outflow obstruction

1. RESIDUAL URINE (fig. 21.11)

If the bladder does not get emptied out completely there is a risk of infection. The patient has the constant feeling that he wants to void (hence frequency). When the volume of residual urine is gross, there is overflow incontinence on the slightest increase of intra-abdominal pressure.

2. HYPERTROPHY OF THE DETRUSOR (fig. 21.12)

Hypertrophy is at first no more serious than having a large biceps, but because the disposition of the muscular wall of the bladder is a basket-work, the network becomes more coarse as hypertrophy gets worse, and the mucosa herniates out between the gaps in the network as vesical pressure increases. It is conventional to assign different names to the various stages of the rake's progress of the hypertrophying bladder: at first the exaggerated criss-cross fibres are called trabeculation: later

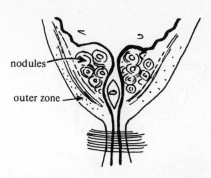

Fig. 21.8. Typical small fibrous prostate. Histologically identical with the big bulky adenoma.

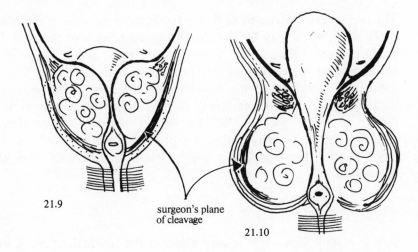

21.9

surgeon's plane of cleavage

21.10

Fig. 21.9. Adenomas pressing the muscle fibres against the remnant of the prostatic acinar tissue to form the 'surgical capsule'.
Fig. 21.10. Adenomas on either side form so-called lateral lobes. Note how the verumontanum is pushed down distally, dangerously near the external sphincter. Hence risk of incontinence after prostatectomy.

little herniations of mucosa are called sacculation: finally when the herniae bulge right outside the bladder, they are recognized as diverticula. The dangers of diverticula are, first that they readily become infected since their content of urine is seldom completely expelled, and secondly their lining of urothelium undergoes squamous metaplasia and carcinoma is more likely to occur.

Fig. 21.11. Residual urine. Possible formation of stones.

  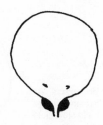 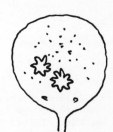

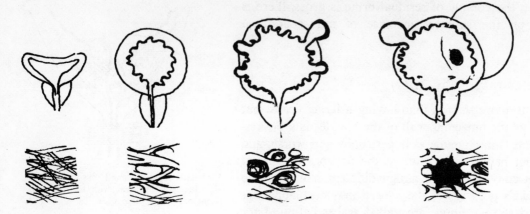

Fig. 21.12. Hypertrophy of the detrusor.

3. BACK PRESSURE ON THE URETERS

The ureters are obstructed as they pass through the wall of the bladder, probably in some way by the hypertrophied muscle of the wall of the bladder itself. Rarely is there reflux from giving way of the ureterovesical valve. As hydronephrosis and hydroureter get worse, so the kidney develops all the physiological sequelae of atrophy of the medulla (fig. 21.13)—i.e. failure to acidify and to concentrate urine, and failure to retain sodium. So the patient becomes dehydrated and acidotic. Part of his dehydration is expressed in a contracted circulating blood volume. If the patient is now operated on, and loses more blood, he may die.

4. INFECTION (fig. 21.14)

Infection may supervene at any stage in the residual urine: it makes renal function temporarily worse through oedema and inflammation, and the ensuing scarring makes it permanently damaged. The presence of infection increases the risk of any form of prostatectomy, makes the kidney inflamed and oedematous, may cause bacteraemia and may lead to epididymitis, cystitis and haematuria.

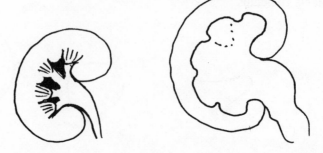

Fig. 21.13. Back pressure on the ureters. As hydronephrosis and hydroureter get worse the kidney develops all the physiological sequelae of atrophy of the medulla.

Chapter 21/*Prostate Gland*

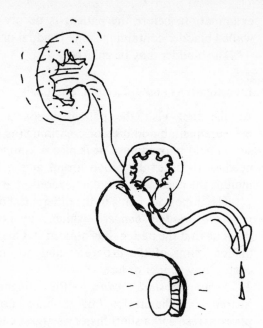

Fig. 21.14. Diagram to show possible areas of involvement when infection occurs.

Clinical features (fig. 21.15)

1   Because of the *outflow obstruction* there is a *poor stream*, especially first thing in the morning: the patient may take a long time to pass water, hence he may avoid a public WC (or get arrested for loitering). As the obstruction gets worse he may go into *acute retention*, an event sometimes precipitated by overdistension of the bladder, or becoming cold.

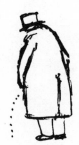

Fig. 21.15.

2   From the *residual urine*, there is a constant desire to empty the bladder, hence the symptom of *frequency*: it is often most bothersome at night. When the bladder becomes really enormous, there is *overflow incontinence*, wet trousers, and lower abdominal distension.

3   If there is *uraemia* and hydronephrosis, there may be confusion, loss of appetite, and loss of weight (fig. 21.16). Anaemia occurs from lack of erythropoietin production by the kidneys. Failure of conservation of salt and water lead to haemoconcentration (hence a falsely high Hb reading at the first test), dehydration, and acidosis.

4   *Infection* may be ushered in with haematuria, rigors (from bacteraemia) and epididymitis.

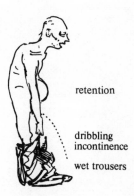

retention

dribbling incontinence

wet trousers

Fig. 21.16.

Local physical signs

The enlarged prostate may be impossible to distinguish on rectal

Chapter 21/*Prostate Gland*

199

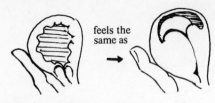

feels the
same as →

Fig. 21.17. Rectal examination of the prostate.

examination, before the patient is deeply anaesthetized, from a thick-walled bladder containing some residual urine (fig. 21.17).

The bladder may be enlarged.

Investigations and differential diagnosis

At the first visit the patient needs a urine culture, haemoglobin measurement, blood urea or creatinine (as a rough test of GFR), and his serum acid phosphatase. It is also a kindness, and saves the patient two needles, to order the blood group at the first visit. Radiography must include the chest Xray, and an excretion urogram.

The important items in the differential diagnosis are:

1 *From bladder cancer*—which may not cause haematuria to be so obvious that the patient has noticed it. One may see a filling defect in the bladder films of the urogram, and one ought always to carry out a cystoscopy sooner or later.

2 *From prostatic cancer*—the diagnosis is impossible without histological diagnosis: but a hard nobbly gland, a raised acid phosphatase and a short history suggest cancer.

3 *From a prolapsed intervertebral disk*—a minor degree of neurogenic disturbance of bladder function can give rise to a clinical picture very much like a benign enlargement of the prostate, and so also can a low disc lesion which irritates the cauda equina. If your prostatic patient also has backache, think of this diagnosis.

4 *From a stricture*—the diagnosis will not be made before cystoscopy, unless the patient admits to a previous urethral inflammation or urological operation.

5 *Other causes of bladder dysfunction*—there is a mixed bag which includes diabetic peripheral neuropathy, anaemia, and depression. Each may manifest itself as frequency and a poor stream.

Treatment of the benign prostate

1. THE COLD CASE

Prostatectomy is indicated if there is residual urine, upper tract obstruction, or severe sacculation in the bladder films. Prostatectomy should rarely be done for symptoms of frequency alone. If there is no objective evidence of outflow obstruction, then one is well advised to wait and see. Many men pass through a phase when their prostate bothers them, and then gets better.

2. ACUTE RETENTION

When acute retention comes on after a long build up of prostatic symptoms then prostatectomy is inevitable. Every patient should be admitted to hospital. There he should be given a large dose of morphine (say 20 mgm), and a warm bath. Sometimes this combination allows him to void, and takes the stress out of the emergency.

More often he cannot void. On his return to bed, a 15 Ch. Foley self-retaining catheter will be passed with strict aseptic precautions. The urine will be drained and the catheter left in, connected to a sterile receiving plastic bag containing 10 ml. of 5% chlorhexidine or some equally effective antiseptic.

The prostatectomy will be performed as soon as may be convenient, i.e. on the next available operating list, so long as the essential preoperative investigations have been performed. These include haemoglobin and blood group, blood urea, and the urine microbiological investigations. Customarily, the prostatectomy was put off until the urogram had been performed: but this is not essential. True, a urogram is desirable, but it can be done during the post-operative period.

3. CHRONIC RETENTION WITHOUT URAEMIA

The patient who comes in with a very large and painless bladder with overflow incontinence, but with a reasonably good renal function as judged by his blood urea, should be treated as an ordinary cold prostatectomy. It is not necessary for the bladder to be drained by preliminary catheterization.

4. CHRONIC RETENTION WITH URAEMIA

Here you are up against an entirely different, and far more serious situation. The patient is certainly not in a good state for prostatectomy, and your first duty is to make him as fit as possible. First, the patient must have an adequate diagnosis made: this includes estimation of his haemoglobin and his electrolytes, and an electrocardiogram.

Then he should be catheterized, with a narrow self-retaining 16 Ch. catheter, connected to a sterile container charged with antiseptic. Decompression should be slow, in the hope of avoiding haemorrhage from the wall of the bladder, which can otherwise be severe, and even complicated by clot retention.

The patient will usually be short of water and salt, and anaemic. Having assessed his electrolyte and water deficiency one must replace the deficiency, preferably by mouth, but sometimes assisting in this with an intravenous infusion containing salt and bicarbonate.

As the extracellular fluid compartment is slowly repleted, you may uncover a serious deficiency of red cells, and it is necessary to monitor the haemoglobin and haematocrit with care, if necessary replacing blood deficiency by a transfusion of whole blood or packed cells.

As the pressure is taken off the kidneys, and you begin to replace the fluid deficit, the patient may go into a serious state of diuresis and salt losing. It may be necessary to give very large volumes indeed by mouth and by vein in order to keep up.

The cardiovascular condition may need expert attention, and one does well to seek the advice of a cardiologist, who may recommend digitalization.

Do not omit to give some thought and care to the mental condition of the patient. He will be a sick and frightened old man, probably more than a little confused by his strange surroundings, perhaps fuddled by drugs and pain. Do not isolate him if he becomes confused, and avoid sedation as a substitute for attention. He needs light, and stimulation, and company; and there is no company he desires so much as that of his family and his friends. Visitors should be encouraged as much as possible.

A little alcohol to the man who enjoys it is a great comfort in his time of need.

There is no place for emergency operation in this group of men.

5. CLOT RETENTION

The benign prostate may bleed so much that clots stop up the outflow from the bladder: this is rare, and requires emergency cystoscopy and evacuation of the clot. Beware the decoy prostate—the big adenoma which masks a carcinoma on the trigone.

6. INFECTION

The patient whose presenting feature is infection should not be operated upon in a hurry. It is far better to spend several days treating the infection, while the bladder is drained, and the patient has developed some natural resistance to the organisms, than to rush in to operate and run the risk of bacteraemia.

CARCINOMA

Aetiology

A varying incidence of carcinoma of the prostate is reported from different countries, perhaps arising from errors in making the diagnosis. It seems not to be increasing, nor to be related to any industrial agent or to smoking. It is not causally related to benign nodular hyperplasia, though the two conditions frequently co-exist (with the possible exception of 'post-sclerotic hypertrophy' in the peripheral tissue of the prostate). Carcinoma is more common in men of Blood Group O, but is not related to their social status or fertility. It is rare both in native Japanese and the men of Japanese ancestry settled in other countries.

Incidence

The incidence depends upon what you mean by carcinoma of the prostate. Small 'latent cancers' can be found in the glands of 14% of 50-year-old men, an incidence which increases to 80% of 80-year olds: but there is confusion as to what these statistics mean. Similar small latent foci of cancer are found in lungs, adrenals, thyroid, colon and stomach, raising the question of the 'critical mass' in the pathogenesis of malignancy.

Site (fig. 21.18)

Cancer seems most often to start off in the peripheral outer zone of the prostate, a zone which really only becomes obvious by the time the inner zone has become full of nodular hyperplasia. The outer zone is the same as the acinar part of the surgical capsule, so that normal prostatectomy for a benign condition leaves behind this peripheral tissue.

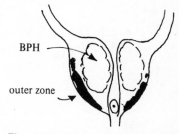

Fig. 21.18. Diagram to show the most common site for carcinoma of the prostate.

Pathology

Macroscopically a carcinoma has no defined edge, and tends to spread as a hard and irregular mass into the neighbouring tissues, encircling the rectum (and sometimes causing obstruction) but seldom penetrating Denonvilliers' fascia.

Histologically a wide spectrum of different degrees of anaplasia are found in the prostate even in the same patient and it is wise to take little notice of classifications based on interpretations of degrees of anaplasia when only a small biopsy has been taken.

Stages

Figure 21.19 shows the standard system of staging currently used. One should take all these staging schemes with a pinch of critical salt: it has been shown that up to 80% of cases thought on clinical grounds to be in Stage I or II turn out to have lymph node metastases: positive peripheral blood cancer cells are found in 80% of Stage II cases at the time of

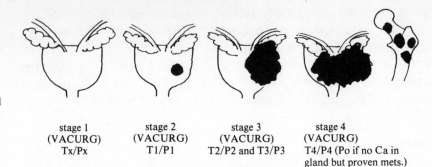

stage 1
(VACURG)
Tx/Px

stage 2
(VACURG)
T1/P1

stage 3
(VACURG)
T2/P2 and T3/P3

stage 4
(VACURG)
T4/P4 (Po if no Ca in
gland but proven mets.)

Fig. 21.19. Clinical and pathological staging of prostatic cancer. (VACURG = Veterans Administrative Collaborative Urologic Research Group. TNM=the proposed international system of the U.I.C.C.).

orchidectomy: 56% of Stage I and II cases turn out to have bone marrow involvement.

Clinical features

Many patients are found to have 'focal carcinoma' of Stage I in the course of routine prostatectomy. Some have a rapidly progressive onset of their prostatism which suggests a more rapidly growing tumour. Others present with pain or a pathological fracture from a distant metastasis, usually in the bone. A few come up with unusual manifestations of prostatic cancer:

1   Some have rectal obstruction caused by encircling of the rectum by tumour spreading out from the gland and around the wall of the rectum, without invading its lumen.

2   A few develop a haemorrhagic condition, as a consequence of unusual fibrinolysins made by the prostatic tumour tissue—a condition which can be remedied by giving epsilon-amino-caproic-acid.

3   In a few men, extraprostatic spread of the tumour compresses and invades the ureters, and they come up in uraemia with bilateral ureteric obstruction.

In addition to the clinical features of outflow obstruction the most useful sign is the finding on rectal examination of a hard or nobbly prostate gland. But one must bear in mind the considerable diagnostic and observer error which is attached to this finding: first, not all hard and nobbly glands are prostatic cancer—many are fibrous nodular hyperplasia, and quite benign: some are tuberculous: some are prostatic stones. Except in the very old man who has other distinct evidence of tumour, it is best to make certain of the diagnosis by means of a biopsy before starting off hormonal treatment.

Investigation

1. *Serum acid phosphatase*

This enzyme is manufactured by healthy prostatic acinar cells, and also by well differentiated carcinoma cells which retain their enzyme systems. If there is an unduly high level of acid phosphatase it signifies an unduly large bulk of differentiated prostatic tissue: but if negative it signifies nothing.

2. *Bone X-rays*

If bone X-rays show sclerotic patches these have to be differentiated from Paget's disease: if they show osteolytic areas, these indicate thinning of cortical bone, which is a late event. Because a bone X-ray shows no obvious metastasis one cannot take this as evidence that all is well. Gamma camera scanning with radioactive isotopes can improve the diagnostic rate of detection of bony metastases.

3. *Biopsy*

If on endoscopy irregularity or fronded tumour can be seen to project into the lumen of the base of the bladder or the urethra, it can be resected and will provide useful histology at the same time as relieving the patient's symptoms. If the lumen seems normal, and most of the suspected hard area of prostate is in the outer peripheral tissue, it can be biopsied by means of a fine-bore Franzen needle which aspirates cells and gives a cytological diagnosis, or by means of the Trucut needle which removes a thin core of tissue for histological diagnosis.

Management

STAGE I

The occult cancer detected by accident in a gland removed by TUR or open prostatectomy for outflow obstruction needs no treatment. Evidence exists to show that life expectancy is as good as for patients with completely benign glands, and that hormonal treatment only makes things worse, by introducing an added risk of cardiovascular side effects.

STAGE II

With the small nodule, again, there is no evidence that anything ought to be done. In some centres, particularly in North America, it is believed that these patients ought to be treated by radical total prostatectomy: but the 15-year survival of such patients is no better than those treated by a policy of 'wait and see' (i.e. give hormones when there are symptoms, but otherwise do nothing).

STAGE III

Here there is evidence that the cancer has spread outside the gland. (As has been already mentioned, careful study of the bone marrow or the lymph nodes shows that many cases really fall into this category even though they seem on rectal examination to be in Stages I or II.) If there are urinary symptoms, then they should be relieved by transurethral resection. If there seems to be local spread outside the gland, there is as yet no clear-cut answer as to the best form of treatment. The choice is between doing nothing except for symptoms; treating the pelvis and local gland with radiotherapy; and giving hormones. So far no statistics indicate which of these policies is the best.

STAGE IV

Here the patient is riddled with metastases, and in pain from those in the bone. Something must be done: it is usual to begin by giving stilboestrol, but for a long time there has been argument about what is the correct dose. At the time of writing the evidence suggests that 1 mgm of stilboestrol three times a day is as good as higher doses, and slightly better than lower ones.

Some patients cannot tolerate oral stilboestrol: if it is phosphorylated (Honvan, Stilphostrol) it can be given intravenously because it is water-soluble, and on arriving in the blood stream is hydrolysed to stilboestrol again. It is still not clear where stilboestrol works, whether in the prostate gland itself, or through the intermediary of a pituitary feedback mechanism. TACE (trichloroanisene) up to 25 mgm daily by mouth gives similar results to stilboestrol without some of its side effects. The main problem however with all these compounds is their increased incidence of cardiovascular complications in the form of coronary thrombosis and stroke, which often make the outlook in years rather worse than if the patient was not treated. Against this must be put the profound and prolonged relief of pain from bony metastases which they provide.

Castration offers a similar result to stilboestrol, and it has the advantage of avoiding the cardiovascular side effects of the hormone. If stilboestrol has failed, orchidectomy seldom helps the patient. Nor does adrenalectomy, though it was given a good trial in the 1950s: but hypophysectomy, either through the transnasal route, or by radioactive Yttrium implantation of the pituitary, offers relief of pain to about two in three patients, though no increase in survival.

General policy

It is well to remember that every man in time gets a cancer of the

Chapter 21/*Prostate Gland*

prostate (in histological terms) but only 0.2% of us die from it: that one should aim to treat the patient and his symptoms, not an Xray or a microscopical slide: that left alone, most cases do rather better than when treated by hormones, radiotherapy or surgery, unless metastases hurt, or growth in the urethra gets in the way of the urine. Never make the cure worse than the disease, and remember that most old men with prostatic cancer die of old age.

FURTHER READING

ANSELL I.D. (1976) Histopathology (of the prostate). *Scientific Foundations of Urology*, eds. Williams D.I. and Chisholm G.D., p. 331. Heinemann, London.

ARDUINO L.J. & GLUCKSMAN M.A. (1962) Lymph node metastases in early carcinoma of the prostate. *J. Urol.*, **88**, 91.

BAGSHAW M.A., RAY G.A., PISTENMA D.A., CASTELLINO R.A. & MEARES E.M. (1975) External beam radiation therapy of primary carinoma of the prostate. *Cancer*, **36**, 723.

BLACKARD C. (1974) Management of cancer of the prostate. *Brit. J. Hosp. Med.*, **11**, 357.

BLACKLOCK N.J. (1976) Surgical Anatomy of the prostate. *Scientific Foundations of Urology*, eds. Williams D.I. and Chisholm G.D., p. 113. Heinemann, London.

BLANDY J.P. (1976) Benign enlargement of the prostate gland. *Urology*, ed. Blandy J.P., p. 859. Blackwell Scientific Publications, Oxford.

BLANDY J.P. (1970) *Transurethral Resection*. Pitman Medical, London.

BYAR D.P., MOSTOFI F.K. & V.A.C.U.R.G. (1972) Carcinoma of the prostate: prognostic evaluation of certain pathological features in 208 radical prostatectomies examined by the step section technique. *Cancer*, **30**, 5.

FARNSWORTH W.E. (1976) Physiology and biochemistry (of the prostate). *Scientific Foundations of Urology*, eds. Williams D.I. and Chisholm G.D., p. 126. Heinemann, London.

KHALIFA N.M. & JARMAN N.D. (1976) A study of 48 cases of incidental carcinoma of the prostate followed 10 years or longer. *J. Urol.*, **116**, 329.

LUND B.L. & DINGSOR E. (1976) Benign obstruction prostatic enlargement: a comparison between the results of treatment by transurethral electroresection and the results of open surgery. *Scand. J. Urol. Nephrol.*, **10**, 33.

MANN T. (1963) Biochemistry of the prostate gland and its secretion. *Biology of the prostate and related tissues Nat. Cancer Inst. Monograph*, **12**, 137.

MOSTOFI F.K. (1970) Benign hyperplasia of the prostate gland. Chap. 27, *Urology*, ed. Campbell M.F. and Harrison J.H. Saunders, Philadelphia.

OATES J.K. (1976) Prostatitis. *Urology*, ed. Blandy J.P., p. 914. Blackwell Scientific Publications, Oxford.

REEVES D.S. (1976) Pharmacology of the prostate. *Scientific Foundations of Urology*, eds. Williams D.I. and Chisholm G.D., p. 147. Heinemann, London.

SHUTTLEWORTH K.E.D. & BLANDY J.P. (1976) Carcinoma of the Prostate. *Urology*, ed. Blandy J.P., p. 926. Blackwell Scientific Publications, Oxford.

SINGH M., BLANDY J.P. & TRESIDDER G.C. (1973) The evaluation of transurethral resection for benign enlargement of the prostate. *Brit. J. Urol.*, **45**, 93.

Chapter 22
The Urethra

SURGICAL ANATOMY

Male urethra (fig. 22.1)

The urethra is a tube made of epithelium of varying character. Near the bladder, it is lined as one would expect, by transitional urothelium. Near the meatus it is lined for two or three centimetres by stratified squamous epithelium. In the middle, from about the level of the external sphincter to just below the glans, it is lined by modified columnar epithelium which is set about with little mucous glands.

Surrounding the epithelial pipe is the erectile tissue of the corpus spongiosum, which is part and parcel of the glans penis. This in turn is enclosed, in its widest part near the base of the penis, by the bulbo-spongiosus muscle.

The narrowest part of the tube is just inside the external meatus. The weakest part of the tube is where it pierces the perineal membrane to join on to the prostatic urethra, and it is at this point that the urethra is most easily torn across in injury.

Fig. 22.1. Anatomy of the male urethra.

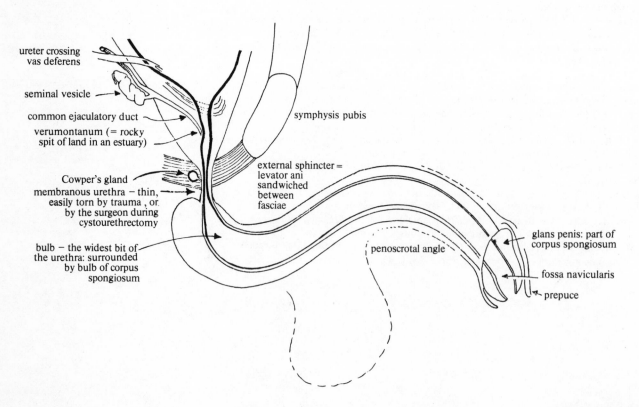

ureter crossing vas deferens

seminal vesicle

common ejaculatory duct

verumontanum (= rocky spit of land in an estuary)

Cowper's gland

membranous urethra – thin, easily torn by trauma , or by the surgeon during cystourethrectomy

bulb – the widest bit of the urethra: surrounded by bulb of corpus spongiosum

symphysis pubis

external sphincter = levator ani sandwiched between fasciae

penoscrotal angle

glans penis: part of corpus spongiosum

fossa navicularis

prepuce

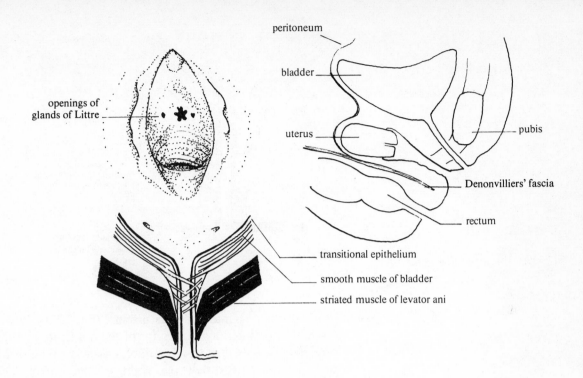

Fig. 22.2. Anatomy of the female urethra.

openings of
glands of Littre

peritoneum

bladder

uterus

pubis

Denonvilliers' fascia

rectum

transitional epithelium

smooth muscle of bladder

striated muscle of levator ani

Female urethra (fig. 22.2)

The female urethra is a similar pipe, running from the bladder to the vagina. Above, where it joins the bladder, the tube is lined usually by urothelium; below, by the modified squamous epithelium typical of the vagina. The level at which these two epithelia meet is very variable, and it is not uncommon to find the 'vaginal' epithelium encroaching on to the trigone.

The tube is surrounded by spongy erectile tissue similar to the corpus spongiosum of the male, and this in turn is enclosed in a double muscular sheath; an inner sleeve derived from the detrusor of the bladder, and an outer sleeve made up of the external sphincter and some of its fibres running down more distally. The entire tube from top to bottom is set about with myriads of little glands secreting mucus.

CONGENITAL LESIONS

Hypospadias and epispadias which are associated with urethral lesions are discussed on pages 164 & 222.

Congenital diverticula occur in the male urethra. They appear to be an attempt to form a double-barrelled urethra, and occasionally complete duplication is found. More often the duplication is partial, and

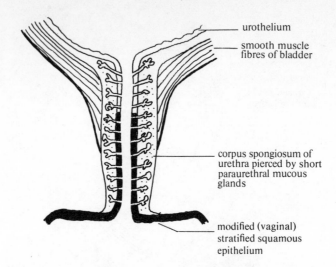

urothelium

smooth muscle fibres of bladder

corpus spongiosum of urethra pierced by short paraurethral mucous glands

modified (vaginal) stratified squamous epithelium

Fig. 22.3. Congenital diverticula.

Fig. 22.4. Anterior diverticulum of male urethra ('anterior urethral valve').

has an opening into the true urethra (fig. 22.3). Boys born with this condition balloon out the cavity of the duplicated urethra as they void, and the contents then slowly dribbles away without their control, so that the parent notices that the child is incontinent. Often an abscess develops in the ballooned-out diverticulum, and when incised, it continues to leak (fig. 22.4).

Diverticula are also found in the female, but it seems more probable that they are secondary to an abscess in the paraurethral glandular tissue.

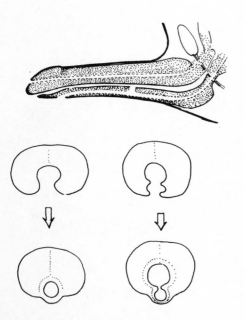

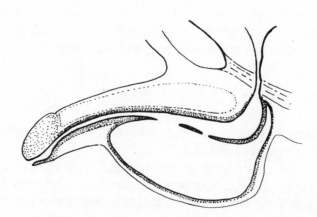

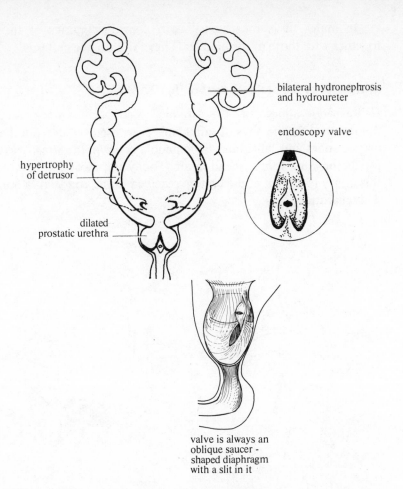

bilateral hydronephrosis and hydroureter

endoscopy valve

hypertrophy of detrusor

dilated prostatic urethra

valve is always an oblique saucer - shaped diaphragm with a slit in it

Fig. 22.5. Congenital posterior urethral valves in male.

Posterior urethral valves only occur in boys (fig. 22.5). There are a pair of sail-shaped valves adjacent to the verumontanum, which are rather like the valves of a vein. Urine cannot get past them without difficulty. Little boys with this condition characteristically 'dirty themselves when they wet' because they have to strain. Even at birth the upper tracts and bladder are found to be enormously hypertrophied. Voiding cystography shows a characteristic picture, and the treatment is simple in theory though difficult in practice. Usually a miniature resectoscope is used to cut the valves, but more recently a tiny diathermy hook, worked under image intensifier control, has been used to do the same job more simply, and with less trauma to the urethra.

TRAUMA

It is fortunate that injuries are rare in the female urethra, and usually heal up with the simplest of surgical repair and catheter drainage.

In males, it is most sensible to consider injuries of the urethra together with those of the bladder. They fall into five patterns.

(i) Injuries to the perineal urethra (fig. 22.6)

Fall-astride injury of the urethra has been known from time immemorial. In the days of sail, ship's crew used to fall from the rigging astride spars and rails: later the manhole cover in the street was a pitfall for the unwary Johnny-head-in-air. Today the most common cause for this injury is a 'kick in the crutch' received in the course of a non-violent demonstration.

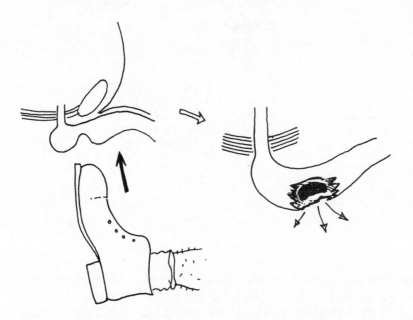

Fig. 22.6. 'Kick-in-the-crutch' injury.

There is a laceration in the bulbar urethra, with tearing of the corpus spongiosum and the lining of the urethra, extravasation of blood, and urine. The danger is that the urine which extravasates into the haematoma in the perineum will be infected, and lead to gangrene. The older surgical literature is full of accounts of the consequences of this gangrene: the skin overlying the fascial compartment enclosed in the confines of Scarpa's fascia would slough (fig. 22.7). Since Scarpa's fascia extends up on to the lower abdominal wall, this would slough too, with horrible and usually fatal consequences for the victim. If they survived the toxic effects of the infection, their testicles, deprived of a covering of skin, remained viable thanks to the testicular blood supply (figs 22.8, 22.9).

Chapter 22/*Urethra*

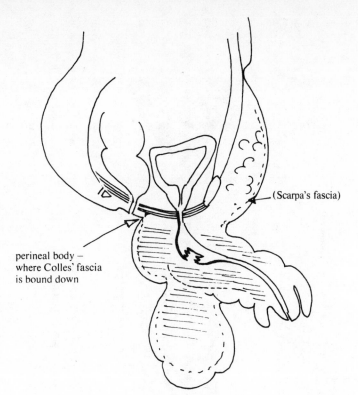

(Scarpa's fascia)

perineal body —
where Colles' fascia
is bound down

Fig. 22.7. Closed injury of the bulbar urethra.

MANAGEMENT

The object of treatment is to prevent extravasation of infected urine, and drain it if it has extravasated. It is not possible or wise to repair the injury. It is better to perform suprapubic drainage and allow the perineal injury to heal on its own, dealing with any later stricture by dilatation or urethroplasty as seems appropriate.

(ii) Torn membranous urethra (fig. 22.10)

After a fracture of the pelvic ring, in which an entire H shaped segment is displaced backwards, carrying the prostate and bladder with it, the membranous urethra is shorn off at the level of the pelvic diaphragm. The bladder neck mechanism is not injured, though it usually goes into spasm, so that at first the patient does not and cannot empty the bladder.

The diagnosis is made by the fact that there is a fractured pelvis, there is escape of blood (often in large amounts) from the urethra, and the patient cannot void.

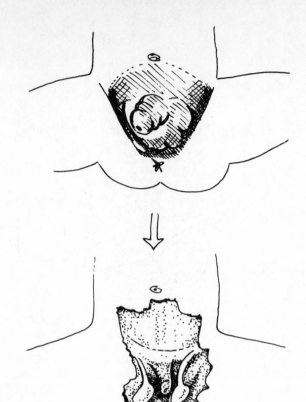

Fig. 22.8. Extravasation under Scarpa's and Colles' fascia.

Fig. 22.9. Diagram to show lower part of abdominal wall sloughed off and the testicles in a field of septic granulations.

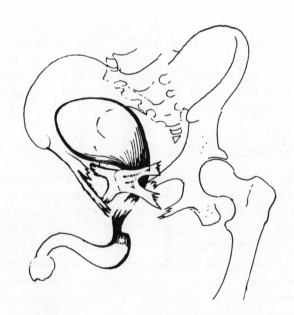

Fig. 22.10. Torn membranous urethra.

Chapter 22/*Urethra*

In a very shocked patient resuscitation may take priority over all else. Later in the day, if the patient is in a better general state, the ideal management is to explore the injury and approximate the severed ends of the urethra over a splinting catheter. But if the patient is too ill, then a suprapubic cystostomy catheter is left indwelling, and formal repair carried out at a later date. If the ruptured membranous urethra is not completely dislocated then it may heal together if the bladder is merely splinted and left alone; and in minor injuries it is possible that this may be better than exploring them as unskilled use of a catheter will aggravate the situation (fig. 22.11).

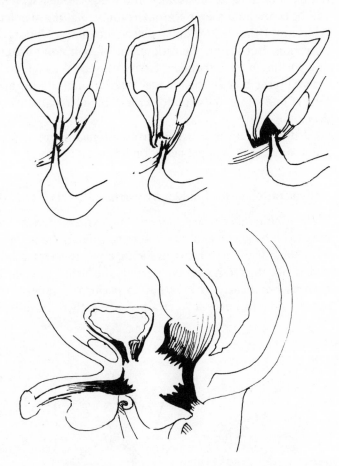

Fig. 22.11. Healing and scarring around a complete tear make a very difficult stricture to treat by urethroplasty.

Fig. 22.12. Down-trousers crush injury with rectal damage.

(iii) Down-trousers crush injury, with rectal damage (fig. 22.12)

Thanks to improved techniques of resuscitation and rescue, more and more men are surviving the shock of severe fractures of the pelvis in which the crush not only tears off the membranous urethra, but may split open the rectum as well. Here the main danger (after loss of blood) is the escape of gas-forming gram-positive rods into the haematoma and the crushed muscle. As soon as possible a colostomy must be performed to divert the faeces, and a suprapubic cystostomy performed to drain the urine. Repair is then carried out in stages: the important principle here is never to attempt a primary repair in the presence of a rectal injury and massive crushing of tissue.

(iv) Rupture of the distended bladder (fig. 22.13)

When a drunkard with a full bladder is run over by a motor vehicle, the full bladder may burst, usually into the peritoneal cavity. As a rule there will be other indications for laparotomy, e.g. the suspicion of closed gut injury, and the laceration in the vault of the bladder is found at this operation. But if not, then the onset of symptoms from the presence of dilute urine in the peritoneal cavity may be very silent. The treatment is to sew up the hole in the bladder, search carefully for associated visceral injury, and close the wound with a bladder catheter and a peritoneal drain.

If the rupture is entirely extraperitoneal there will be no peritonitis, and if drained, it will get better on its own.

(v) Laceration of the bladder by fractured pelvis (fig. 22.14)

More commonly, when there is an extraperitoneal laceration of the bladder, it has been caused by a sharp spike of bone cutting into the wall of the bladder. There is always a huge pelvic haematoma in such a case, and if a catheter has been passed, the urine is very bloody. In such patients one nearly always has to perform a laparotomy because it is not possible to know for certain whether there have been other visceral

Fig. 22.13. Intraperitoneal rupture of the bladder occurs when the bladder is distended. It usually bursts at the apex into the peritoneal cavity.

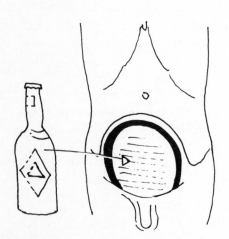
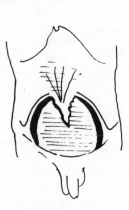
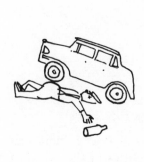

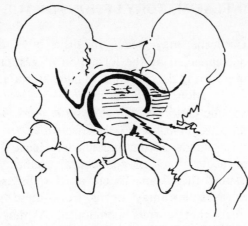

Fig. 22.14. Extraperitoneal rupture of the bladder.

injuries. The tear in the bladder is sutured and the wound closed with a catheter and appropriate drainage.

MANAGEMENT OF LOWER URINARY TRACT INJURIES

The patient is admitted with a history of an injury. The following drill may assist in the management: first, one must find out if he has passed water. If the patient has voided and the urine is clear, one can be fairly sure that the bladder and urethra are all right.

If there is any blood at the external meatus, you can be equally sure that all is not all right.

When the patient is resuscitated, and preferably in the operating theatre with full aseptic precautions—a good time for this is when the orthopaedic team are sewing up lacerations and setting associated fractures—a *soft* rubber Foley catheter no larger than 16 Ch. should be *gently* advanced up the urethra using a non-touch technique. If the catheter enters the bladder and *clear* urine comes out, there is unlikely to be any damage to the bladder or urethra, and the catheter may be removed. If the urine is bloodstained, the catheter should be left *in situ* connected to sterile closed drainage.

If there is the slightest difficulty in passing the catheter, stop. Get help. A urologist should be summoned who will probably perform a suprapubic cystostomy. If the patient's general condition is good, he may explore the pelvis with a view to repairing the lacerated membranous urethra, or at least approximating its ends over a splinting catheter: or he may find some other indication to proceed to a laparotomy.

When in any doubt, do not pass a catheter. There is no urgency about draining the urine, and nothing should be done before the general condition of the patient has been improved. The bladder, leaking or not, can be left alone for 24 hours if necessary.

INFLAMMATORY LESIONS OF THE URETHRA

Urethritis may occur in little boys about the age of 7, and is accompanied by the formation of granulomatous polypi in the bulbar urethra and the symptom of haematuria. It is best left alone.

In adults urethritis may be primary—due to gonorrhoea or non-specific urethritis. The *Neisseria gonorrhoeae* inhabits the paraurethral mucous glands, so it only affects that part of the urethra where there are these glands, i.e. the middle part. Hence it is here that endoscopy during an acute attack of gonococcal urethritis reveals little holes with pus issuing therefrom. Later, as the disease gets worse, abscesses and extravasation may occur from these paraurethral glands into the surrounding corpus spongiousm. As they heal up, they are followed by fibrosis, and so cause a stricture.

It is possible that a similar pathological process can follow infection of these glands by the virus *Chlamydia* (a cause of non-specific urethritis).

Secondary urethritis is seen after instrumentation and secondary to disease in the upper tract, so that one may have to consider some primary pathology in the bladder, prostate or even kidney, if a urethritis does not respond to the usual chemotherapy recommended by the venereologist. The man with a urethral discharge should always be referred to an expert in that field: the penalty for not detecting syphilis may be madness in later life.

Urethral stricture

The end result of urethral inflammation, whether caused by urethritis or trauma, is to heal by a scar, which results in narrowing of the lumen of the urethra i.e. a stricture (fig. 22.15).

Strictures occur in certain well-defined zones. They may occur at the meatus, or rather just inside it, following instrumentation, especially when a catheter has been left inlying for any length of time. They occur in the middle of the urethra, either from pressure necrosis of the urethral wall from a catheter, just at the penoscrotal junction, or along the entire length of the middle of the urethra as far back as the bulb, from gonococcal urethritis. Finally they occur in the region of the prostatic urethra in consequence of the healing which takes place after a rupture of the membranous urethra.

Treatment of urethral stricture is in the first instance by regular, gentle, and skilful *bouginage*, using graduated steel or plastic bougies (see page 269). If this fails, then one may slit the narrow region from within with an endourethral knife—*internal urethrotomy*. But this generally gives only short-lived relief, and it is better to proceed to some

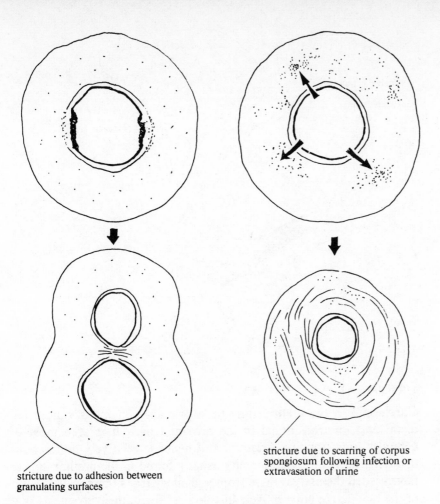

stricture due to adhesion between granulating surfaces

stricture due to scarring of corpus spongiosum following infection or extravasation of urine

Fig. 22.15. Diagram of urethral strictures.

form of *urethroplasty*, a plastic procedure in which full thickness skin is inlaid into the narrow part of the urethra to keep it permanently enlarged (see page 303).

Complications of stricture (fig. 22.16)

Periurethral abscess is common as the result of damming-up of secretions proximal to a stricture. It bursts and forms a fistula between the urethra and the scrotal skin.

A fistula, always secondary to a stricture and an abscess, may have several orifices, and make several tracks which wander around under the skin of the scrotum. When there are many of these fistulae, the condition is called a 'watering-can perineum': it is still common in Africa where neglected gonococcal stricture is frequently encountered.

Stones may form in the pockets of periurethral abscesses, as a result of the presence of stagnant infected urine.

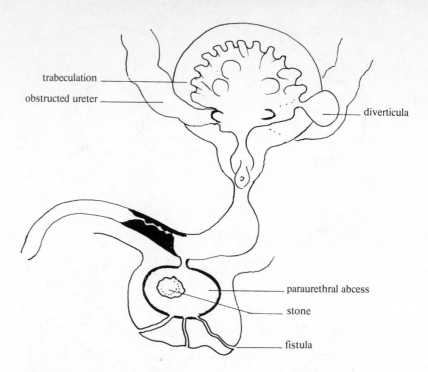

trabeculation

obstructed ureter

diverticula

paraurethral abcess

stone

fistula

Fig. 22.16. Complications of a urethral stricture.

URETHRAL CARCINOMA

Carcinoma in the urethra may be a primary squamous cancer in the distal part, or transitional in the proximal part. It is seen most often behind a long-standing stricture, and hence is relatively more common in Africa. In Britain the tumours usually found in the urethra appear to have seeded themselves there from a primary transitional cell carcinoma in the bladder. Whatever their histological form, their prognosis is very bad, since such a thin layer of tissue separates the tumour from the rich vascular plexus of the corpus spongiosum, that systemic spread is usually early.

FURTHER READING

ATTWATER H.L. (1943) The history of urethral stricture. *Brit. J. Urol.*, **15**, 39.
CASS A.S. (1976) Bladder trauma in the multiple injured patient. *J. Urol.*, **115**, 667.
BLANDY J.P. (1975) Injuries of the urethra in the male. *Injury*, **7**, 77.
BLANDY J.P. (1976) Urethral stricture and carcinoma. *Urology*, ed. Blandy J.P., p. 1014. Blackwell Scientific Publications, Oxford.
BLANDY J.P., WADHWA S., SINGH M. & TRESIDDER G.C. (1977) Urethroplasty in Context. *Brit. J. Urol.*, **48**, 111.
HOPE-STONE H.F. (1975) Carcinoma of the penis. *Proc. Roy. Soc. Med.*, **68**, 777.
JACKSON D.H. & WILLIAMS J.L. (1974) Urethral injury: a retrospective study. *Brit. J. Urol.*, **46**, 665.
MITCHELL J.P. (1975) Trauma to the urethra. *Injury*, **7**, 84.
OATES J.K. (1976) Sexually transmitted diseases. *Urology*, ed. Blandy J.P., p. 980. Blackwell Scientific Publications, Oxford.
SINGH M. & BLANDY J.P. (1976) The pathology of urethral stricture. *J. Urol.*, **115**, 673.

Chapter 23
The Penis

The penis is constructed of three distensible spongy sacs, the twin corpora cavernosa and the corpus spongiosum which surrounds the urethra and ends in an expansion—the glans (fig. 23.1).

Distension of the sacs produces a rigid erection because they are surrounded with a dense thick fascia (Buck's fascia). The spongy spaces of the two corpora cavernosa intercommunicate, and contrast introduced into one enters and distends the other. The corpus spongiosum is virtually separate, though a few small vessels pass across to the cavernosa (fig. 23.2).

On section each of the corpora cavernosa has a large artery running down its middle. Outside Buck's fascia is the dorsal vein of the penis, under it the deep dorsal vein flanked by a dorsal artery and nerve.

At rest blood is shunted from branches of the penile veins (fig. 23.3). During erection 'polsters' close off these A-V shunts, while channels into the cavities of the corpora open up, allowing blood to distend the spongy tissue. Note that the corpus spongiosum which surrounds and keeps open the urethra during ejaculation is served by a separate system from the corpora cavernosa: in priapism, the spongiosum is flaccid, and only the cavernosa are erected. In flaccidity the blood is bypassed through arteriovenous anastomoses directly into the veins. Erection is under the control of the pudendal nerves (S2/3).

Ejaculation (fig. 23.4), a complex process which requires an intact last two lumbar sympathetic ganglia, has two phases. In the first the seminal vesicles 'pump up' by ten or so strokes, and in the second they fire off, pushing before them the 0.5 ml or so of inspissated sperm stored

Fig. 23.1. Cross-section of the penis, and diagram to show position of corpus spongiosum.

Fig. 23.2. Note how during erection the larger and stronger corpora cavernosa are well anchored to the medial aspects of the ischial rami.

Fig. 23.3. (a) blood flow to penis during flaccid state.

(b) blood flow to penis during erection.

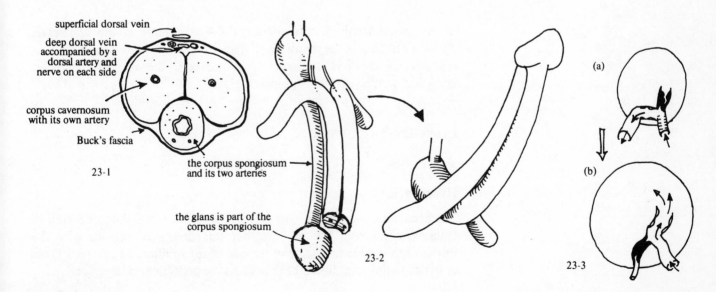

superficial dorsal vein

deep dorsal vein accompanied by a dorsal artery and nerve on each side

corpus cavernosum with its own artery

Buck's fascia

23-1

the corpus spongiosum and its two arteries

the glans is part of the corpus spongiosum

23-2

(a)

(b)

23-3

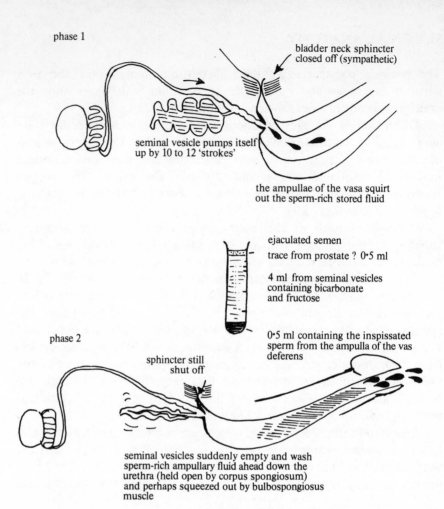

phase 1

bladder neck sphincter
closed off (sympathetic)

seminal vesicle pumps itself
up by 10 to 12 'strokes'

the ampullae of the vasa squirt
out the sperm-rich stored fluid

ejaculated semen

trace from prostate ? 0·5 ml

4 ml from seminal vesicles
containing bicarbonate
and fructose

0·5 ml containing the inspissated
sperm from the ampulla of the vas
deferens

phase 2

sphincter still
shut off

seminal vesicles suddenly empty and wash
sperm-rich ampullary fluid ahead down the
urethra (held open by corpus spongiosum)
and perhaps squeezed out by bulbospongiosus
muscle

Fig. 23.4. Mechanism of ejaculation.

in the ampullae of the vasa deferentia. The volume in the vesicles is
about 4 ml. Hence the majority of sperm in the ejaculate are in the first
0.5 ml. As the vesicles expel their contents, the internal sphincter
contracts and the external sphincter relaxes.

CONGENITAL LESIONS

Hypospadias

The explanation generally given for hypospadias is a failure of fusion of
embryonic folds in the midline, but this does not explain why the
median raphe goes to one or other side of the midline. In severe degrees
of hypospadias one should bear in mind the possibility of intersex.

222   Chapter 23/*Penis*

Hypospadias is classified according to its degree: the meatus may lie just below and behind the pit on the glans penis (glandular), on the corona (coronal), or much further back (penoscrotal and perineal) (fig. 23.5).

Associated with the unusual placing of the meatus there is a shortening of the urethra, and a fibrous cord which bowstrings the penis downwards (chordee). The prepuce exists only as a frill on the dorsum of the penis.

Neonates with this condition must not be circumcised. Sometimes there is an associated narrowing of the external meatus, though this is less common than it seems—most of the tiny meatuses which one sees are really perfectly adequate. But a true pinhole meatus may need to be slit open.

There are many operations in use for hypospadias. The usual

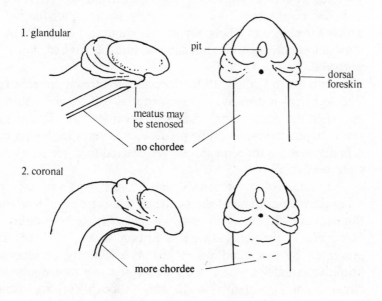

1. glandular

pit

dorsal foreskin

meatus may be stenosed

no chordee

2. coronal

more chordee

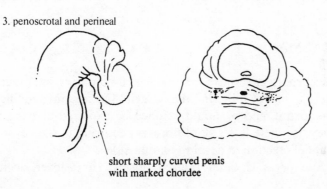

3. penoscrotal and perineal

short sharply curved penis with marked chordee

Fig. 23.5. Hypospadias.

operation performed in Britain is that devised by Denis Browne and is done in two stages. The first stage, in which the chordee is excised, the penis straightened, and the meatus dropped even more proximally, is done at about 18 months to 3 years old. The second stage, in which a buried strip of skin is rolled in to make a complete new urethra is done about 6 months later, so that the whole procedure is finished with before the child goes to school.

Phimosis

Ritual circumcision as part of stone age tribal initiation rites have nothing whatever to do with modern surgery. Those religions which practice infantile circumcision do so for reasons of faith, not health, though it is common to attempt to rationalise the first by the second.

Real phimosis, where the foreskin cannot be retracted to permit complete cleansing of the glans, rarely occurs after the natural age at which foreskin and glans separate—about 2 years. When separation does not occur, then circumcision should be advised, but not before 2 years old.

Attempts to fiddle with the foreskin, to stretch or retract it forcibly, lead to a real narrowing of the preputial orifice, and cause ballooning out when the child voids, and recurrent infection. Napkin rash, due to ammoniacal dermatitis of the prepuce, also leads to this phimosis, but it is better that the foreskin should get scarred than the true meatus of the glans penis.

Neonatal circumcision does protect against the chance of subsequent carcinoma of the penis: of this there is no shadow of doubt. But neonatal circumcision carries a mortality and morbidity of its own: carcinoma of the penis is rare in Britian, and in any case seems to be prevented by soap and water just as effectively as circumcision. In primitive countries where soap and water are rare commodities, then circumcision is probably worth while, though in those societies where this ritual is performed, the real motives stem from very ancient tribal and religious considerations into which reason does not enter.

TRAUMA

The corpora cavernosa may be fractured during intercourse. The lesion consists of a split in the tough fascia surrounding the corpus cavernosum, and it should at once be explored and the rent sewn up. Otherwise there is a risk of fibrosis occurring in the corpus, resulting in failure of erection to develop on that side.

The penis is often injured during zip-fastener accidents, and in consequence of industrial and traffic trauma. As much skin must be conserved as possible, and even if the penis is entirely denuded, it can be covered in scrotal skin or free grafts.

Subcutaneous injections of silicone and paraffin have been administered by mentally peculiar patients or their equally odd doctors in an attempt to make the organ more useful in intercourse. Eventually an ugly foreign body granuloma occurs, calling for reconstructive surgery.

INFLAMMATION

The glans penis is of course the classical site for the Hunterian primary chancre of syphilis, due to inoculation of the skin by *Treponema pallidum*. A dull red papule appearing at very variable intervals after the relevant coitus, gradually enlarges, ulcerates, and then scabs. The local lymph nodes are enlarged. Dark field examination of the juice expressed from the ulcer shows the spirochaetes.

Other lesions which may resemble a chancre include herpes genitalis—usually multiple soft vesicles which become secondarily infected: soft chancre—caused by *Haemophilus ducreyi*: Granuloma inguinale: Lymphogranuloma venereum: and infected scabies. The diagnosis and treatment of these ulcers is a specialized matter, and the penalty for ineffectual amateur treatment is disastrous. Essentially the diagnosis depends upon repeated dark field examination and repeated serological testing. Whatever it looks like, one should always suspect a syphilitic chancre in a genital lesion.

Balanitis

Straightforward balanitis in the uncircumcised male who cannot get his foreskin back to clean away the underlying smegma is common, especially in hot climates where the macerated skin readily gets secondarily infected. After clearing up the initial infection, circumcision allows the glans to become more cornified and dry, and so resist infection.

Balanitis xerotica obliterans

A whitish, sometimes weeping change in the skin on the prepuce or the glans, often extending around and down the external meatus for a centimetre or more, of unknown aetiology, *Balanitis xerotica obliterans* is the local and usually the sole manifestation of the skin condition known as *lichen sclerosus et atrophicus*. It gives rise to stenosis of the meatus, and an irretractable and rather sore prepuce. Circumcision deals with the foreskin, but the narrow meatus may need further meatoplasty to keep it open.

Allergic dermatitis

A cutaneous allergic inflammation due to the antioxidants present in rubber condoms or other contraceptive devices and chemicals, may give rise to severe reactions on the penis.

Peyronie's disease (fig. 23.6)

François de la Peyronie first described this condition in 1743: it consists of the deposition of hard scar tissue in the fascia surrounding the corpus cavernosum on one or both sides, and in the septum separating them. Nobody knows what causes it: it is sometimes found associated with equally inexplicable scarring in the hands, lobes of the ears, and retroperitoneal tissue. Nobody knows how to treat it. At the time of writing cortisone injections, ultrasound, radiotherapy, excision and grafting, diathermy, para-aminobenzoic acid and even procarbazine have been used. Controlled studies are rare, and when attempted, show no improvement over the naturally slow tendency of the lumps to dissolve away in a time course measured not in months but in years. It causes pain on intercourse, and because the distensible erectile tissue

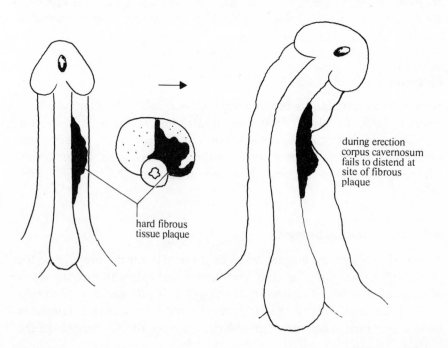

hard fibrous
tissue plaque

during erection
corpus cavernosum
fails to distend at
site of fibrous
plaque

Fig. 23.6. Peyronie's disease.

Chapter 23/*Penis*

does not fill out during erection, the penis bends, sometimes so markedly as to make intercourse painful for the patient's sexual partner, if not for himself.

CARCINOMA

Cancer of the penis is common in Africa, rare in the West. It is generally related to want of cleanliness and prevented by circumcision or washing. It is possible that penile cancer may be initiated or promoted by other local lesions including the scars of soft chancre or syphilis.

Pathology

Penile cancer is a squamous cell carcinoma, it occurs in various degrees of dedifferentiation, the most benign form being allied to the benign penile wart or *condyloma acuminatum*. The giant benign wart named after Buschke and Loewenstein is important, though not common, since it responds very well to local excision without mutilation or sacrifice of the penis.

Spread and staging

The penile cancers which are seen are seldom in their earliest stage (Stage I) in which the cancer is confined to the foreskin or coronal sulcus or glans itself. When seen in such an early stage the outlook is excellent, but it is important to be prepared to take a biopsy of any suspicious-looking lesion in this region, only delaying the procedure to check with a dark field that it is not a chancre.

Treatment at this stage may be either by local amputation or, if facilities exist, by local radiotherapy. The latter gives less deformity, and is no less effective.

In the second stage (Stage II) the tumour has begun to invade the shaft of the penis, and so the spongy tissue of the corpora cavernosa and spongiosum is infiltrated with growth. In such a case a wide amputation should be performed, taking the line of excision well away from the edge of the visible and palpable growth. If necessary the amputation may have to include the testes. In this stage the local nodes are often very indurated and inflamed, but it is better to wait for inflammatory changes to subside before considering node dissection.

In the third stage (III) the tumour is associated with biopsy-proven but operable lymph nodes in the groins, and in Stage IV the condition is hopeless, with invasion of the perineum and irremovable lymph nodes.

In Stages III and IV the outlook is bad. In the early stages sufficiently radical amputation combined with irradiation of the nodes and (very reluctantly—and as a last resort) excision of the inguinal lymph nodes, gives fair results.

Recently it has been shown that some of these squamous cell cancers melt away with the systemic antimitotic agent *bleomycin:* this is an interesting substance which seems to attack keratin, so that hair falls out, and has serious side effects including fibrosis of the lungs.

DISORDERS OF ERECTION AND EJACULATION

Priapism

It is not clear yet exactly what goes wrong with the erection mechanism during priapism. It comes on after intercourse, especially (it is said) if prolonged or unusually vigorous, though no writer has cared to define what he means by this: it occurs more often in males with the sickle cell trait; it is seen in leukaemia, and in patients on intermittent dialysis as a bizarre sequel of over-heparinization.

One sees the corpora cavernosa stiff and distended, but the corpus spongiosum flaccid, as well as the glans penis. The condition is painful.

Innumerable methods of treatment have been tried. John Hunter pointed out that the blood in a priapism was not clotted, and thrombosis has nothing to do with its pathology. Anticoagulants do no good, nor do attempts to block the sympathetic or parasympathetic nerves. Heparin washouts offer temporary benefit only. The only successful therapy is urgent and immediate surgery: the saphenous vein is anastomosed to a window cut in the fascia of one or other corpus cavernosum (fig. 23.7).

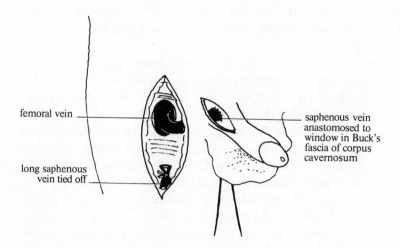

femoral vein

long saphenous vein tied off

saphenous vein anastomosed to window in Buck's fascia of corpus cavernosum

Fig. 23.7. Corpus–saphenous bypass for priapism.

The blood escapes through the venous bypass and the erection subsides. If the corpus-saphenous shunt is performed within the first day of the onset of priapism one may expect recovery of function: if left later than this most patients are left with a damaged erectile system, and permanent impotence.

Impotence

A very careful history must be taken when a patient complains of impotence. The condition falls into the following six categories:

(I) PERFORMANCE FALLS SHORT OF EXPECTATION

Some men consider that ejaculation three times a night 7 nights a week is normal, and if performance falls short of this, they seek the advice of a physician. It is always wise for your professional sympathy to be untinged with envy. There is no treatment. Do not be bullied into prescribing androgens.

(II) EJACULATION NORMAL: COITUS NO GOOD

It is common for a patient to admit that he can masturbate perfectly well, and have nocturnal emissions, but cannot make love to climax with his wife, or sexual partner. Clearly there is nothing wrong with the mechanism: the reasons must be sought in a psychosexual disturbance. Treatment is best left to one who specializes in it. The prognosis is excellent in good hands but, as in other delicate operations, the amateur should not meddle.

(III) EJACULATION NOT REACHED: ERECTION NORMAL

Failure to reach ejaculation may be seen in lesions of the lower lumbar sympathetic ganglia, or in men on ganglion-blocking agents. Be careful to distinguish this from retrograde ejaculation.

(IV) RETROGRADE EJACULATION

Here, as a result of congenital or acquired slackness of the 'internal sphincter', or as a result of some disorder of the sympathetic, the ejaculate at orgasm passes into the bladder. Attempts to repair the bladder neck are unsuccessful, but the semen can be recovered, washed, concentrated, and used in artificial insemination to father children.

(V) FAILURE OF ERECTION

This may be due to organic causes, e.g. diabetes, vascular and neurogenic lesions. Or it may be a consequence of psychosomatic problems, of which depression is the most common, and the one which responds most easily to treatment. In managing such a patient it is wise to examine the femoral pulses carefully to detect a disturbance of blood flow, to perform a neurological examination to detect other manifestations of nervous disorder, and test the urine for sugar. Having excluded these common organic problems the patient is best served by seeking the advice of a psychiatrist.

(VI) EJACULATIO PRAECOX

Ejaculation occurs before the patient has completely penetrated. This occasions considerable marital discord. It is often associated with a degree of emotional distress which suggests that there is more to the problem than meets the eye. Many patients find that if they try to make love a little later, the trigger is not set so delicately. Others need sympathetic counselling about the techniques of civilized love-making. This symptom presents in a whole spectrum of variations, of which one aspect is the failure of the husband to give his wife an orgasm—from which much psychological mischief flows. Discussion and explanation of the details of love-making often gives a more rewarding result than the hasty prescription of some pill or other in an effort to avoid embarrassment. If the patient cannot discuss these things with his doctor, to whom else can he turn? If the doctor is ignorant or inhibited, he should refer the patient to a colleague who is not. Even in this allegedly permissive age, it is tragic to see how frequently patients have not been able to discuss their troubles with anyone who will listen.

FURTHER READING

BLANDY J.P. (1968) Circumcision. *Hospital Medicine*, **2**, 551.

BLANDY J.P. (1976) Penis and Scrotum. *Urology*, ed. Blandy J.P., p. 1049. Blackwell Scientific Publications, Oxford.

BLANDY J.P. (1976) Male infertility and impotence. *Scientific Foundations of Urology*, eds. Williams D.I. and Chisholm G.D., p. 187. Heinemann, London.

BLANDY J.P. (1976) Sexual problems in Urology. *Psychosexual Problems*, ed. Crown S. Academic Press & Grune & Stratton, London.

KIPLING M.D. (1976) Occupational considerations in carcinoma of the urogenital tract. *Brit. J. Hosp. Med.* **15**, 465.

OATES J.K. (1976) Sexually transmitted diseases. *Urology*, ed. Blandy J.P., p. 980. Blackwell Scientific Publications, Oxford.

Oates J.K. & McClean A.N. (1972) Diagnosis of genital ulceration. *Brit. J. Hosp. Med.*, **7**, 37.

Raz S. & Kaufman J.J. (1976) Small-Carrion prosthesis operation for impotence: improved technique. *Urology*, **7**, 68.

Scott F.P., Bradley E.W. & Timm G.W. (1973) Management of erectile impotence. *Urology*, **2**, 80.

Chapter 24
The Testicle and
Seminal Tract

By tradition the term 'testicle' includes the testis and the epididymis.

SURGICAL ANATOMY (fig. 24.1)

The testis is situated in the scrotum, anterior to the epididymis, and slung from the abdominal wall by its spermatic cord. Around the testis there is a thin space containing a trace of fluid—the cavity of the tunica vaginalis. The testicular artery is a branch of the aorta at the level of the renal arteries, which curves round lateral to the inferior epigastric vessels to pass from the retroperitoneal tissue into the groin and down the inguinal canal. There is a rich venous drainage from the testicle: within the internal spermatic fascia a plexus of veins is in communication with a second plexus outside the fascia, both may become enlarged to form a varicocele.

The testis is made up of tubules containing the sperm-forming cells, which drain into the rete testis, and thence, through the vasa efferentia, into the upper end of the epididymis. The epididymis is a long coiled tube from whose lower end the coil begins to straighten out and form the vas deferens (fig 24.2). The vas deferens passes along the posterior aspect of the spermatic cord, hugging the abdominal wall, and curves around the inferior epigastric vessels, to dive down into the pelvis and enter the crack between bladder and prostate, piercing the prostate to reach the ejaculatory duct on the side of the verumontanum. A diverticulum of the vas deferens is the seminal vesicle, a coiled up sac subdivided into compartments like a honeycomb.

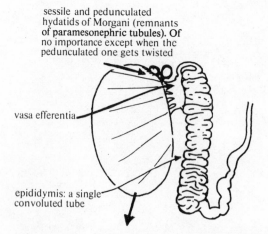

sessile and pedunculated hydatids of Morgani (remnants of paramesonephric tubules). Of no importance except when the pedunculated one gets twisted

vasa efferentia

epididymis: a single convoluted tube

Fig. 24.1. Surgical anatomy of the testis.

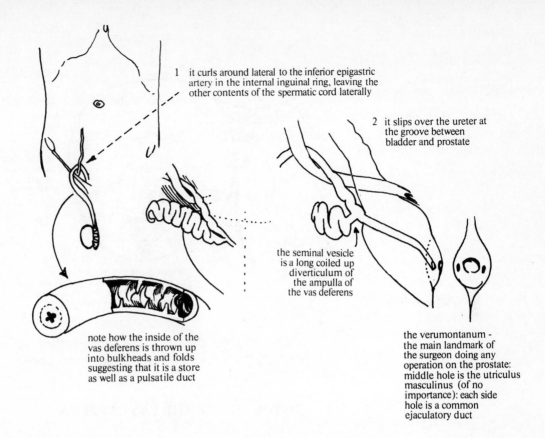

1 it curls around lateral to the inferior epigastric artery in the internal inguinal ring, leaving the other contents of the spermatic cord laterally

2 it slips over the ureter at the groove between bladder and prostate

the seminal vesicle is a long coiled up diverticulum of the ampulla of the vas deferens

note how the inside of the vas deferens is thrown up into bulkheads and folds suggesting that it is a store as well as a pulsatile duct

the verumontanum - the main landmark of the surgeon doing any operation on the prostate: middle hole is the utriculus masculinus (of no importance): each side hole is a common ejaculatory duct

Fig. 24.2. Anatomy of the vas deferens.

HISTOLOGY OF THE TESTIS (fig. 24.3)

The testicular tubules have a basement membrane in which are found two kinds of cell: there are Germinal cells, giving rise to generation after generation of gametes, and finally ending up with tailed spermatozoa. In attendance upon the germinal cells are the Sertoli cells—tall willowy cells, which appear to serve the office of groom and attendant to the developing sperms, and probably play an important role in the final shaping of the mature spermatozoon.

Packed in between the testicular tubules are the Leydig or interstitial cells. These more darkly staining cells are thought to manufacture testosterone.

HISTOLOGY OF THE EPIDIDYMIS

Although the epididymis probably has to reabsorb about 80% of the sperm which pass down its long convoluted canal, its structure is rather simple. The tube is lined by pseudostratified columnar epithelium, with

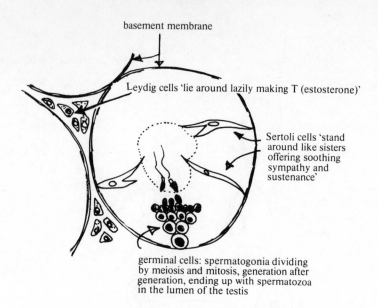

basement membrane

Leydig cells 'lie around lazily making T (estosterone)'

Sertoli cells 'stand around like sisters offering soothing sympathy and sustenance'

germinal cells: spermatogonia dividing by meiosis and mitosis, generation after generation, ending up with spermatozoa in the lumen of the testis

Fig. 24.3. Histology of the testis.

microvilli protruding into the lumen (called stereocilia). These do not beat like true cilia and their function is not known.

HISTOLOGY OF THE VAS DEFERENS

The most striking feature of the vas is its thick muscular coat. The epithelium is similar to that of the epididymis, and similarly lined with stereocilia. As the vas nears the seminal vesicle its wall becomes more and more convoluted and honeycombed, until, like the seminal vesicle itself, it is rather like a collection of sacs—reflecting its function as a store for sperm.

CONGENITAL ANOMALIES OF THE TESTICLE

Undescended testicle

The development of the testis begins in the genital ridge, adjacent to the mesonephros in the foetal abdominal cavity. The developing testis takes over the mesonephric Wolffian duct to use it as its gonadal duct—vas deferens and seminal vesicle, hence the occasional anomalous entry of the ureteric branch of the mesonephric duct into the seminal vesicle.

Around the time the boy baby is to be born, the developing testicle emerges down the inguinal canal, being guided in its course by a lump of jelly—the gubernaculum—which appears to distend the tissues in

Chapter 24/*Testicle and Seminal Tract*

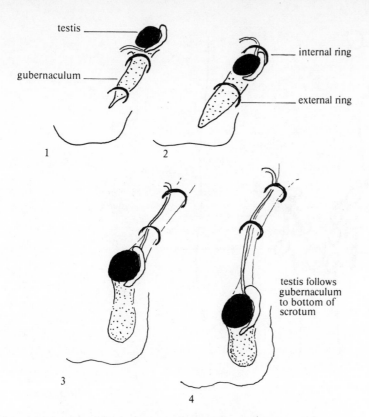

testis

gubernaculum

internal ring

external ring

testis follows
gubernaculum
to bottom of
scrotum

1 2 3 4

Fig. 24.4. Descent of the testicle.

front of it, and carry the testicle into the scrotum. As it passes down into the scrotum, the gubernaculum and testis carry a projection of the peritoneal cavity on their anterior surface—the processus vaginalis (fig. 24.4).

At birth, and for some time afterwards, there may be an identifiable processus vaginalis along the front of the spermatic cord. In adult life this is where indirect inguinal herniae appear, and there is endless discussion as to whether herniae are caused by strain to follow this least line of resistance, or whether there is always a patent cavity in those patients who subsequently get a hernia.

In the adult testis the lower end of the peritoneal extrusion forms the cavity of the tunica vaginalis, hence its anterior relationship to the testicle.

Two things may go wrong with this development. Either there may be an *error of direction*, and gubernaculum and testis go off course, ending up in the abdominal wall, the perineum, or the thigh to form ectopic testicles—abdominal, perineal, or crural; or on the other hand, the testicle may get *held up along the normal course of descent*,

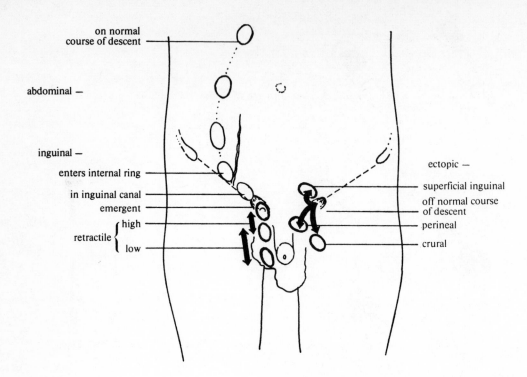

on normal
course of descent —

abdominal —

inguinal —

enters internal ring —

in inguinal canal —

emergent —

retractile { high — / low —

ectopic —

superficial inguinal

off normal course
of descent

perineal

crural

Fig. 24.5. The undescended testicle.

somewhere between the posterior abdominal wall and the bottom of the scrotum (fig. 24.5).

This second variety of anomaly is incomplete descent, and is classified according to how far the testicle can move i.e. it may be abdominal, inguinal, emergent, or retractile. Retractile testes fall into two further subgroups, and these are of major importance: first, there is the low retractile testis of the normal little boy, second the high retractile testis which needs an operation to get it into the scrotum.

Low retractile testes are normal. Nearly every little boy around the time of 5, when he first goes to school, has a very vigorous cremaster muscle, which will draw the testis up into the lower part of the abdomen just outside the external inguinal ring, at the least sign of danger: and this includes the cold bony fingers of an examining school medical officer. Hence the high incidence of 'undescended testicles' in routine school medical examinations. Examined later in a warm and relaxed environment (the bath is best of all) the testis is allowed by its cremaster to fall down slackly into the scrotum.

High retractile testes cannot be got down into the scrotum, and even under profound anaesthesia, the furthest that they can be placed is at the neck of the scrotum. It is sometimes very difficult to be sure without repeated examination into which category to place the child.

Complications of undescended testicle are three, and all are important: first, there is an increased risk of malignancy: perhaps of the order of 1 : 1,000. Bringing the testicle down into the scrotum by orchidopexy does not elimate this danger, but it allows the malignancy to be noticed by the patient so that treatment may be carried out in time, whereas malignancy in the intra-abdominal testicle is impossible to diagnose at an early stage.

The second danger is that of infertility: the undescended testis is notoriously apt not to produce sperm. The reason is not clear, but is thought to be in some way related to a difference in temperature between the abdominal cavity and the scrotum. Definite evidence of histological atrophy of the tubules can be detected by the age of 6 so that if a testis is to be brought down, it should be brought down before that age.

The third danger is that of torsion of the undescended testicle: this is related to the voluminous covering of tunica vaginalis often associated with maldescent.

MANAGEMENT OF THE MALDESCENDED TESTIS

If a testis is not in the scrotum or 'low retractile', by the age of 2, there is no evidence that it will ever go down spontaneously. Nor is there any evidence that giving gonadotrophic hormones will persuade anything other than a low retractile testis to go into the scrotum and stay there.

The first thing to do is to make the diagnosis: if the testis is ectopic, it needs orchidopexy, and the only difficulty is to decide when to do it. Perhaps it is just as well to wait until the child is dry, and as well to get it over before he goes to school. The age of 5 is generally advised today but recent electron-microscopical evidence suggests that the damage may be done by the age of 3.

If the testicle is on the normal line of descent, but higher than the low retractile position, it should be treated in exactly the some manner: i.e. subjected to orchidopexy between the ages of 3 and 5.

When both testes are undescended, there is all the more reason to perform the operation without undue delay. Certain difficulties however complicate the picture.

Sometimes the testicle cannot be found in the inguinal canal at operation: what then? There is every reason to advise a laparotomy to find the abdominal testis, and bring it into the groin if possible, rather than leave it where it is with the risk of malignant change going undetected. When the cord is so short that one cannot bring the testis into the scrotum it ought to be brought down as far as possible, and the site re-explored a year or so later when the cord may have lengthened.

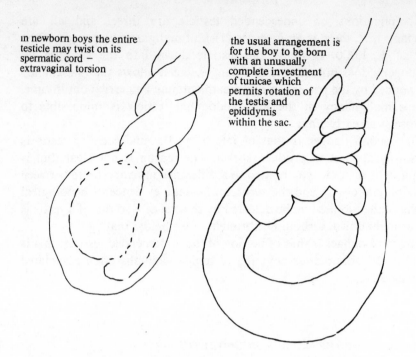

in newborn boys the entire testicle may twist on its spermatic cord – extravaginal torsion

the usual arrangement is for the boy to be born with an unusually complete investment of tunicae which permits rotation of the testis and epididymis within the sac.

Fig. 24.6. Torsion of the testis.

The operation is called orchidopexy (see page 305). At the same time as orchidopexy, a coexisting hernial sac can be removed.

Torsion of the testis (fig. 24.6)

If there is a complete investment of the testis by the visceral layer of tunica vaginalis, then it forms a narrow pedicle upon which the testicle and epididymis may twist within the parietal tunica vaginalis: like a light-bulb in its socket. This occurs at any age, though it is most often seen around puberty. There are often preceding attacks of severe pain in the testicle, coming on suddenly, and as suddenly relieved. The attacks may wake the boy, or they may come on during the day. Twisting the pedicle impairs the venous drainage from the testis, and it then becomes congested, swollen and very painful. Later it will get infarcted, unless untwisted. In an emergency one should try to untwist the testicle by hand, seeing if it is possible to shift it round within the tunica. As soon as possible the testicle should be operated on: one may be fortunate and be able to save the testis by untwisting it in time. The other side should also be explored and fixed, since the anomalous arrangement of the tunica is often bilateral.

The common mistake is to think that the warm swollen testis is a case of epididymitis, and to treat it with antibiotics. Nothing could be more negligent.

Chapter 24/*Testicle and Seminal Tract*

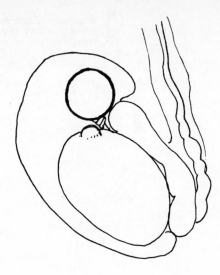

Fig. 24.7. Torsion of the appendix testis.

Torsion of the appendix testis (fig. 24.7)

There are two useless tiny cysts, remnants of Müllerian duct origin, lying on the top of the testicle. One is usually sessile, the other has a little pedicle, and so it may twist. One may find a black pea-sized lump under the scrotal skin after an episode of severe pain. The cysts are 'hydatids of Morgagni'. The inflammation around a twisted hydatid of Morgagni may be out of all proportion to the size of the little lump.

Varicocele

In some boys around puberty the veins draining the left testicle become exceedingly large, bulky, and varicose. If they hurt they should be removed. Otherwise they may be left alone, with one exception: if they are associated with an impaired sperm production, then removing the veins may improve the sperm count, so careful examination for a varicocele is important in investigation of the infertile husband. Secondary varicocele may (rarely) appear when a renal tumour grows into and blocks the testicular vein on the left side as it enters the renal vein.

Hydrocele (fig. 24.8)

1. PRIMARY

Some hydroceles are congenital, and represent the remaining bulky part

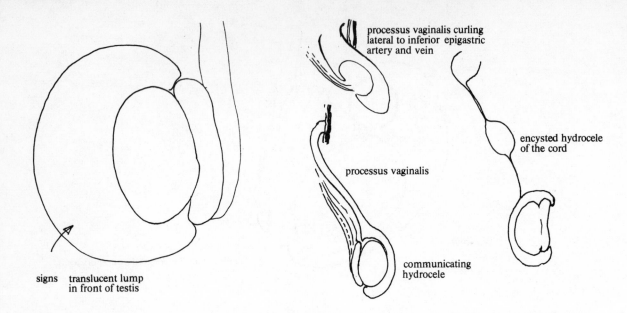

processus vaginalis curling
lateral to inferior epigastric
artery and vein

encysted hydrocele
of the cord

processus vaginalis

communicating
hydrocele

signs   translucent lump
in front of testis

Fig. 24.8. Hydrocele and its variants.

of the processus vaginalis. If they communicate with the peritoneal cavity (i.e. fill up with fluid at the end of the day or have a cough impulse) they should be operated upon. Otherwise they usually go away in about 18 months, and need to be explored only if they persist.

2. SECONDARY

Other hydroceles are acquired, from trauma, neoplasm or inflammation. But the majority are 'idiopathic'. The explanation for their origin is still not very clear: it is said that the testis has no lymphatics of its own, and the hydrocele fluid serves as lymph, to be taken up in the lymphatics of the parietal layer of the tunica vaginalis. If these become blocked, then there is an accumulation of lymph in the hydrocele cavity. This of course in no way explains how the lymphatics come to be blocked, unless there is coexisting disease of the retroperitoneal lymphatics as one sees in filariasis and post-radiation scarring.

Small hydroceles can be left alone, but only after aspirating them to allow the testis to be carefully examined to make sure there is no underlying carcinoma.

Large hydroceles may be aspirated at intervals, they always fill up again, and sooner or later the patient will probably want an operation to cure it for good (see page 308). Hydroceles may be classed as 1. Congenital—fetal remnant. 2. Traumatic—following effusion of blood. 3. Inflammatory—secondary to infection. 4. Neoplastic—

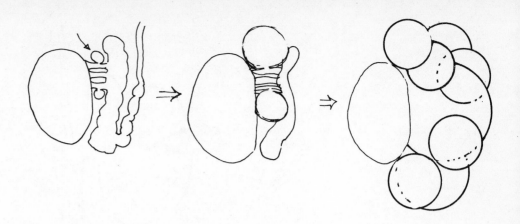

secondary to tumour. 5. Obstructive—in heart failure, filariasis and in other instances where retroperitoneal lymphatics are blocked.

Fig. 24.9. Cysts of the epididymis.

Cysts of the epididymis (fig. 24.9)

It is believed that cysts of the epididymis begin as diverticula of the vasa efferentia testis, and so contain seminal plasma and a few sperm. They can appear at any age, usually in middle life, and are best not meddled with. As they grow they get troublesome, presenting as multilocular cysts behind the testis. Brilliantly translucent, they are never malignant. If they get so large that the patient (or his tailor) starts to complain, it is worth removing them. Do not aspirate them: they have many loculi, the aspiration is painful, seldom complete, and often followed by a haematoma which makes things worse. Leave them alone or remove them complete. It is important to remember that removal of these cysts may lead to sterility, through inadvertent injury to the tubules of the vasa efferentia.

When the fluid contains so many sperm that it appears milky, these cysts are sometimes called *spermatoceles*.

TRAUMA TO THE TESTICLE (fig. 24.10)

The testis is easily injured at sport or at work, and the lesion is usually a split in the visceral layer of the tunica vaginalis, through which blood and testicular tubules spill like cotton wool. A huge painful hydrocele containing blood (haematocele) follows. If left alone, it gradually

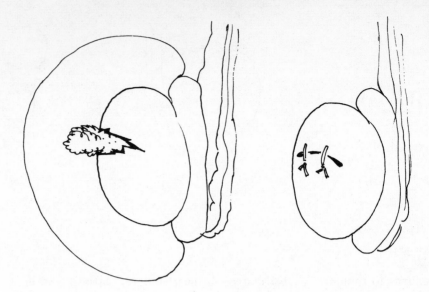

Fig. 24.10. Testis trauma.

resolves and the injured testis is left with a fibrous contracted scar. To preserve testicular function it should be explored as an emergency. The split tunica is sewn up and blood is evacuated. When dealing with such a case, remember that there may be a coexisting tumour of the testicle—about one in five tumours first present after injury, and it has been suggested that their bulk makes them more accident-prone.

INFLAMMATION

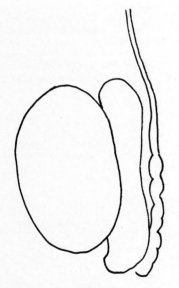

Fig. 24.11. Orchitis.

Acute orchitis may occur in a variety of virus infections, notably mumps in the adult male (never before puberty). Coxsackie and other viruses may cause the same kind of pathology and the inflammation may be followed by testicular atrophy. Rare examples are seen of haematogenous infection lodging in the testicle (fig. 24.11). Distinguish from cremaster spasm (fig. 24.12) and 'lover's nut' (fig. 24.13).

Acute epididymitis (fig. 24.14) may be blood borne, but more often it is secondary to urinary infection, the organisms getting into the epididymis through the lumen of the vas deferens. Secondary to urinary infection, there is an acute inflammation of the epididymis, which becomes red, swollen, and tender. A secondary hydrocele and scrotal swelling may obscure the picture and make a distinction from tumour or torsion impossible (fig. 24.15a & b). In such a case exploration is absolutely necessary: only if it is quite obvious that it is the epididymis

Chapter 24/*Testicle and Seminal Tract*

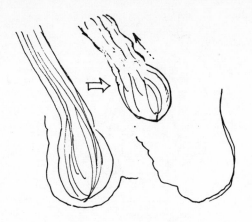

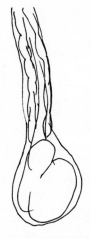

Fig. 24.12. Cremaster spasm. Painful exaggeration of the normal retraction of the cremaster may give rise to severe pain. Patient will note that testis jumps up into the superficial inguinal pouch. Treat by dividing cremaster fibres.

which is swollen, or if there is urinary infection, can one afford not to take the patient to the operating theatre. Remember too that some acute inflammations of the epididymis are caused by tuberculosis, and so it is wise always to have the urine examined by three early morning specimens sent for Ziehl–Neelsen stain and Loewenstein–Jensen culture for tubercle bacilli.

Chronic epididymitis may occur secondary to long-standing inflammation in the region of the prostate, and in some men it grumbles on without any causative organisms ever coming to light. Possibly this is a *chlamydia* infection, but the cause is seldom remediable and one may end having to divide the vasa, or even in others to remove the epididymis *in toto*.

Chronic epididymitis is a feature of genital tuberculosis (fig. 24.16). It has a characteristic beaded craggy feel, and may form a sinus on to the scrotal skin. Treatment consists of early exploration and excision (to establish the diagnosis), followed by a protracted course of anti-tuberculous chemotherapy. One should seek for co-existing genitourinary tuberculosis, but it is by no means always present. One can sometimes isolate the tubercle bacilli from the semen. Associated with the tuberculosis of the epididymis there is nearly always a series of tubercles along the course of the vas deferens, one may find the seminal vesicle involved, and also the prostate gland, which, on endoscopy, has a characteristic scooped-out appearance.

Gumma was reported in the testicle with great frequency in the last century when it was important to make the clinical diagnosis, because it improved with mercury. Today it is very rare, so rare that when in doubt the testicle should be removed, since tumour is a much more probable diagnosis.

Non-specific inflammation caused by extravasation of sperm may take place either in the tissues of the testis or the epididymis; the galea capitis (helmet of the head) of the sperm is made of waxy material

Fig. 24.13. 'Lovers Nut'. Common complaint in casualty department of severe pain in testicle, radiating to groin, possible to iliac fossa. Often mistaken as acute appendicitis. Exact aetiology unknown, probably tense distended veins brought on by sexual excitement not relieved by climax.

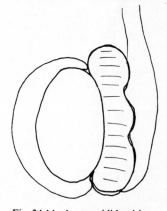

Fig. 24.14. Acute epididymitis.

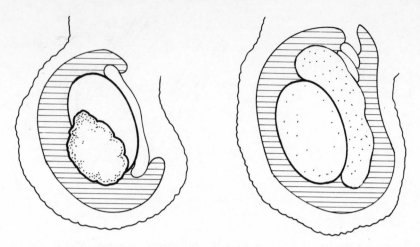

Fig. 24.15. Secondary hydrocele may make distinction from a tumour or torsion impossible.

similar to the waxy envelope of the tubercle bacillus, and equally able to take up acid fuchsin. It evokes a foreign body giant cell reaction resembling tuberculosis, called sperm granuloma.

Gonorrhoea

Today in the UK gonorrhoea is a very rare cause of acute epididymitis. In Mittemeyer's large series (1966) only 4.1% had had GC within a fortnight of the appearance of the epididymitis. Rodin (1969) saw only one in 1,214 cases of gonorrhoea which was followed by epididymitis.

Granulomatous orchitis is a separate entity, probably an autoimmune reaction to antigens liberated by a previous attack of *Escherichia coli* infection. It presents as a hard testicular lump which cannot be distinguished from a malignancy.

TESTICULAR NEOPLASMS

The cause of testicular tumour is not known. About 500 new cases occur every year in Britain, or about 20 cases per million males at risk. It is more rare in African Negroes than Caucasians. The age incidence is to some extent dependent upon the histology. All testicular tumours are rare before puberty, and when they occur, behave more innocently than in adults. Teratomas occur with a peak incidence at 18 to 20 years, seminomas a decade later. In extreme old age one may encounter lymphoma in the testicle. For practical purposes, the only safe rule to remember is that any solid lump in the testicle is a tumour until proved otherwise. If you are in doubt, explore it.

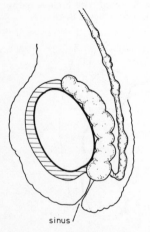

sinus

Fig. 24.16. Genital tuberculosis.

Chapter 24/*Testicle and Seminal Tract*

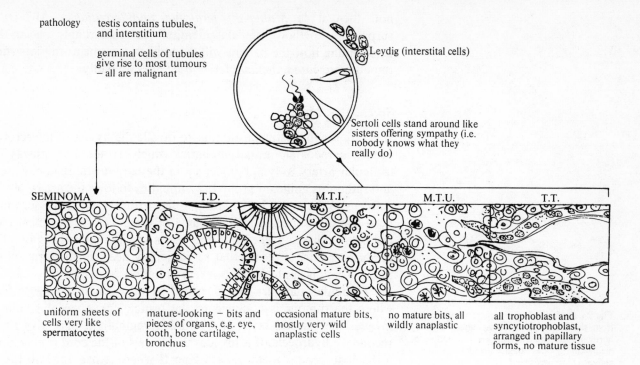

pathology testis contains tubules, and interstitium

germinal cells of tubules give rise to most tumours – all are malignant

Leydig (interstital cells)

Sertoli cells stand around like sisters offering sympathy (i.e. nobody knows what they really do)

SEMINOMA   T.D.   M.T.I.   M.T.U.   T.T.

uniform sheets of cells very like spermatocytes

mature-looking – bits and pieces of organs, e.g. eye, tooth, bone cartilage, bronchus

occasional mature bits, mostly very wild anaplastic cells

no mature bits, all wildly anaplastic

all trophoblast and syncytiotrophoblast, arranged in papillary forms, no mature tissue

Pathology of germinal cell tumours (fig. 24.17)

Fig. 24.17. Tumours of the testis.

Seminoma arises from the grandmother germinal cell—the spermatocyte. It is formed of sheets of rather uniform cells. It has a uniform grey cut section, and it spreads like all testicular tumours, mainly by the lymphatics but sometimes by the vessels.

Teratomas arise from the younger generations of germinal cells, and may give rise to any tissue at all: they are classified according to their degree of differentiation. The most well differentiated (*Teratoma differentiated*)—T.D.—have no 'malignant' looking tissue in sight: there are cysts and areas of bone and cartilage and well-differentiated epithelium. Macroscopically it is often full of cysts, and this polycystic disease was at one time thought to be an innocent condition, a mistake which time and metastases corrected.

The most malignant teratomas contain pure wild trophoblast and syncytiotrophoblast: these are *Teratoma trophoblastic*—T.T. which spread like wildfire through the vascular tissues, and have a tragically brief prognosis.

Between these two extremes are the common teratomas encountered in clinical practice. They are subdivided according to whether the pathologist can find any well-differentiated parts amongst the more anaplastic tissue. If he can find even the least trace of a mature looking tissue, the tumour is *Malignant teratoma intermediate*—M.T.I. If not, then it is *Malignant teratoma undifferentiated*—M.T.U. This surprising method of classification is remarkably accurate in determining how the patient will respond to treatment: the *intermediate* tumours are cured, the *undifferentiated* ones do badly.

Spread (fig. 24.18)

It is rare for the testicular tumour to invade the tissues of the scrotum; it usually spreads along its lymphatics which retrace the pathway of the testicular artery to lymph nodes up in the para-aortic region. A second, and rather insignificant group of lymphatics follows the artery of the vas deferens to the nodes in the internal iliac group. Only if the scrotum has been wantonly incised in the course of diagnosis or treatment can the testicular cells gain access to the nodes in the inguinal region. This is important, since it means that radiotherapy need not be directed to the groin, which is apt to develop severe radiation dermatitis.

Testicular tumours are classified in three clinical stages: Stage I where the tumour is confined to the testicle for a variable time. If it invades the visceral layer of the tunica vaginalis it may give rise to a secondary hydrocele. If it invades the vessels of the cord it may give rise to haematogenous metastases; Stage II where it has got into the para-

Fig. 24.18. Spread of testicular tumours: (a) from the testis via the lymphatics in para-aortic nodes, (b) from para-aortic nodes to mediastinal nodes, thence to thoracic duct and into bloodstream.

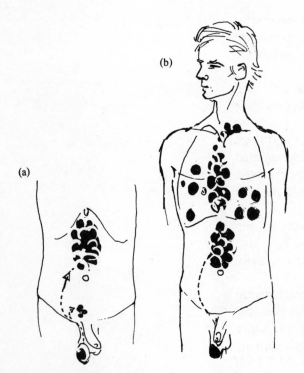

note inguinal lymph nodes
not involved unless previous
surgery done in groin, e.g.
hernia or orchidectomy

Chapter 24/*Testicle and Seminal Tract*

aortic nodes; and Stage III where it has got beyond them, to the mediastinal nodes, or into the peripheral vascular tree by way of the thoracic duct or the testicular veins. In choriocarcinoma and a small group of the others, there is direct haematogenous spread.

Clinical features

The young man with a testicular tumour is in the prime of life. He may notice a lump in the testis, or pain, or just a curious sensation. It is at this stage that one would wish that the diagnosis could always be made, for at this stage the disease is curable. About 20% of these patients will have had a recent *injury* to the testis, and in about a similar 20% there will be local redness, oedema and pain suggesting an *inflammation*. Hence the need to be extra cautious in handling the patient with recent trauma or with what appears at first sight to be 'epididymitis'. A few men come up with features related to hormonal secretion: gynaecomastia may be due to pituitary gonadotrophin secretion related to any type of germinal cell tumour, or to a Sertoli cell tumour (which is extremely rare). Leydig cell tumours (which are also very rare) may occur in prepubertal boys, and give rise to premature virilization thanks to their secretion of testosterone.

Treatment

The testicle is removed through an inguinal incision, the cord being clamped at the internal ring. At this operation an attempt is made to stage the tumour by feeling for para-aortic lymph nodes, a diagnosis which is subsequently checked with a lymphangiogram. Radiotherapy is given to the retroperitoneal tissues in all cases, and if one knows that the para-aortic nodes are involved, the lymphatics of the mediastinum are irradiated as well. In advanced cases chemotherapy can not only prolong life but sometimes seems to offer a permanent cure.

MALE INFERTILITY

In more than half the infertile couples who seek advice, it is the male partner who is responsible. Therefore many doctors feel that, before subjecting the wife to innumerable gynaecological investigations, a simple semen analysis should be done first. There are many different types and causes of infertility, and it will probably be helpful to consider these in the order in which one sets out to investigate the man who has been referred with suspected male infertility.

General assessment

The general examination should detect evidence of endocrine deficiency or bizarre intersex abnormalities. One should bear in mind the possibility of Klinefelter's syndrome in the tall man with thin arms and minute soft testes. At this first interview it is wise to enquire tactfully whether erection, penetration, and ejaculation appear to be in order. Test the urine for sugar.

Local physical examination

With the patient standing up, examine his testes for evidence of a varicocele and for herniae, and undescended testes. Note carefully the size of the testes, the presence or absence of the vasa deferentia, and any tell-tale scar in the groin of previous hernia surgery at which the vas may have accidentally been injured.

Semen analysis

The bulk of the normal semen comes from the seminal vesicles, which push ahead a minute amount of sperm rich fluid issuing from the vas deferens. About 4 ml come from the seminal vesicles, about 0.5 ml from the vasa deferentia, and only a drop or two from the prostate gland.

Semen coagulates within about 20 minutes, and then liquifies again in the next hour. The analysis takes into account the following:

1 *Volume.* If the semen is very scanty in volume this usually means disease in the vesicles, e.g. diabetes or tuberculosis. If in doubt one can estimate the fructose in the semen, since fructose is secreted by the vesicles. The seminal vesicular fluid is controlled by androgens, and may be boosted by giving them.

2 *Sperm density.* There is a wide range of normal density: about 50×10^6 sperm/ml being the median figure, and less than 5 million being rather likely to be infertile.

3 *Motility.* The vigour with which the sperm lash their tails and swim around the slide varies greatly, and appears to be related to androgen-dependent factors: it can be stimulated by giving androgens. Sluggish or absent movement may signify androgen deficiency, or the presence of plasma anti-sperm antibodies which appear in the semen and stop the sperm moving properly.

4 *Morphology.* Despite the quality control processing in the epididymis, about 20% of sperms seen in the slide have bizarre morphological forms, with double heads and other monstrous appearances. In severe oligospermia the abnormal forms are relatively more common.

As a result of the semen analysis, the patients are now seen to fall into different groups:

a Normal sperm density, but still infertile.
b Fewer than·5 to 10 million sperm/ml.
c No sperm at all.

(A) NORMAL SPERM DENSITY, BUT INFERTILE

In some of these men it has been possible to show that their sperms present in perfectly good numbers cannot achieve pregnancy because there are antibodies which immobilize or kill them. In some cases it has been possible to wash off these antibodies, resuspend the sperms in buffered saline, and inject them directly into the wife's cervix to produce a pregnancy.

In other cases no cause can be found for the ineffectualness of these sperms. In some perhaps there is some indiagnosable defect or an inimical factor present in the wife's cervical mucus or uterus. They remain an enigma.

(B) FEWER THAN 5 TO 10 MILLION SPERM/ML

Oligospermia is next investigated by a testicular *biopsy*. This will reveal whether or not there are many germinal cells in the production line capable of being stimulated. If there are (see below), then one can give androgens: this will cause a substantial increase in sperm density in about 40% of men, and Chlomiphen may yield a similar response. If the tubules are hopelessly damaged there is (as yet) no known treatment.

(C) NO SPERM AT ALL

Here the trouble may be in the factory, or in the delivery system. The only way one can tell is to explore the testicle. This will reveal a block or defect in the delivery system; or a disorder of the testicular tubules.
1   *Blockage* can sometimes be seen as soon as the testicle is exposed to the light of day. One may find a complete absence of vas deferens, or it can be seen not to join on to the epididymis. In some cases there is a gap between the middle and lower third of the epididymis. In other cases the blockage is not so obvious, and one may then perform a vasogram (fig. 24.19), injecting contrast medium up and down the vas to outline the epididymis and the rest of the vas and seminal vesicle. Cut down on the vas: cannulate it with a No. 2. 'intracath' and inject 1 ml Hypaque towards the testis, and 2 ml towards the bladder. Expose films. This will show whether there is any blockage between the vas, the vesicles, and ejaculatory duct, and the vas and the epididymis. In obstructed cases

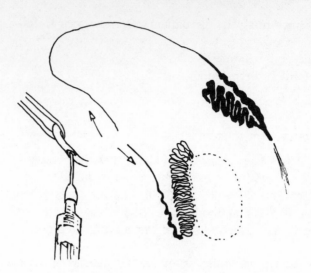

Fig. 24.19. Vasography.

one can sometimes by-pass the block by appropriate surgical anastomoses.

2   If there is no block then one must perform a testicular biopsy and, in practice, it is usual to perform a testicular biopsy even when a block has been found since blockage may coexist with other damage to the tubules. The testicular biopsy may show one of five histological patterns:

Testicular biopsy (figs 24.20, 24.21)

1 There may be normal tubules. If one finds normal tubules and no sperm, and no block can be shown in the vasogram, it is possible that the trouble lies at the level of the vasa efferentia testis, which (at present) cannot be outlined by methods of investigation currently available. Normal tubules are commonly found when there is a blockage, and offer a hopeful prognosis after bypass surgery.

2 There may be no germinal cells. Germinal cell aplasia is found in undescended testes brought down too late. There are plenty of Sertoli and Leydig cells, but not a spermatogonium in sight. The condition is, so far, hopeless.

3 There may be spermatogonia, but none of their progeny. This is called germinal cell arrest; and may be a milder form of 2. It carries a bad prognosis, but is not entirely hopeless. It seems likely that one might eventually be able to find the deficiency which stops the spermatogonia from completing their work.

4 The 'sloughing effect': here the tubule is filled with a jumbled up collection of spermatids, spermatocytes, and immature sperms. This can

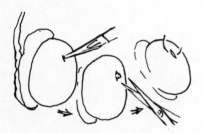

Fig. 24.20. Testicular biopsy.

Chapter 24/*Testicle and Seminal Tract*

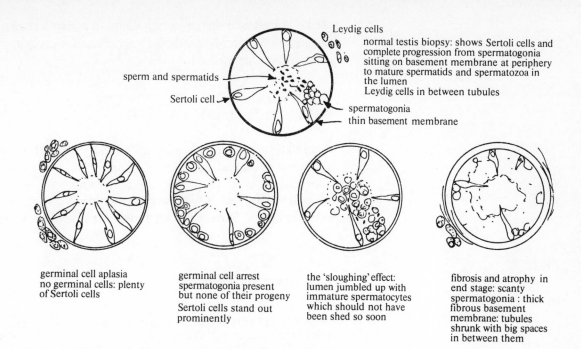

Leydig cells

normal testis biopsy: shows Sertoli cells and complete progression from spermatogonia sitting on basement membrane at periphery to mature spermatids and spermatozoa in the lumen
Leydig cells in between tubules

sperm and spermatids

Sertoli cell

spermatogonia
thin basement membrane

germinal cell aplasia
no germinal cells: plenty
of Sertoli cells

germinal cell arrest
spermatogonia present
but none of their progeny
Sertoli cells stand out
prominently

the 'sloughing' effect:
lumen jumbled up with
immature spermatocytes
which should not have
been shed so soon

fibrosis and atrophy in
end stage: scanty
spermatogonia : thick
fibrous basement
membrane: tubules
shrunk with big spaces
in between them

Fig. 24.21. Testicular biopsy.

be secondary to blockage, and it can be reversed. Patients who respond to androgen or chlomiphen therapy seem to have this kind of testicular morphology.

5 Fibrosis and atrophy. This is 'end-stage testicular disease'. Tubules are narrow, fibrosed, and largely empty of all but a few dead-looking germinal cells and scanty Sertoli cells. Nothing can be done. This picture may follow mumps or ischaemia.

TREATMENT

If there is a remediable block, a bypass can be performed (fig. 24.22). If there is a varicocele, it should be removed. If there is the 'sloughing effect' or normal tubules in the testis, then stimulation either with androgens or chlomiphen may be beneficial.

If there is a good semen volume, but low sperm density, the semen may be gently centrifuged (not too quickly or else the sperms may be broken up). This will yield a small volume of sperm-rich concentrate, which can be taken up in a small syringe and injected through the cervical os into the uterus or cervical canal of the wife at the time of her predicted ovulation. AIH in this way with centrifuged sperm can be occasionally successful.

The method may be modified by first washing the sperm (centrifuging and resuspending them twice or three times in buffered

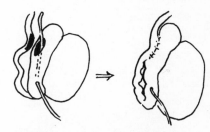

Fig. 24.22. Bypassing blocked tubules.

sterile saline), and then injecting them. In patients shown to have positive plasma anti-sperm antibodies successful pregnancies have been achieved by this method.

WHAT TO TELL THE PATIENT

Although in general it is wise to tell the patient the truth as far as you can perceive it, and you must be frank when you think the chances are hopeless so as to allow the couple to make up their mind about an adoption, it is well to be careful to temper the wind to the shorn lamb and dilute your frankness with a measure of gentleness and sympathy.

FURTHER READING

ALLEN T.D. (1976) Disorders of sexual differentiation. *Urology*, **7**, Supp. 1.

BARNES M.N. *et. al.* (1973) One thousand vasectomies. *Brit. Med. J.*, **4**, 216.

BLANDY J.P., HOPE-STONE H.F. & DAYAN A.D. (1970) *Tumours of the Testicle*. Heinemann, London.

BLANDY J.P. (1976) Male infertility and impotence. *Scientific Foundations of Urology*, eds. Williams D.I. and Chisholm G.D., p. 187. Heinemann, London.

BLANDY J.P. (1976) Testicular neoplasms and The Seminal Vesicles. *Urology*, ed. Blandy J.P., p. 1203 and 1231. Blackwell Scientific Publications, Oxford.

BLANDY J.P., CHAPMAN R., POLLOCK D. & MOLLAND E.A. (1976) The management of tumors of the testis. *Controversy in Surgery*, eds. Varco and Delaney. Saunders, Philadelphia.

DEL VILLAR R.G., IRELAND G.W. & CASS A.S. (1972) Early exploration in acute testicular conditions. *J. Urol.*, **108**, 887.

DICKINSON S.J. (1973) Structural abnormalities in the undescended testis. *J. Pediatr. surg.*, **8**, 523.

GROSS M. (1969) Rupture of the testicle: the importance of early surgical treatment. *J. Urol.*, **101**, 196.

JOHNSTON J.H. (1976) Intersex. *Urology*, ed. Blandy J.P., p. 1138. Blackwell Scientific Publications, Oxford.

LEADER A.J., AXELRAD S.D., FRANKOWSKI R. & MUMFORD S.D. (1974) Complications of 2,711 vasectomies. *J. Urol.*, **111**, 365.

CHAPMAN R.H. & WALTON A.J. (1972) Torsion of the testis and its appendages. *Brit. Med. J.*, **1**, 164.

KRARUP T. (1976) Torsion of the testis: a follow-up of 48 patients. *Scand. J. Urol. Nephrol.*, Supp. **33**, 16.

LINGARDH G., DOMELLÖF L., ERIKSSON S. & FAHRAEUS B. (1975) Dysplasia of the testis and epididymis. *Scand. J. Urol. Nephrol.*, **9**, 1.

MACLEOD J. (1971) Human male infertility. *Obstet. Gynec. Surv.*, **26**, 335.

MITTEMEYER B.T., LENNOX K.W. & BORSKI A.A. (1966) Epididymitis: a review of 610 cases. *J. Urol.*, **95**, 390.

MOSTOFI F.K. & PRICE E.B. (1973) *Tumors of the Male Genital System*. Atlas of Tumor Pathology, 2nd Series. U.S. Armed Forces Inst. Pathol., Washington.

PUGH R.C.B. (ed.) (1976) *Pathology of the Testis*. Blackwell Scientific Publications, Oxford.

SCORER C.G. & FARRINGTON G.H. (1971) *Congenital deformities of the testis and epididymis*. Butterworth, London.

WHITAKER R.H. (1976) Congenital disorders of the testicle, and Benign Disorders of the Testicle. *Urology*, ed. Blandy J.P., pp. 1153 and 1179. Blackwell Scientific Publications, Oxford.

WONG T.W., STRAUSS F.H. & WARNER N.E. (1973) Testicular biopsy in the study of male infertility: (1) Testicular causes of infertility; (2) Post testicular causes of infertility. *Arch. Path.*, **95,** 151 and 160.

YEATES W.K. (1976) Male infertility & Vasectomy. *Urology*, ed. Blandy J.P., pp. 1243 and 1271. Blackwell Scientific Publications, Oxford.

Chapter 25
The Common Operations of Urological Surgery

It is futile for the medical student to become too fascinated by the details of surgical operations; yet they are fascinating, and it will not be long before he is a house-surgeon, and will be expected to get the patient ready for an operation and look after him afterwards. This brief outline of some of the more common operative procedures aims to emphasize the important aspects of pre- and post-operative care, as well as explain what it is that the surgeon is trying to do in the operating theatre.

DIATHERMY

Although every surgeon uses surgical diathermy to some extent, it is in the field of urological surgery that the most progress has perforce had to be made in the design and exploitation of this device. In urological operating theatres the diathermy machine is one of the most important pieces of equipment: it gives out a very considerable amount of energy, and unless treated with respect and care, can be an exceedingly dangerous weapon. For this reason every student ought to know at least something about how it works.

It will be recalled that the first electric battery—the single cell of Volta—when connected to a frog's leg, made it jump. When cells were piled together in series, the leg jumped more violently—as was demonstrated by Galvani as a physiological curiosity. Thanks to Michael Faraday, who devised the dynamo, it was possible to produce a current which rapidly alternated: now the frog's leg jumped each time the current was interrupted, and if the dynamo was revolved sufficiently quickly, a series of rapid twitches resulted in sustained contraction—tetanus, or 'faradic' contraction.

If one increases the rate of alternation of the current above 10,000 cycles a second (and a dynamo itself is no good for this purpose, one needs a sparkgap circuit or a thermionic valve) then a critical point is reached at which a muscle will no longer twitch, and a nerve is no longer depolarized. Hence there is no pain and no movement, and it now becomes possible to pass a huge current through the body without any apparent effect.

To pass such a current terminals must be applied to the skin, and under these terminals there is always some electrical resistance, and therefore some heating effect. If the terminal is very large—i.e. the 'earth plate' of the ordinary surgical diathermy machine—the rise in temperature under the plate is negligible. But if the terminal is very small—e.g. a needle electrode or a resectoscope loop—then the tissues under the electrode can get very hot indeed. This heating effect which occurs as the current strength is stepped up is the basis of surgical diathermy.

Coagulation and cutting

At first the heat warms the tissues: later they are boiled, going white and opaque—like a poached egg. It is this white coagulation which is used for haemostasis, since it curdles the walls of small blood vessels, makes them crinkle up, and coagulates the blood trapped in them. Further increase in the current causes the tissues to become roasted or fried, and even to catch fire. This 'black' coagulation which is often seen in general surgical open operations, is a misuse of diathermy, since haemostasis is not improved by all the smoke and noise. One can slowly divide tissues with a narrow electrode using the coagulating current, but the work is slow, causes considerable local destruction by heating the surrounding tissues, and the electrode constantly becomes coated with carbon and sticks in the wound.

If the current is still further increased there is an entirely new phenomenon: an arc is struck at the end of the electrode. A ring of sparks can be seen. This halo of spark disrupts the tissues, cutting them as cleanly as a knife. The energy of the current is expended in the cutting, and there is hardly any local heating. Cutting is clean: there is no carbonization of the loop, and it does not drag in the tissues. Nor does it provide any haemostasis.

In the past a great mystery was made over the difference between the cutting and the coagulating current. The reason for this is a matter of historical accident. The great pioneer of neurosurgery, Harvey Cushing, had his friend Bovie make him a spark-gap machine, with which Cushing was able to get perfect haemostasis of the small vessels of the brain by white coagulation, but it was never strong enough to strike an arc in air, and certainly not under water.

Later on, Wappler, a celebrated instrument maker of New York, devised a thermionic valve which would give out a very big current at very high frequency. With this current it was now possible to strike an arc, and get clean cutting of tissues, even under water. But the pioneer urologists who used the new Wappler endotherm were horrified to find that although it was cutting well, it did not stop the bleeding. Most of them had been used to Bovie's old spark-gap machine, and had been using it to coagulate bladder tumours at cystoscopy—which it did quite well. So they devised makeshift systems whereby they could feed valve-cutting current or spark-gap coagulating current into their instruments at will believing that it was some peculiar property of the different wave forms which made the currents cut or coagulate. If only they had realized, they could have achieved the same ends by using their valve current at a lower setting. Since few surgeons understood anything about electricity they persuaded their instrument makers to build them machines with both a rather weak spark gap circuit and a very powerful valve circuit housed in the same machine. The latest diathermy instruments are solid-state valve instruments, which offer a continuous range of current settings.

The safety of any of these very powerful diathermy currents depends on the current finding its way back to earth through the earth electrode. Tragically often, the wire connecting the earth plate to the machine is broken, or has not been connected. In such circumstances current will find its way back to earth through the most convenient path it can: if the arm is in contact with a metal part of the operating table, the current will pass along that pathway to earth. This is perfectly safe if the contact takes place over a wide area, for then the rise in temperature will be no greater than it would be under the diathermy plate: but if the contact is a small area, then all the current will pass through that small part, and it will be first poached, then roasted, and perhaps set on fire. Although in modern operating theatres there are precautions and warning lights which should prevent such an accident taking place, it is only by informed understanding of the nature of the danger that accidental diathermy burns can be prevented.

ENDOSCOPIC PROCEDURES

Indications

Virtually every patient with urethral or bladder pathology will have to be examined endoscopically. In many cases the treatment can be carried out at the same time.

Fig. 25.1a. Cystourethroscopy.

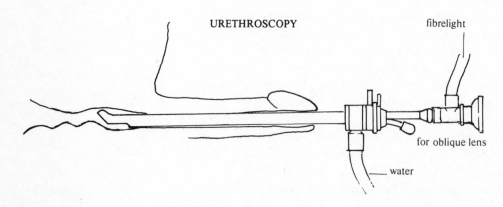

Preparation

One should know what organisms are growing in the urine before endoscopy in view of the slight risk of bacteraemia.

Anaesthesia

Minor procedures may be performed with local anaesthetic using a hibitane-xylocaine gel. Anything which involves diathermy, the removal of a piece for biopsy, or the assessment and staging of a carcinoma requires a deep general anaesthetic with *full relaxation*. Cystoscopy is not a field for a quick gas-and-asphyxia type anaesthetic.

Procedures

1. CYSTOURETHROSCOPY (fig. 25.1)

The urethra must be examined at the time of cystoscopy, using a foroblique lens. A clear view requires a clean lens, a bright light, and a

Fig. 25.1b.

CYSTOSCOPY

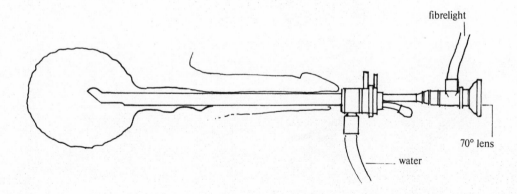

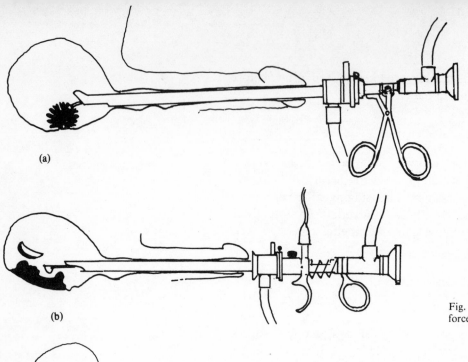

(a)

(b)

Fig. 25.2. (a) Biopsy with cystoscopic forceps, (b) biopsy with resectoscope.

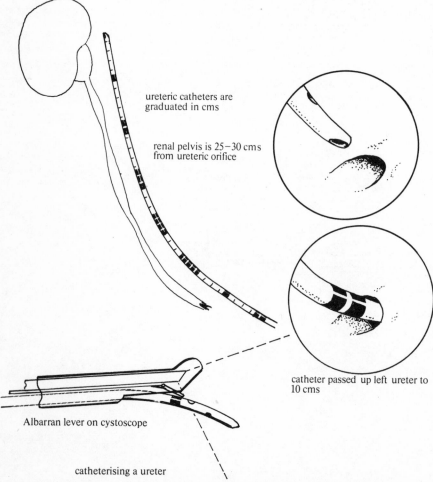

ureteric catheters are graduated in cms

renal pelvis is 25−30 cms from ureteric orifice

catheter passed up left ureter to 10 cms

Albarran lever on cystoscope

catheterising a ureter

Fig 25.3. Catheterizing a ureter.

Chapter 25/*Common Operations*

flow of sterile irrigating fluid (water or glycine). To examine the interior of the bladder the 30° lens is removed and replaced by a 70° lens.

2. BIOPSY (fig. 25.2)

Biopsy forceps can be slipped down the lumen of the cystoscope. A sharp pair of cups tears off a fragment of bladder wall or tumour. This may bleed, and the bleeding may be controlled with diathermy. Alternatively the biopsy may be taken with the resectoscope loop.

3. CATHETERIZING THE URETERS (fig. 25.3)

With the aid of a catheter slide with Albarran lever one may pass fine catheters up the ureter to the kidney and inject contrast medium, or wedge a bulb-ended catheter (named after Chevassu or Braasch) into the ureteric orifice and inject contrast: this manoeuvre—ureterography— gives better delineation of the ureter and is useful in conditions where there is obstruction or a disorder of ureteric motility (fig. 25.4). Ureterography is done with image intensification control and the surgeon can watch what is going on on a television monitor.

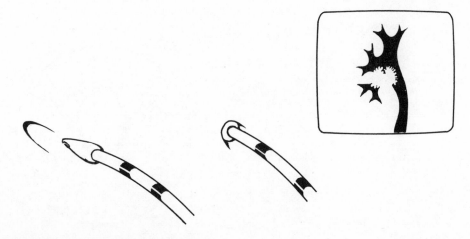

Fig. 25.4. Ureterography has largely replaced the conventional retrograde pyelogram. A bulb-ended Chevassu catheter is gently jammed into the ureteric orifice and hypaque injected while the patient is screened on the image intensifier.

4. CLOSED CYSTODIATHERMY (fig. 25.5)

A fine electrode may be passed up the catheter slide. By means of the Albarran lever on the slide the end of the electrode is brought into contact with a small tumour, or a bleeding area, and the 'coagulating' current applied. This is very useful for small tumours. A modification of this method makes use of a large ball electrode either fixed to the top of the cystoscope or put down the resectoscope sheath. The 'big ball' or Kidd electrode allows deep coagulation of larger tumours over a wider area and is quick and safe.

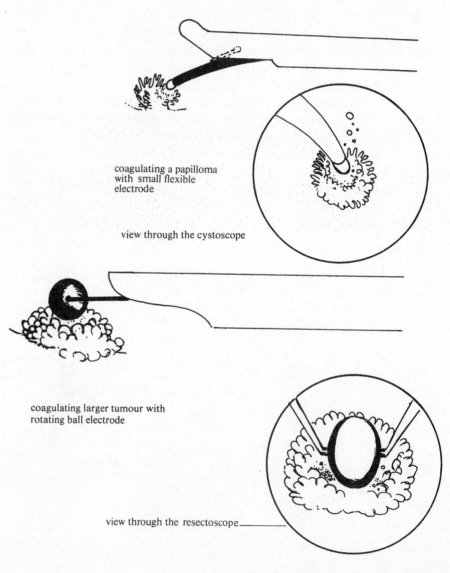

coagulating a papilloma
with small flexible
electrode

view through the cystoscope

coagulating larger tumour with
rotating ball electrode

view through the resectoscope

Fig. 25.5. Closed cystodiathermy.

Chapter 25/*Common Operations*

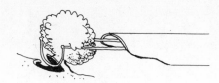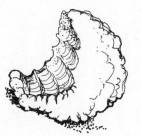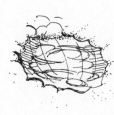

a small bladder tumour can be completely resected using the resectoscope in one bite

a larger tumour is resected piecemeal down to bladder muscle

Fig. 25.6. Transurethral resection.

5. TRANSURETHRAL RESECTION (fig. 25.6)

For a bladder tumour the resectoscope offers rapid and exact removal of superficial growths right down to the bladder muscle. The pieces which are removed afford excellent histological material. The surgeon must have a diathermy machine which allows an arc-cutting current as well as a coagulating (heating) current to do effective resection.

6. LITHOLAPAXY (fig. 25.7)

This ancient urological operation is still useful today; it allows the surgeon to crush a stone in the bladder with the lithotrite, and evacuate the bits with an Ellik evacuator and a resectoscope sheath. Completeness of removal is checked by looking into the bladder afterwards with the irrigating telescope.

DILATION OF STRICTURES

Indications

Virtually all strictures can be dilated, and if dilatation gives rise to little pain, and does not have to be done too often, this can remain the permanent method of treatment.

Preparation

No special precautions other than knowing the urine microbiology.

Chapter 25/*Common Operations* 261

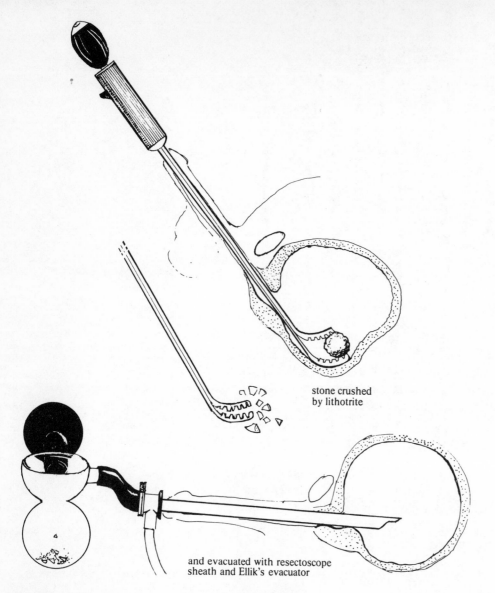

stone crushed
by lithotrite

and evacuated with resectoscope
sheath and Ellik's evacuator

Fig. 25.7. Litholapaxy.

Anaesthesia

Local or general.

Position

The patient is best placed supine rather than in the cystoscopy position.

Method

For most strictures a curved 'sound' or 'bougie' is used. The minor

Chapter 25/*Common Operations*

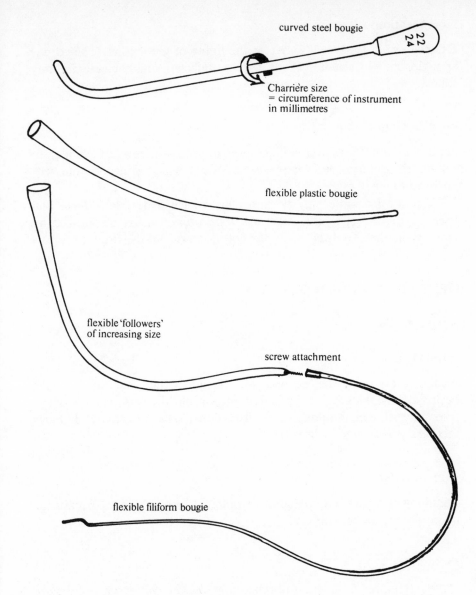

curved steel bougie

22
24

Charrière size
= circumference of instrument
in millimetres

flexible plastic bougie

flexible 'followers'
of increasing size

screw attachment

flexible filiform bougie

Fig. 25.8. Different types of 'bougie' used in dilation of strictures.

variations in their design are of little importance. The steel sound allows the surgeon great control and delicacy of touch (fig. 25.8). The flexible bougie is more difficult to handle, but occasionally more useful. Neither should be painful. The instrument is introduced with the tip downwards, then rotated to follow the curve of the urethra. It may need to be 'lifted' gently through the external sphincter where a little resistance will be encountered if the patient is anxious, or the local has been ineffective. Never should the bougie be forced.

Complications

Clumsy use of the sound may tear the lining of the urethra. The corpus spongiosum will bleed and may become infected, and bacteraemia may follow.

Modifications

1. Use of a filiform (threadlike) bougie with a screw attachment to graduated sounds of flexible plastic or steel is useful in negotiating very narrow bougies.
2. A concealed knife may be attached to such a flexible filiform and used to slit the stricture—*internal urethrotomy*. This is followed by leaving a catheter indwelling to prevent re-stenosis of the stricture.

OPERATIONS ON THE KIDNEY

Simple Nephrectomy

INDICATIONS

Nephrectomy may be needed for benign conditions which have destroyed the kidney, for infective pyelonephritic contracted kidneys prior to transplantation, and for hopelessly destroyed kidneys secondary to calculous disease.

PREPARATION

Breathing exercises: group and cross match 1 litre of blood. Check urine microbiology and sensitivity.

ANAESTHESIA

Profound anaesthesia, with full relaxation, and an endotracheal tube are needed in view of the risk of opening the pleura.

POSITION

The patient is placed in the lateral position, the loin arched over inflatable cushions or the 'bridge' of the operating table which may in addition need to be 'broken' (fig. 25.9). (Extreme arching of the patient may squash the inferior vena cava and lead to impaired venous return and hypotension. The remedy is to unbreak the table and let the bridge down.)

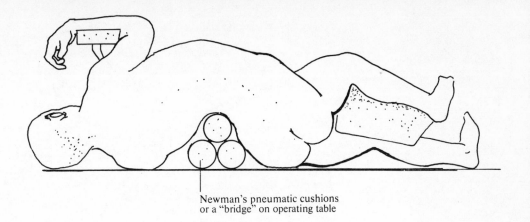

Newman's pneumatic cushions
or a "bridge" on operating table

INCISION

The kidney is routinely approached through a loin incision; of this there are several variants (fig. 25.10). The author prefers to strip the periosteum off the 12th rib, entering the perinephric space through the rib bed, without resecting the rib. The pleura may be opened in doing this.

Fig. 25.9. Operating position for simple nephrectomy.

Fig. 25.10. Loin incision used in approaching the kidney.

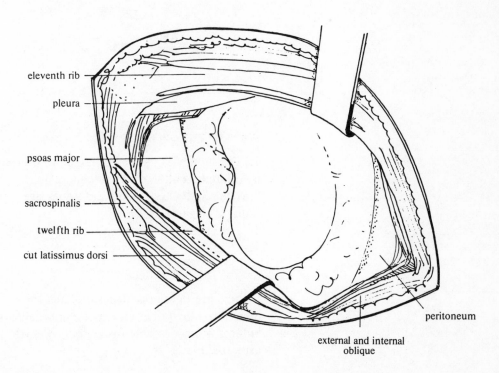

eleventh rib

pleura

psoas major

sacrospinalis

twelfth rib

cut latissimus dorsi

peritoneum

external and internal oblique

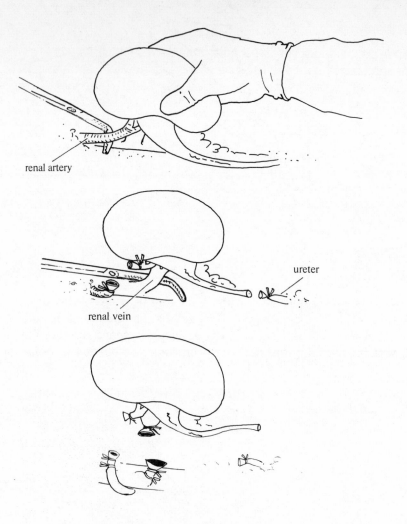

renal artery

ureter

renal vein

Fig. 25.11. Stages of the operation in simple nephrectomy.

STEPS OF THE OPERATION (fig. 25.11)

1. The kidney is dissected free from surrounding adhesions taking care not in injure colon, cava, and duodenum.
2. The renal artery, vein, and ureter are separately ligated, using catgut if the case is infected.
3. The incision is closed in layers with catgut.

VARIANTS ON THE OPERATION

If there are dense perinephric adhesions—e.g. after previous surgery or infection—then the kidney is approached under its capsule. If the kidney is very much distended by hydronephrosis, the contents are aspirated first.

TUBES AND DRAINS

No drain is needed in an uncomplicated uninfected case so long as there has been good haemostasis. In other cases a tube drain to a sterile bag is left in.

POST-OPERATIVE CARE

Nothing by mouth until bowel sounds return and flatus passes. Continue the intravenous drip until then. Breathing and coughing exercises as soon as the patient is round. Up the next day, general condition permitting. Sutures removed 10th day, drain out 24 or 48 hours.

COMPLICATIONS

Early—collapse and infection of the basal segments of the lung, pneumothorax if air not aspirated as the wound closed and the pleura opened. Reactionary haemorrhage can occur if a ligature slips off the renal artery, but more commonly occurs from a muscular vessel. Ileus is common, and may last three of four days if there has been much difficulty in dissecting out the kidney from its bed.
Late—wound infection and subphrenic abscess. Sinus from the use of non-absorbable ligature. Hernia may occur in the wound, especially when the 12th rib is resected. Arteriovenous aneurysm has been reported if the artery and vein are not ligated separately.

Transabdominal nephrectomy

INDICATIONS

Carcinoma of the kidney. Polycystic kidneys. As part of nephro-ureterectomy.

PREPARATION

As above.

ANAESTHESIA

As above.

POSITION ON TABLE

Supine, perhaps with a sandbag under the buttocks on the side of the tumour.

INCISION

If the patient is short and fat, a transverse incision. If the patient is long and thin, a long paramedian incision.

STEPS OF THE OPERATION (fig. 25.12)

1. Laparotomy is performed.
2. The colon and duodenum are reflected medially, dividing their peritoneal reflection.
3. The renal vein is mobilized and retracted upwards, but not tied.
4. The renal artery, lying under the vein, is ligated in continuity.
5. Now the renal vein is doubly ligated and cut.
6. The renal artery is dissected cleanly, double ligated and cut.
7. Now the entire kidney, inside its 'box' of Gerota's fascia, together with the suprarenal, is removed *en bloc*.
8. The wound is closed after repositioning the colon, but without repairing the peritoneum.

TUBES AND DRAINS

In a straightforward case, no drain is needed. If there has been incomplete haemostasis or infection, a drain is left in for up to 48 hours.

POST-OPERATIVE CARE

Nasogastric suction and i.v. fluids until ileus resolves. Early mobilization. Breathing and coughing exercises.

COMPLICATIONS

As for nephrectomy, plus intestinal obstruction, burst abdomen, etc.

Operations for renal stones

INDICATIONS

Any stone too big to go down the ureter, unless there are strong medical contraindications.

PREPARATION

Culture and sensitivity of urine. 1 litre of blood.

Fig. 25.12. Stages of the operation in transabdominal nephrectomy.

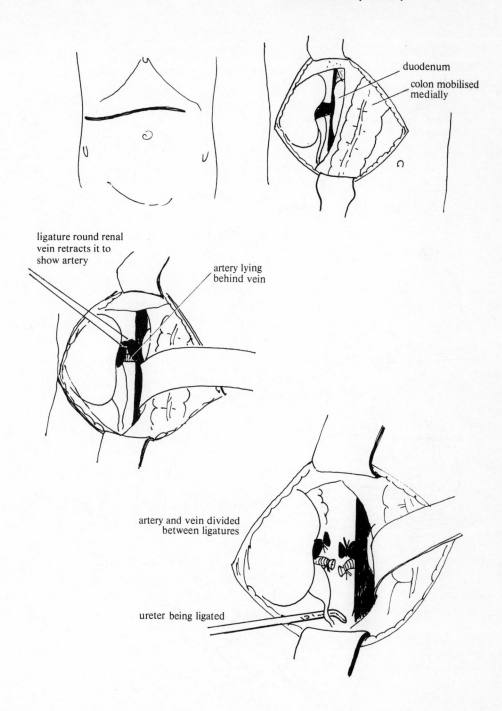

duodenum

colon mobilised medially

ligature round renal vein retracts it to show artery

artery lying behind vein

artery and vein divided between ligatures

ureter being ligated

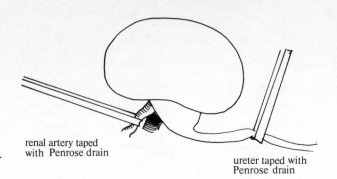

Fig. 25.13. Preparation of kidney for removal of stone.

renal artery taped
with Penrose drain

ureter taped with
Penrose drain

Fig. 25.14. Stages of extended pyelolithotomy.

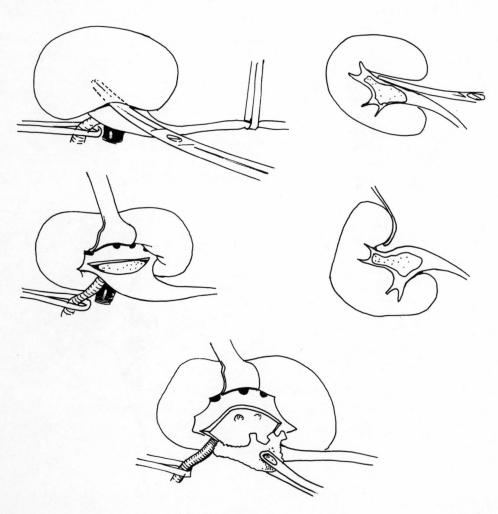

ANAESTHESIA   as for simple nephrectomy.

INCISION

STEPS OF THE OPERATION (fig. 25.13)

1. Dissect the kidney from its surroundings.
2. Secure a tape around the renal artery and ureter.
3. If the stone is in the pelvis, enter Gil-Vernet's tissue plane, retract the parenchyma, incise the pelvis, and extract the stone (fig. 25.14).
4. If the stone has large mushroom extensions into the outlying calices, and the caliceal tissue is thinned out (as it usually is), an incision is made through the ballooned-out calix on to the stone; it is broken off, and extracted, while the main body of the stone is removed through the pelvis (fig. 25.15).
5. If the outlying mushroom stone is covered by a thick vascular layer of healthy kidney tissue the renal artery is temporarily occluded with a bulldog clamp, ice-cold sterile saline is run into the pelvis and over the

Fig. 25.15. Removal of mushroom-shaped stones.

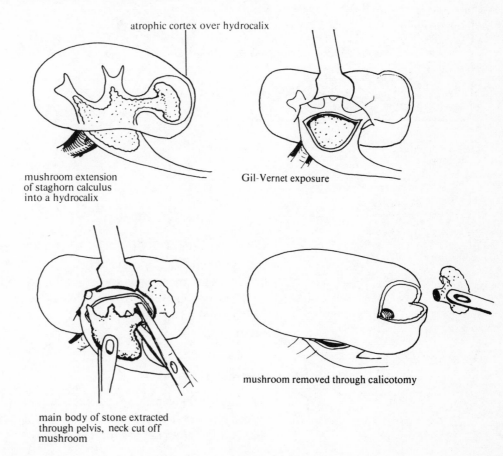

atrophic cortex over hydrocalix

mushroom extension
of staghorn calculus
into a hydrocalix

Gil-Vernet exposure

main body of stone extracted
through pelvis, neck cut off
mushroom

mushroom removed through calicotomy

Chapter 25/*Common Operations*

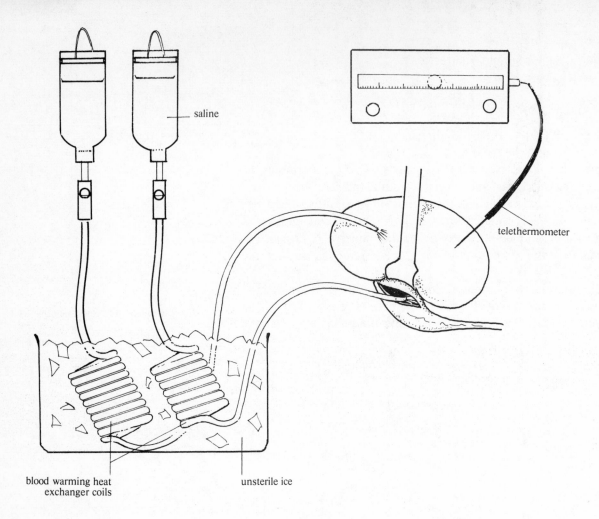

saline

telethermometer

blood warming heat
exchanger coils

unsterile ice

Fig. 25.16. Simple technique for renal
hypothermia

surface to cool it to 20°C(fig. 25.16). The renal parenchyma is incised,
the stone removed, and the parenchyma closed.

6. Xrays are taken *in situ* to make sure all bits of stone are removed.

7. The incision in the pelvis is closed.

8. The wound is closed with a tube drain to the outside of the renal
pelvis.

TUBES AND DRAINS

The kidney may be drained, in addition, with a nephrostomy in cases
where the renal function is especially precarious. Post-operative care
and complications are as for nephrectomy.

Chapter 25/*Common Operations*

Fig. 25.17. Anderson Hynes pyeloplasty.

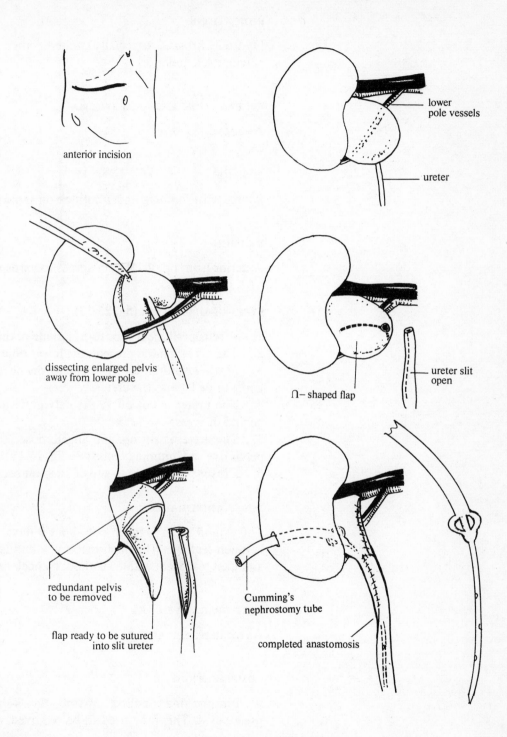

anterior incision

lower pole vessels

ureter

dissecting enlarged pelvis away from lower pole

∩– shaped flap

ureter slit open

redundant pelvis to be removed

flap ready to be sutured into slit ureter

Cumming's nephrostomy tube

completed anastomosis

Pyeloplasty

Hydronephrosis, especially where the obstruction lies at the pelviureteric junction.

PREPARATION AND ANAESTHESIA

As above.

POSITION

Supine with sandbag under buttock on same side.

INCISION

Anterior from tip of 12th rib across towards umbilicus.

STEPS OF OPERATION (fig. 25.17)

1.   A retroperitoneal exposure is made of the renal pelvis.
2.   The ureter and, if present, the lower pole vessel, are taped.
3.   Marker sutures are inserted to define the U-shaped flap which is going to be let into the ureter.
4.   The ureter is cut off at the pelviureteric junction and led out from behind the vessel.
5.   The ureter is slit up, and anastomosed to the U-shaped flap of renal pelvis over a Cummings tube (see fig. 25.17).
6.   Closure with drain to site of anastomosis.

TUBES AND DRAINS

The wound drain is taken out about 4 days, or even more delay if there is much leakage. The nephrostomy splinting tube is left in for 10 days, and then removed, with or without a check nephrostogram before.

POST-OPERATIVE CARE

As for nephrectomy

COMPLICATIONS

A urinoma may collect around the kidney and form a calcified pseudocyst. This may need to be removed, and should be prevented by adequate drainage. Clots may go down the ureter and obstruct it. Delayed complications include stone formation and the development of a similar hydronephrosis on the other side.

Nephrostomy

INDICATIONS

Nephrostomy may be needed as a temporary measure to allow the patient to get over some temporary injury or obstruction to the ureter, or as a means of permanent diversion when nothing else will do.

PREPARATION

It may be necessary to give a resonium enema in the anuric patient to bring down the serum potassium: or even to dialyse the patient to make him fit for an operation.

ANAESTHESIA

One may occasionally have to do this under local infiltration anaesthesia: but it is not a minor operation, and one ought always to try to obtain the assistance of an experienced anaesthetist.

POSITION

Lateral, as for nephrectomy.

INCISION

A short incision forward from the tip of the 12th rib.

STEPS (fig. 25.18)

1. The peritoneum is reflected forwards, and the distended kidney gently pulled backwards until the renal pelvis is reached.
2. The renal pelvis is opened between stay sutures.
3. A forceps is passed retrogradely through the thinned out renal parenchyma: it seizes a nephrostomy tube and draws the tube through the parenchyma into the renal pelvis.
4. In cases where permanent drainage is likely to be needed, a ring-nephrostomy ('Tresidder's method) is used: a long tube with a side hole cut in it half way along is brought in and out of the kidney (see fig.) This

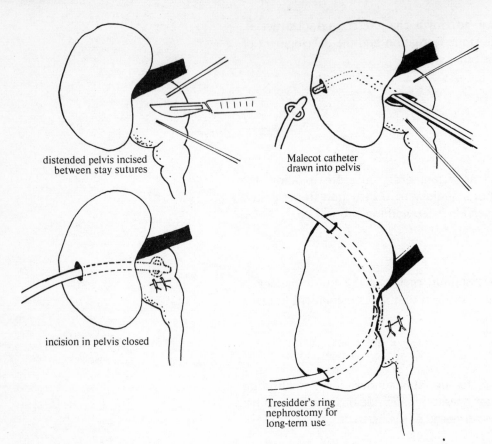

distended pelvis incised
between stay sutures

Malecot catheter
drawn into pelvis

incision in pelvis closed

Tresidder's ring
nephrostomy for
long-term use

Fig. 25.18. Nephrostomy.

allows easy replacement of the old tube, by simply stitching the new one to its end.

POST-OPERATIVE CARE

Beware the diuresis which sometimes follows relief of obstruction.

COMPLICATIONS

Secondary haemorrhage may occur around the tube from vessels in the renal parenchyma especially when the tube is being removed. If the tube is not changed sufficiently often encrustation and stone formation will occur. Urinary infection is inevitable.

Transplantation

INDICATIONS AND PREPARATION

These are a matter of great importance and are carried out in collaboration with the physician in charge of the patient.

Chapter 25/*Common Operations*

ANAESTHESIA

An anaesthetist with special experience is necessary.

POSITION

The patient is supine.

INCISION

A curved muscle-cutting incision is made in the right or left iliac fossa.

STEPS OF THE OPERATION (fig. 25.19)

1.   The peritoneum is displaced back from the vessels in the iliac fossa. The common iliac artery and its bifurcation are defined.
2.   The internal iliac artery is ligated and cut near its branches, its proximal end being occluded with a bulldog clamp. Its lumen is irrigated with heparinized saline.
3.   The external iliac vein is dissected clear of its adventitia, taking care to ligate any small tributaries which may be encountered. The vein is doubly occluded and a window is cut in it.
4.   The donor kidney is brought from the ice: the renal artery is sutured with everting running continuous arterial sutures to the internal iliac artery.
5.   The vein is sutured similarly.
6.   The patient is given the calculated dose of hydrocortisone and azathioprine intravenously.
7.   The renal vein clamps are removed: then the arterial: and any small points of bleeding attended to with a recovery suture or two.
8.   The ureter is anastomosed using a short submucosal tunnel into the bladder over a Gibbon catheter which is secured to the skin with a stitch.
9.   The wound is closed with a sterile closed-system drain.

POST-OPERATIVE CARE AND COMPLICATIONS

These are too specialized to be detailed here, but some of the more important ones may be noted:
1.   Anuria from renal failure in the donor kidney consequent upon antemortem ischaemia in the dying patient.
2.   Rejection.
3.   Obstruction to the ureter.
4.   Renal artery thrombosis or haemorrhage.
5.   Burst kidney—a manifestation of oedema and rejection.

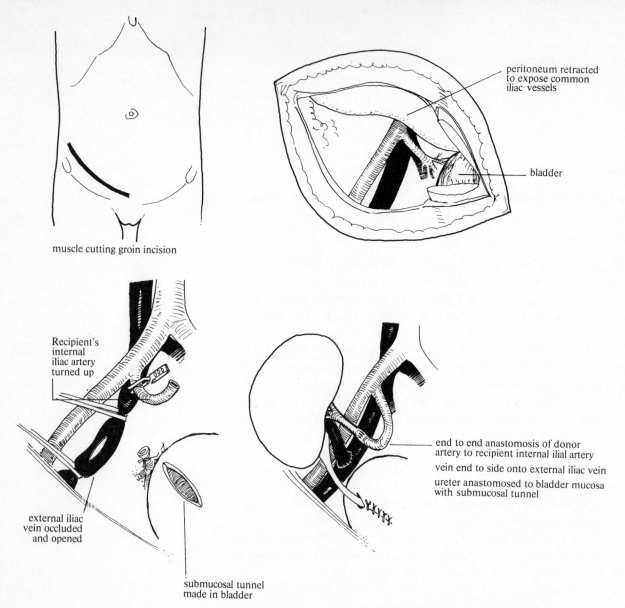

muscle cutting groin incision

peritoneum retracted
to expose common
iliac vessels

bladder

Recipient's
internal
iliac artery
turned up

external iliac
vein occluded
and opened

submucosal tunnel
made in bladder

end to end anastomosis of donor
artery to recipient internal ilial artery

vein end to side onto external iliac vein

ureter anastomosed to bladder mucosa
with submucosal tunnel

Fig. 25.19. Renal transplantation.

6. Urinoma—from leakage of urine around the kidney.
7. Leak from rejection damage to the ureter, or ischaemic necrosis of
its end.

Removal of a donor kidney from a cadaver

INDICATIONS

The kidneys from any patient who has not got hypertension, cancer, or
widespread infection, are suitable.

Chapter 25/*Common Operations*

Permission must be obtained from the next of kin of the dying patient: it helps if the patient has signed a card to indicate his willingness to be a kidney donor, but in law one must ask the next of kin. If the next of kin cannot be found, then one must obtain the permission of the hospital administrator or secretary who is the legal possessor of the body. It is wise also to check with the police in accident cases to make sure that no murder charge lies in connection with the cadaver, otherwise the lawyers may claim that death was caused by removal of the kidneys or that vital forensic evidence was disturbed.

Removal of the donor kidneys is difficult and delicate and needs complete aseptic precautions, and should be done in an operating theatre. The skin is prepared and the wound draped.

INCISION (fig. 25.20)

A long midline or transverse incision may be used according to the build of the patient. The colon is retracted medially to expose the renal vessels. A cuff of aorta and cava is taken on each side, or the entire segment of aorta and cava removed *en bloc*. The kidneys are immediately flushed through with ice-cold sterile rheomacrodex or Collins solution, and then attached to a suitable perfusion machine if one is available.

The wound is closed with a running suture and a dressing applied.

OPERATIONS ON THE URETER

Removal of a stone in the ureter

INDICATIONS

If the stone is stuck, too large to go down, or the urine is infected.

PREPARATION

A plain Xray is taken *en route* to the theatre.

POSITION

1. A stone in the upper third of the ureter is approached as for a kidney, in the lateral position, through a short 12th rib tip incision.
2. In the middle third (the easy part) of the ureter it is approached

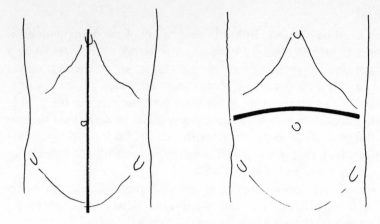

use a vertical or transverse incision

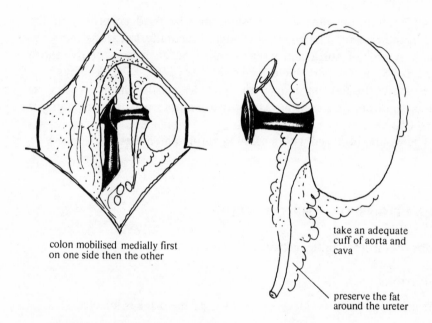

colon mobilised medially first
on one side then the other

take an adequate
cuff of aorta and
cava

preserve the fat
around the ureter

Fig. 25.20. Cadaver donor nephrectomy.

through a transverse abdominal incision sited over the stone, with the patient in the half-lateral position.

3. In the lower third of the ureter the Pfannenstiel incision is used.

STEPS OF THE OPERATION

1. *Upper and middle third* (fig. 25.21)

The ureter is approached extraperitoneally, and the stone felt with the

Chapter 25/*Common Operations*

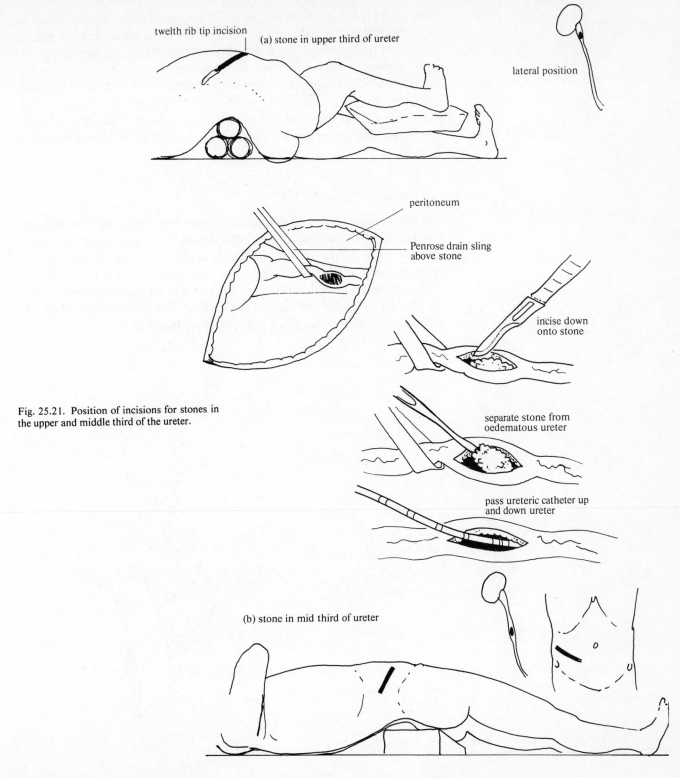

twelth rib tip incision

(a) stone in upper third of ureter

lateral position

peritoneum

Penrose drain sling above stone

incise down onto stone

separate stone from oedematous ureter

pass ureteric catheter up and down ureter

Fig. 25.21. Position of incisions for stones in the upper and middle third of the ureter.

(b) stone in mid third of ureter

finger tip as it lies in the ureter which is displaced forwards and tends to stay attached to the back of the peritoneum. A penrose drain is placed around the ureter, above the stone, to stop it from slipping upwards.

The stone is then cut down upon directly, the knife grating on the calculus, which is then eased out of the ureter with a Watson–Cheyne dissector. A catheter is slipped up and down the ureter to make sure that it is clear. The wound is closed with a drain down to the incision in the ureter, but the ureter itself is not sutured for fear of giving rise to a stricture.

2. *Lower third* (fig. 25.22)

The operation is identical, except that to find the ureter one first finds the bifurcation of the common iliac artery, and then feels down the ureter until the stone is located. In low stones it is essential to cut the superior vesical vessels to allow the ureter to be mobilized. If this is done, the rest of the operation is as described above. There is seldom any need to open the bladder provided the vessels are divided. The wounds are all closed with catgut with a drain down to the opening in the ureter.

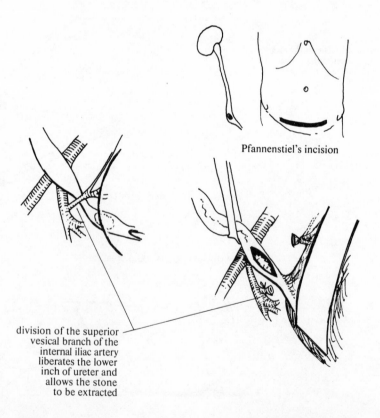

Pfannenstiel's incision

division of the superior vesical branch of the internal iliac artery liberates the lower inch of ureter and allows the stone to be extracted

Fig. 25.22. Pfannenstiel's approach for removal of stone in lower third of ureter.

Chapter 25/*Common Operations*

The drain is left in for 4 days, then inched out a little more each day. This is one exception to the rule that 'a drain is left in until it stops draining'.

COMPLICATIONS

A collection of urine may form around the ureter if the drain is removed too quickly. Ileus is not uncommon. Sometimes the drain site goes on leaking urine for a long time. If the fistula persists for more than two weeks further radiographs should be taken to make sure that a small piece of stone has not been left in the ureter. Sometimes the fistula will only stop if one passes a catheter up past it and leaves it in for a few days.

Reflux-preventing operations

There are many different reflux-preventing procedures. The most usual one is the technique described by Leadbetter and Politano.

INDICATIONS

Intractable reflux in children with intractable infection.

PREPARATION

Blood is grouped and serum saved. The appropriate antibiotic cover may be given.

ANAESTHETIC

General.

INCISION

Pfannenstiel.

STEPS OF THE POLITANO–LEADBETTER OPERATION (fig. 25.23)

1. The bladder is opened between stay sutures.
2. The ureteric orifice is circumcized.
3. The ureter is drawn into the bladder, dividing the tissues which attach the ureter to the muscle of the bladder wall.
4. A new hole is made through the wall of the bladder.
5. A tunnel is made under the bladder mucosa.

6. The ureter is led through the new hole and down the submucosal tunnel to be re-attached to its old position, or even advanced some way towards the bladder neck.

7. The ureter may be splinted: a catheter is certainly passed up it to make sure there is no kink outside the wall of the bladder.

8. The bladder is closed over a Malecot catheter.

TUBES AND DRAINS

If a ureteric splint has been used it is removed after 5 or 6 days. The suprapubic catheter is removed after 8 days.

COMPLICATIONS

Stenosis of the ureter occurs in 2 to 3% of cases, and may be due to

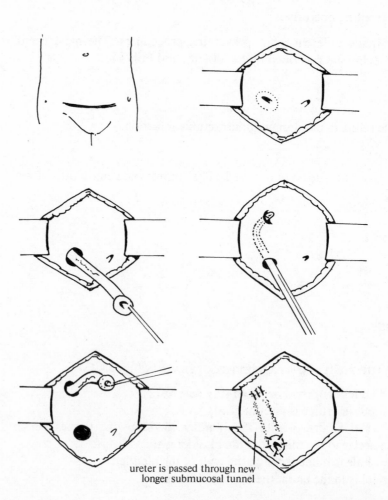

Fig. 25.23. The Politano-Leadbetter operation.

ureter is passed through new longer submucosal tunnel

Chapter 25/*Common Operations*

kinking outside the bladder. The operation occasionally fails to stop reflux. There may be ischaemic necrosis of the lower end of the ureter if it has been trimmed too severely.

These are legion: if the ureter is very dilated, it may be necessary to make it narrower: this is done over an indwelling catheter, and a long strip is cut out off the ureter, taking care to preserve its blood supply.

The Boari flap operation (fig. 25.24)

INDICATIONS

In cases where the ureter has to be joined again to the bladder, but there is an unbridgeable gap: e.g. after accidental surgical injury to the lower end of the ureter, or radiation damage.

PREPARATION

ANAESTHESIA   } as for a stone in the lower third of the ureter.

INCISION

Fig. 25.24. The Boari flap operation.

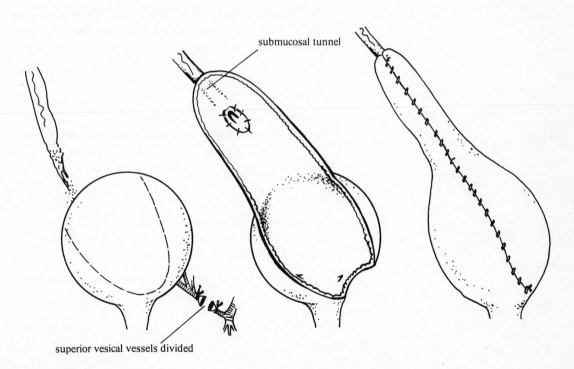

submucosal tunnel

superior vesical vessels divided

1.   The bladder is dissected off its peritoneal reflection.
2.   The superior vesical vessels on the side opposite to the ureter to be implanted are cut between ligatures.
3.   The injured ureter is dissected free and its end trimmed and spatulated.
4.   Marker sutures are placed in the bladder wall to mark out the U-shaped flap.
5.   The flap is then cut, little by little, taking care to secure haemostasis by underrunning the arteries in the wall of the bladder whenever they are cut across.
6.   A short tunnel is made in the upper end of the Boari flap.
7.   The ureter is led through the tunnel over a suitable splinting Gibbon catheter.
8.   The flap is closed with catgut to form a complete tube.

TUBES AND DRAINS

The wound is drained: a splinting Gibbon catheter is secured to the skin: a Malecot is left in the bladder.

POST OPERATIVE CARE

The bladder catheter is left until last. The wound drain is removed at 48 hours: the splinting Gibbon catheter at 10 days, and the bladder catheter on the 12th day.

COMPLICATIONS

The ureter or the Boari flap may slough, leading to a leak and a wound fistula. Otherwise the complications are those of any bladder operation.

Nephroureterectomy (fig. 25.25)

INDICATIONS

Cancer of the renal pelvis or ureter: some cases of tuberculosis.

PREPARATION

1 litre of blood.

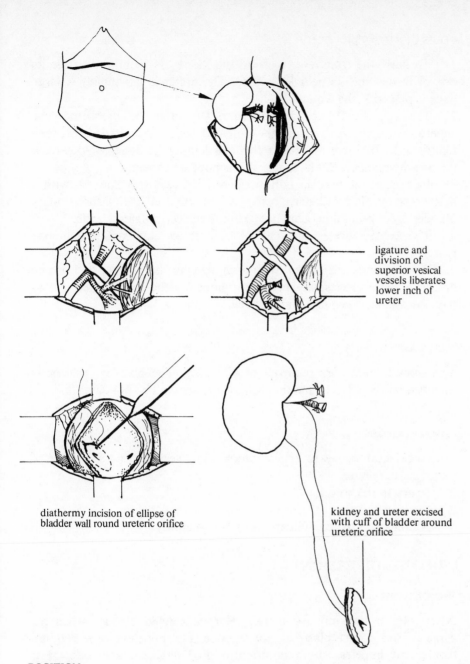

ligature and
division of
superior vesical
vessels liberates
lower inch of
ureter

diathermy incision of ellipse of
bladder wall round ureteric orifice

kidney and ureter excised
with cuff of bladder around
ureteric orifice

Fig. 25.25. Nephroureterectomy.

POSITION

Supine with a sandbag under the affected side under the buttock.

INCISIONS

1 Transverse upper abdominal incision as for the anterior transabdominal nephrectomy.
2 Pfannenstiel.

1.   Through the transverse incision the kidney is mobilized inside its box of fascia and its pedicle divided. The ureter is left intact. A large pack is placed in the wound.

2.   Through the Pfannenstiel incision the ureter is mobilized: the superior vesical vessels on the affected side are divided between ligatures. In tuberculosis, the ureter can simply be dissected out from outside the bladder. But in cancer this is not safe enough.

3.   In cancer, the bladder is now opened between stay sutures: with a diathermy needle the ureteric orifice and a small ellipse of surrounding bladder is cut out, taking care not to injure the contralateral ureter.

4.   The kidney, ureter, and cuff of bladder are now removed in one piece.

5.   Both wounds are closed, with a catheter in the bladder and a tube drain to the extravesical space, but none to the kidney bed unless haemostasis has been less than perfect.

TUBES AND DRAINS

The wound drains are removed at 48 hours. The bladder catheter is removed on the 8th day and the wound stitches on the 10th day.

COMPLICATIONS

1.   Accidental injury to the common iliac vessels, in the course of removing the ureter.

2.   Injury to the bowel.

3.   Prolonged ileus.

4.   All the expected complications of nephrectomy.

URINARY DIVERSION

INDICATIONS

After total cystectomy for cancer. For contracted bladder when for some reason a cystoplasty is not feasible. For hopeless vesicovaginal fistula and hopeless urethral stricture. For neurogenic bladder. For vesical exstrophy.

CHOICE OF METHODS

1.   Stomas or external urinary fistulae

The choice lies between nephrostomy, ureterostomy, or an intestinal conduit. Nephrostomy needs an indwelling tube which always becomes infected and usually forms stones, and is the least good of all methods. Ureterostomy tends to stenose down, and is difficult to fit with a collecting device. The advantages of intestinal conduits depend more than anything upon the excellent appliances which can be attached to an ileal or colonic stoma.

Ileal conduit (fig. 25.26)

This is the most usual method.

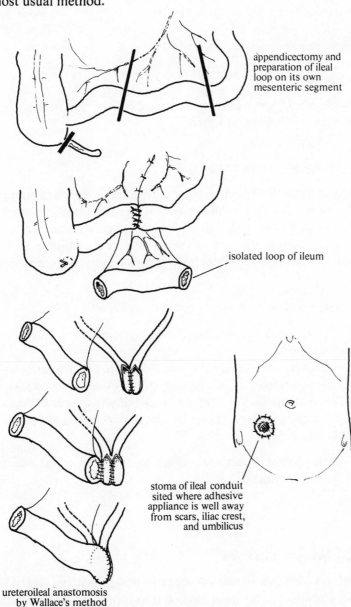

appendicectomy and preparation of ileal loop on its own mesenteric segment

isolated loop of ileum

ureteroileal anastomosis by Wallace's method

stoma of ileal conduit sited where adhesive appliance is well away from scars, iliac crest, and umbilicus

Fig. 25.26. An ileal conduit.

A good bowel mechanical clearance is to be preferred to preoperative attempts to sterilise the bowel.

ANAESTHESIA

General

POSITION

Supine

INCISION

Paramedian, or transverse—according to the reason for which the diversion is being performed.

STEPS OF THE OPERATION

The ureters are dissected, freed up, and their ends anastomosed together. An isolated loop of small bowel is prepared, and intestinal continuity established by end to end anastomosis. The ureters are then anastomosed to one end of the bowel and the other is brought out onto the skin through a circular hole. It is usual to splint the ureters.

COMPLICATIONS

1. Ileus is prolonged, and accompanied by a degree of intestinal obstruction.
2. Urinary peritonitis may follow leakage of the anastomosis.
3. Wound infection is common, from bowel contamination.
4. Burst abdomen is common, especially in cancer patients.
5. Intestinal obstruction by band or volvulus may require re-exploration.

One should remember that some major complication occurs in at least 30% of these cases.

2. Urinary reservoirs

Several attempts have been made to design urinary reservoirs, but none is satisfactory. The usual method is to form a ureterosigmoidostomy.

Ureterosigmoidostomy (fig. 25.27)

INDICATIONS

Continent rectal sphincter for urine, and no previous irradiation.

PREPARATION

Mechanical cleansing by enemas of the bowel.

ANAESTHESIA

General

Fig. 25.27. Ureterosigmoidostomy.

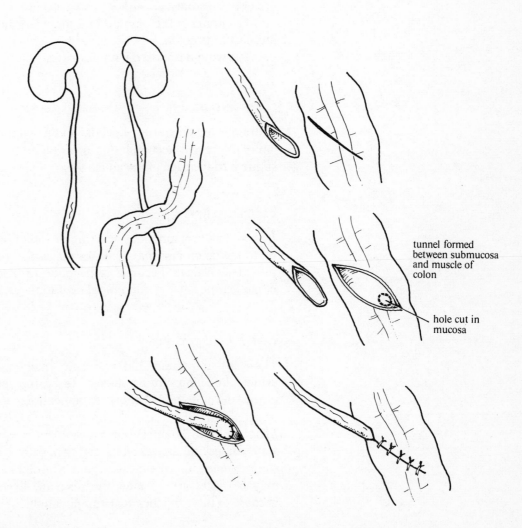

tunnel formed
between submucosa
and muscle of
colon

hole cut in
mucosa

Supine

According to the underlying pathology

1. The ureters are freed up and brought to the edge of the sigmoid.
2. A short oblique tunnel is cut in the muscle of the sigmoid down to but not through the mucosa which pouts out.
3. A small hole is cut in the mucosa, to which the spatulated end of the ureter is anastomosed without using a splint.
4. The ureter is then buried in a tunnel formed by the edges of the cut muscle of the colon.
5. The wound is closed with drainage.

A drain is led down to the pelvis: and a rectal tube left in for the first 48 hours to prevent accumulation of urine in the rectum. It is advisable to suture it to the edge of the anus.

If there has been previous scarring or radiation the ureters will not heal on to the colon and may leak. Leakage also occurs if the lower ends of the ureters have become ischaemic. In addition there are all the complications of any abdominal operation—e.g. ileus and obstruction.

These are important and common: many patients develop recurrent urinary infections from reflux of faeces up the ureters to the kidneys: others develop biochemical complications from the reabsorption of urine from the colon causing *hyperchloraemic acidosis*, and *hypokalaemia*. To offset this each patient is encouraged to drink a lot of water, empty the bowel often, and take extra bicarbonate and potassium supplements. In patients in whom a prolonged survival is expected it may be necessary to alter the form of diversion to an ileal conduit because of these biochemical complications.

OPERATIONS ON THE BLADDER

Simple cystostomy

INDICATIONS

To remove a stone too large to be dealt with by litholapaxy.
To deal with a bladder tumour, diverticulum, or foreign body.

PREPARATION

Urine culture. Blood group and keep serum.

ANAESTHESIA

Profound general anaesthesia

POSITION

Supine

INCISION

Pfannenstiel or vertical lower abdominal midline or paramedian.

STEPS OF OPERATION (fig. 25.28)

1. Having made the Pfannenstiel approach to the bladder, the peritoneum is reflected upwards.
2. Two stay sutures are placed in the muscle of the bladder, and it is opened between them. The urine is aspirated.
3. Whatever has to be done inside the bladder is done, and
4. The bladder is closed in two layers (this is not of critical importance and one layer will do if the bladder is thin and atrophic).
5. The bladder is drained with either a suprapubic catheter or an indwelling self-retaining Foley catheter.
6. The wound is closed with a small extravesical drain.

TUBES AND DRAINS

The wound drain is removed in 48 hours. The bladder catheter is removed on the 8th day. Wound sutures on the 10th day.

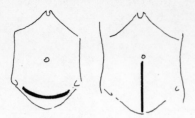

the incision may be Pfannenstiel's or a vertical midline or paramedian one

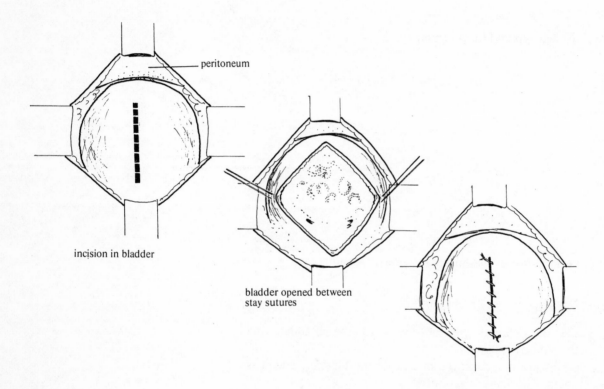

peritoneum

incision in bladder

bladder opened between stay sutures

Fig. 25.28. Surgical steps of suprapubic cystostomy.

COMPLICATIONS

Clot retention: if the disorder inside the bladder should bleed the bladder will fill up with blood clot: this can be evacuated with an Ellik evacuator and the resectoscope sheath. It is seldom necessary to re-open the wound.

Persistent fistula: if this occurs, then there must be outflow obstruction. Try to get the fistula closed by replacing the urethral catheter, and wait until the fistula has been dry for 48 hours before removing the catheter.

Chapter 25/*Common Operations*

Partial cystectomy

INDICATIONS

Rare isolated bladder tumours on the vault.

PREPARATION

Blood and urine culture.

ANAESTHESIA

Position and incision as for simple cystostomy.

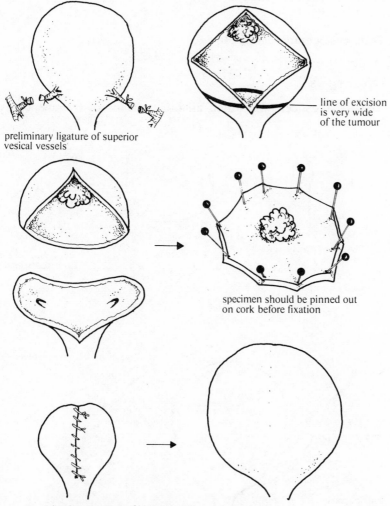

preliminary ligature of superior vesical vessels

line of excision is very wide of the tumour

specimen should be pinned out on cork before fixation

the tiny remnant of bladder will hypertrophy to the former normal size within 2-3 months

Fig. 25.29. Partial cystectomy for tumour.

1. After making the Pfannenstiel incision, the bladder is dissected from the peritoneal covering.
2. Suitable stay sutures are inserted well clear of the tumour to be removed. The bladder is opened.
3. The tumour is removed with a very wide margin, taking care not to trespass upon the ureteric orifices.
4. The bladder is closed with two layers of catgut, over an indwelling catheter.

POST-OPERATIVE CARE AND COMPLICATIONS

As for simple cystostomy.

Total cystectomy (fig. 25.30)

INDICATIONS

Recidivist cancers for which all other means of treatment have been

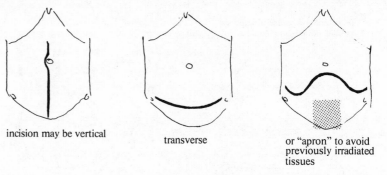

incision may be vertical   transverse   or "apron" to avoid previously irradiated tissues

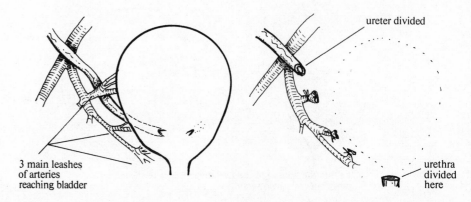

3 main leashes of arteries reaching bladder

ureter divided

urethra divided here

Fig. 25.30. Total cystectomy.

tried: multiple 'papillomatosis' which cannot be dealt with by closed diathermy, distension, or intracavitary chemotherapy.

PREPARATION

1. The bowel must be mechanically cleansed by enemas.
2. The patient must be psychologically prepared and understand what is demanded of the method of diversion which is chosen.
3. At least 2 litres of cross-matched blood must be available.

ANAESTHESIA

Skilled profound general anaesthesia, preferably with controlled hypotension.

INCISION

Vertical or transverse lower abdominal incisions are used.

STEPS OF THE OPERATION

1. The peritoneum is opened and explored to determine whether there are distant metastases, and whether the bladder is operable or not.
2. The superior vesical vessels are cut between ligatures on one side, allowing the bladder to be pulled over and upwards, giving access to the second leash of vessels coming off the internal ilac artery and vein, and in some patients, to the third and deepest group.
3. This is repeated on the opposite side.
4. Both ureters are divided.
5. The urethra is divided below the prostate and turned up.
6. The bladder is now removed, leaving the rectum.
7. After stopping the bleeding, especially from under the pubic arch from the penile veins, the ureters are sutured to the method of diversion selected for the patient—usually (nowadays) an ileal conduit.
8. The wound is closed with precautions against dehiscence.

COMPLICATIONS

Prolonged ileus demands intensive fluid and electrolyte replacement therapy. Wound infection and burst abdomen are common. Pulmonary complications occur because of pain and difficulty in coughing. Total cystectomy carries a 10 to 20% operative mortality and a 50% major complication rate. To all the hazards of a major pelvic operation are added those of the urinary diversion.

ADDITIONAL PROCEDURES

It is often necessary to remove in addition to the bladder the uterus and tubes, the urethra, and sometimes the rectum.

OPERATIONS ON THE PROSTATE

Three methods are in common use today. Transurethral resection, retropubic, and transvesical prostatectomy.

Transurethral resection

INDICATIONS

A benign or malignant gland causing obstructive symptoms and signs, under—say—80 gm in size (a figure which depends upon the skill and experience of the surgeon).

PREPARATIONS

Two pints of blood. Urine microbiology.

ANAESTHESIA

General, preferably with moderate controlled hypotension.

POSITION ON TABLE

The cystoscopy position, with the legs not too drawn up.

STEPS OF THE OPERATION (fig. 25.31)

All the adenoma is removed from inside the prostatic surgical capsule.

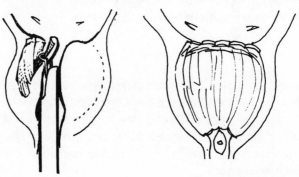

Fig. 25.31. Transurethral resection.

Chapter 25/*Common Operations*

Bleeding is stopped. Chips are evacuated, and the bladder is left with an indwelling irrigating catheter.

ADVANTAGES

Safe and relatively painless for the patient, probably lower mortality rate in high risk patients with cardiovascular and cerebrovascular disease.

DISADVANTAGES

Difficult to do, hard to learn and teach. Very difficult in glands of more than 50 to 60 gms in size, but majority of glands are under 30 gms and TUR is suitable for more than 90% of prostates.

COMPLICATIONS

As for all methods of prostatectomy see below.

Millin or retropubic prostatectomy (fig. 25.32)

INDICATIONS

As above. Any size of gland can be dealt with by this operation, which has the great advantage that it is easy to do and needs no special equipment.

PREPARATION AND ANAESTHESIA

As above.

INCISION

After preliminary cystoscopy a Pfannenstiel incision is made.

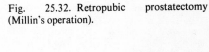

Fig. 25.32. Retropubic prostatectomy (Millin's operation).

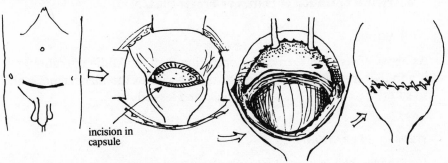

incision in capsule

1. The prostatic capsule is incised transversely near the junction with the bladder.
2. The two 'lateral lobes' are shelled out with scissors and finger tip.
3. The 'middle lobe' and bladder neck fibres are removed with diathermy needle or scissors.
4. Bleeding is stopped by suture ligature of the main vesssels in the corner of the capsular incision—this is the important step which makes the operation so safe and reliable.
5. The capsule is closed over an indwelling catheter.

ADVANTAGES

Easy operation. The larger the gland the easier it is because the plane of cleavage between the adenoma and the surgical capsule gets easier to define.

DISADVANTAGES

High risk of pulmonary embolism. Higher mortality in high-risk patients. Occupies hospital beds for twice as long as TUR.

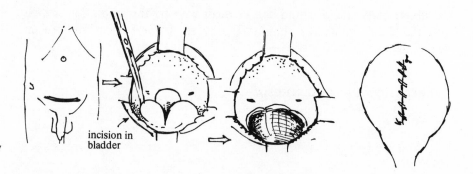

incision in
bladder

Fig.   25.33. Transvesical   prostatectomy (Harris or Freyer operation).

Transvesical operation of Harris or Freyer (fig. 25.33)

INDICATIONS

As above. This is an even easier operation than the Millin operation, but it affords very indifferent access to the arteries at the bladder neck and so suture ligature becomes less precise and less effective.

STEPS OF OPERATION

1. The bladder is opened (see simple cystostomy).

2. A pair of scissors or finger is forced into the plane of cleavage between the adenoma and the capsule at the bladder neck, and the adenomatous 'lobes' are torn out of the capsule.

3. An attempt is made to stop the bleeding.

4. The bladder is closed over a catheter.

ADVANTAGES

Easy operation and allows surgeon to deal with other trouble in the bladder such as a cancer, a diverticulum or a stone.

DISADVANTAGES

Poor control of haemorrhage. Prolonged need for post-operative catheterization. A poor operation, and one not favoured by urologists.

COMPLICATIONS

Inadvertent damage to the sphincter is common and bleeding complications seen frequently.

The complications of prostatectomy

1. Bleeding: there is more bleeding as the adenomas get bigger.
Loss of blood is unpredictable so one should always have 2 units of blood available.

2. Infection—in wound or urine, may be followed by bacteraemia.

3. Pulmonary embolism and deep vein thrombosis is common after the Millin and transvesical operation, rare after TUR.

4. Impotence occurs sometimes after all methods, but more often after open ones.

5. Infertility. After all methods ejaculation tends to push the semen back into the bladder where the bladder neck no longer closes in coordination with the emptying of the vasa and vesicles. This is by no means inevitable or complete, and cannot be taken as a reliable contraceptive.

6. Osteitis pubis—one can get an infarct of the cartilage of the symphysis pubis, which gets secondarily infected, after any of the open methods.

7. Urethral stricture occurs in 2 to 3% of all methods, but is slightly more apt to occur after transurethral surgery.

8. Incontinence occurs as a rule when the external sphincter has been injured.

9. Recurrence of adenoma—may occur after any technique whereby healthy acini have been left behind in the 'capsule'.

10. Carcinoma may also occur in the peripheral tissue left behind.

OPERATIONS ON THE URETHRA

The method of dilating urethral strictures was referred to on page 270 where the technique of internal urethrotomy was also mentioned.

Modern techniques of urethroplasty are still in a developmental stage and it is not possible yet to be didactic about their indications and complications, nor should the medical student trouble to learn about them. However, they are being performed more and more often, and their principles may be of interest.

Meatal and anterior strictures

These respond very well to meatoplasty (fig. 25.34).

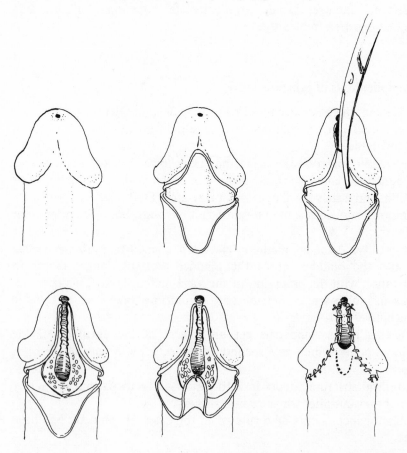

Fig. 25.34. Meatoplasty.

Penile strictures

Formerly these were dealt with in a two-stage method (fig. 25.35). More recently an isolated island skin patch can be let into the strictured urethra, which, because it has its own blood supply on a pedicle of dartos, survives like a pedicled patch of skin anywhere else in the body in spite of infection.

Posterior strictures (fig. 25.36)

One can form a long pedicle ∩-shaped flap of skin from the loose skin of the scrotum. This can be used to make a two-stage urethroplasty: or by modifying the flap to give a dartos pedicled patch, one can make a one-stage patch urethroplasty for high urethral strictures (fig. 25.37).

Fig. 25.35. Methods of dealing with penile strictures.

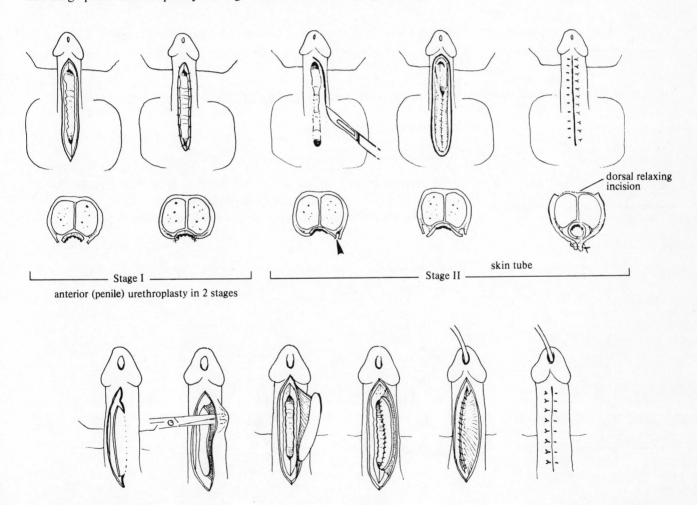

dorsal relaxing incision

skin tube

Stage I ——— Stage II

anterior (penile) urethroplasty in 2 stages

anterior (penile) urethroplasty in 1 stage (method of Leadbetter and Orandi)

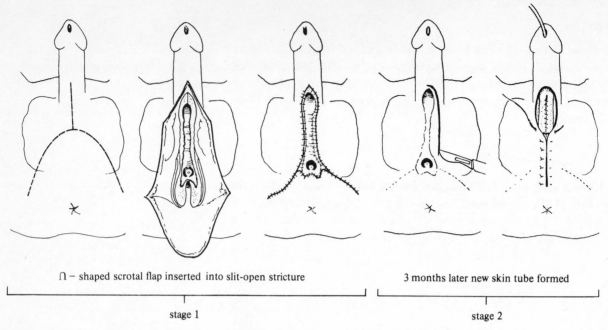

∩ – shaped scrotal flap inserted into slit-open stricture   3 months later new skin tube formed

stage 1   stage 2

Fig. 25.36. Method of dealing with posterior strictures—two stage scrotal flap urethroplasty for stricture of the posterior urethra.

Fig. 25.37. One stage island patch urethroplasty for posterior strictures, a modification of the standard two-stage ∩-shaped flap method.

OPERATIONS ON THE TESTICLE

Orchidopexy (fig. 25.38)

INDICATIONS

All ectopic testes: all those on the normal course of descent which cannot be gently got into the bottom of the scrotum.
The operation should preferably be done before the age of 6.

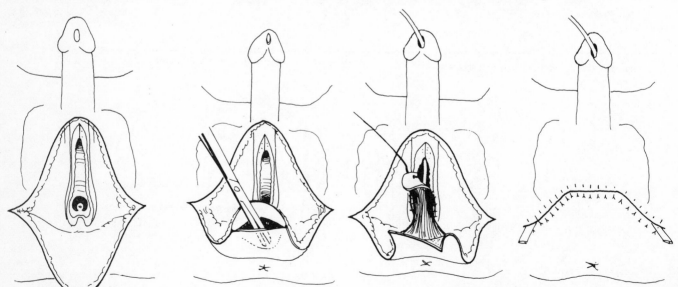

Chapter 25/*Common Operations*

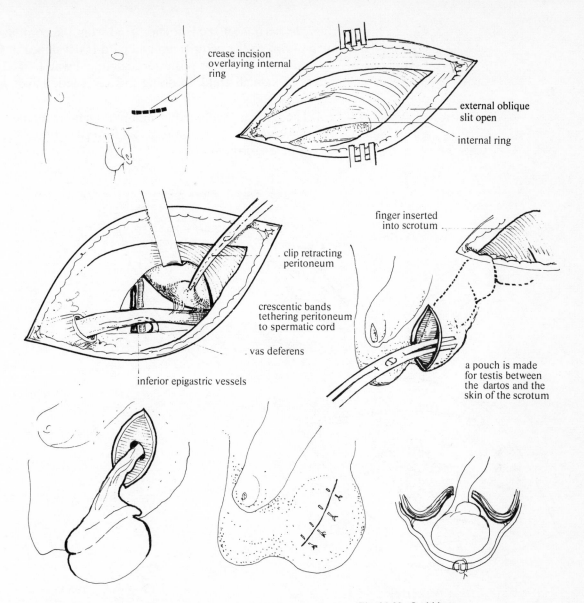

crease incision
overlaying internal
ring

external oblique
slit open

internal ring

clip retracting
peritoneum

crescentic bands
tethering peritoneum
to spermatic cord

vas deferens

inferior epigastric vessels

finger inserted
into scrotum

a pouch is made
for testis between
the dartos and the
skin of the scrotum

Fig. 25.38. Orchidopexy.

PREPARATIONS

The skin, when hairy, should be shaved.

INCISION

An incision in the line of the skin crease gives excellent access and good
cosmetic results.

STEPS OF THE OPERATION

1.   The external oblique is opened along the line of its fibres.

Chapter 25/*Common Operations*

2. The peritoneal sac is found, freed from the cord, and lifted up. The plane between the peritoneum and cord is developed until the finger can be thrust as high as the posterior abdominal wall to the level of the renal artery in a small child. In doing this crescentic bands of adhesions are divided.

3. The testis is then freed from any remaining attachments around the external ring, and placed into a sac formed between the dermis and the dartos in the scrotum.

Fig. 25.39. Orchidectomy.

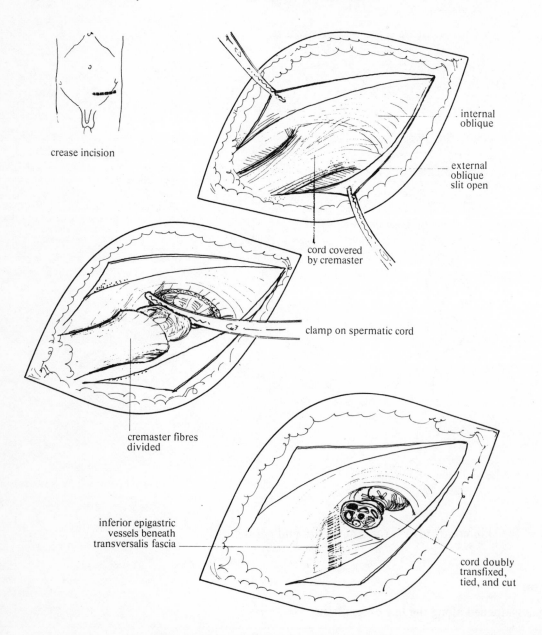

crease incision

internal oblique

external oblique slit open

cord covered by cremaster

clamp on spermatic cord

cremaster fibres divided

inferior epigastric vessels beneath transversalis fascia

cord doubly transfixed, tied, and cut

Chapter 25/*Common Operations*

Orchidectomy (fig. 25.39)

INDICATIONS

Malignant tumour of the testicle. Other hopelessly damaged benign conditions (infected hydroceles, tuberculosis etc.).

STEPS

1. The external oblique is incised in the line of its fibres.
2. The cord is doubly transfixed and ligated at the level of the internal inguinal ring.
3. The testicle is removed and the wound closed. No drain is needed but haemostasis must be scrupulous.

Biopsy of the testis (fig. 25.40)

Through a scrotal incision the tunica vaginalis is nicked with a sharp pointed knife, until a few tubules protrude. They are snipped off and put into Bouin's fixative. One 4-0 catgut suture closes the hole.

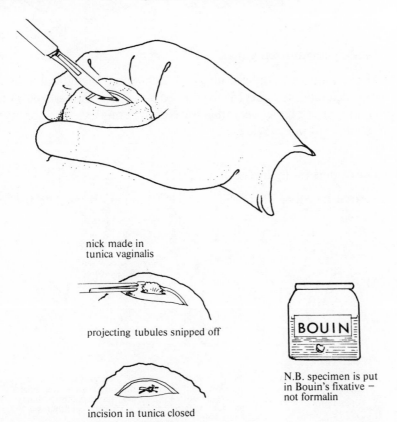

nick made in
tunica vaginalis

projecting tubules snipped off

incision in tunica closed

N.B. specimen is put in Bouin's fixative – not formalin

Fig. 25.40. Testicular biopsy.

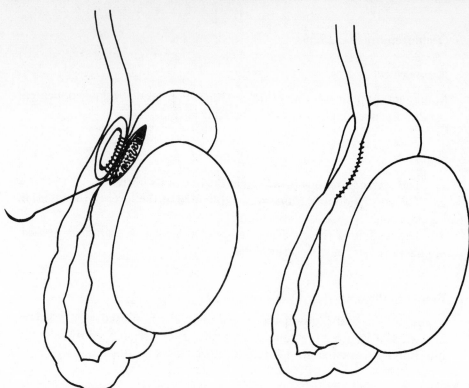

Fig. 25.41. Epididymovasostomy: a side-to-side anastomosis is made between the vas deferens and the connective tissue covering of the epididymis. A magnifying loupe is useful, and many surgeons use a fine nylon or polyethylene splint.

Epididymovasostomy (fig. 25.41)

Using a fine polyethylene intracath as a splint, the lateral hole cut in the vas deferens is sutured to the edges of a similar incision in the epididymis, taking very fine sutures of stainless steel or nylon. The splint is left in for 5 days.

Operations for hydrocele (fig. 25.42)

Fig. 25.42. Operations for hydrocele.

Scrotal incision. The surplus sac is trimmed off and the frill oversewn

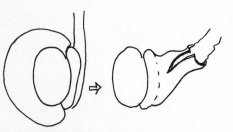

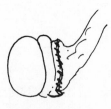

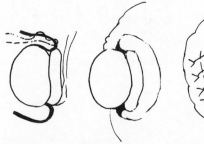

Jaboulay or 'bottle operation'— the sac is everted and sutured to the spermatic cord

excision of surplus sac is often added to the Jaboulay operation

Mr Peter Lord's operation: through a short scrotal incision the fluid is emptied out: then with a series of catgut sutures the surplus tunica is bunched up all round and behind the testis and epididymis — advantage − less haematoma

for haemostasis. alternatively the frill can be bunched up in a series of rucks by 'purse string' sutures placed one after the other (Lord's operation).

COMPLICATIONS

Haematoma is common: if small, leave it alone, if large, evacuate it.

FURTHER READING

BLANDY J.P. (1971) *Transurethral Resection*, p. 18. Pitman Medical, London.
Gow J.G. (1976) Urological Technology. Chap. 1, *Urology*, ed. Blandy J.P. Blackwell Scientific Publications, Oxford.
MITCHELL J.P. & ALDER V.G. (1975) The disinfection of urological endoscopes. *Brit. J. Urol.*, **47**, 571.
MITCHELL J.P. (1976) Endoscopes in use. *Scientific Foundations of Urology*, eds. Williams D.I. and Chisholm G.D., p. 421. Heinemann, London.
MITCHELL J.P. & DOBBIE A.K. (1976) Surgical Diathermy in urological practice. *Scientific Foundations of Urology*, eds. Williams D.I. and Chisholm G.D., p. 440. Heinemann, London.

Glossary of Urological Eponyms and Jargon

Albarran, Joaquin (1860–1912). Cuban urologist working in Paris: described pedunculated 'middle lobe' of prostate: invented the Albarran lever on the catheterizing cystoscope.

ampulla. Latin, a flask.

Anderson–Hynes. Method of pyeloplasty devised by James Christie Anderson, urologist, Royal Hospital Sheffield and Wilfred Hynes, Plastic surgeon, United Sheffield Hospitals. (See: *Hydronephrosis*, Anderson, London, Wm. Heinemann Medical Books. 1963.)

Avicenna (1037). Abu Ali El Hussein Ibn Sina. Iranian physician. Used soft catheters of leather, and of silver. (See Hanafy, M.H. *et al.* (1976) *Urology*, **8**, 63.)

balanitis. Greek, βάλανος, the glans penis, xerotica obliterans (Greek dry; Latin, obliterating).

Behçet, Hulûsi. (1889–1948) Turkish dermatologist. Described a syndrome including ulceration of mouth, genitalia, uveitis, iridocyclitis.

Belfield, W.T. American urologist who probably did the first open prostatectomy intentionally. (See: Belfield, W.T. (1887) *J. Amer. med. Ass.*, **8**, 303).

Bellini, Lorenzo (1643–1704). Anatomist of Pisa. Described, among many other things, the straight collecting tubules of the renal papilla.

Benedict, Stanley Rossiter (1884–1936). Biochemist of Cornell University, USA. Described test for sugar in the urine.

Bertin, Exupère Joseph (1712–81). Associate anatomist at the Academy of Sciences in Paris.

Bigelow, Henry Jacob (1818–90). Surgeon of Boston, USA. (See: Bigelow, H.J. (1879) Lithotrity by a single operation. *Boston Med. Surg. J.* (later *New Eng. J. Med*) **98**, 259 and 291.)

Bilharz, Theodor Maximilian (1825–62). German physician working in Cairo who first described *Schistosoma haematobium;* hence Bilharziasis.

Boari, Achille (1894). Italian urologist who devised bladder flap procedure for bridging gap at lower end of ureter.

bougie. French, candle (wax 'bougies' were often used to dilate urethral strictures).

Bouin, Paul (1870). Histologist of Strasbourg. Described fixative for testicular biopsies containing picric acid, acetic acid and formalin.

Bowman, Sir William (1816–1892). Ophthalmic surgeon of London, described the capsule of the glomerulus and recognized that it was extruded from the end of the renal tubule.

Braasch, W.F. Urologist of the Mayo Clinic, described many urological conditions and invented many instruments, of which the bulb-ended ureteric catheter is best known today.

Bricker, Eugene, M., Professor of Surgery, Washington University School of Medicine, St. Louis. Described ileal conduit. (See: Bricker E.M. (1950) Bladder substitution after pelvic evisceration *Surg. Clin. N. Amer.*, **30**, 1511.)

Bright, Richard. (1789–1859) Guy's Hospital Physician.

Browne, Sir Denis (1892–1967). Paediatric surgeon at Great Ormond Street Hospital for Children. Invented operation for hypospadias. (See: *Post. Grad. med. J.* (1949), **25**, 367.)

Brown–Buerger. One of the best cystoscopes was devised by Tilden Brown and Leo Buerger. (See: A new combination observation catheterizing and operating cystoscope. *New York Med. J.*, Aug. 25, 1917.)

von Brunn A. (1841–1895). Professor of Anatomy, Göttingen. Described cell nests in chronic cystitis. (See *Arch. Mikr. Anat.* (1893) **41**, 294.)

Buck, Gordon (1807–77). New York surgeon who described the deep fascia of the corpora cavernosa of the penis.

calix. Greek κύλιξ, cup, 'confused by modern scientific writers with Graeco-Latin *calyx* and written calyx' (O.E.D.).

calyx. Greek κάλυξ, from root καλύπτειν. Often confused with calix. The whorl of leaves forming the outer covering of the flower while in the bud.

Carr, R.J. Contemporary radiologist, Bradford. Described his tiny concretions, worked with Henry Hamilton Stewart in studying the 'stone nest theory' of calculus formation.

Charrière, Joseph (1803–76). Instrument maker of Paris, made instruments for Civiale (1792–1867) and many other celebrated French surgeons. Made the first effective lithotrite. Devised the French (logical) metric system of catheter sizes, the number signifying the circumference of the instrument in millimetres.

Chevassu, M. Urologist of Paris. Made many contributions including a useful bulb-ended catheter for the ureter: his thesis (Paris, 1906) first clearly distinguished between seminoma and teratoma and urged early and radical orchidectomy.

chordée. A painful downward concavity of the penis. Originally associated with inflammation of the corpora cavernosa from gonorrhoea (chaudepisse cordée) it is now used more often

310 *Glossary*

for the bend associated with hypospadias.

Clutton, Henry (1888). The curved steel bougies named after him were copied from those recommended by Otis (q.v.) and Clutton never pretended otherwise.

Colles, Abraham (1773–1843). Professor of Surgery in Dublin. Described the tough layer of superficial fascia of the perineum. (A treatise on Surgical Anatomy, Edinburgh, 1811.)

Collings, C.W. Early exponent of TUR: knife named after him. (See: *J. Urol.* (1926) **16,** 545.)

coudé. French, elbowed—a shape of catheter invented by Mercier of Paris.

Cowper, William (1666–1709). Anatomist and surgeon of London who described the glands sandwiched in the levator ani behind the bulbar urethra.

Culp, Ormond. Chief of Urology, Mayo Clinic.

Cushing, Harvey Williams (1869–1939). Surgeon of Boston: the father of modern neurosurgery.

Denonvilliers, Charles Pierre (1808–72). Surgeon and Anatomist of Paris: remembered for the fascia formed by fusion of the layers of peritoneum between rectum and prostate. (See: L'anatomie du Perinée. *Bull. Soc. Anat. Paris* (1836) **12,** 106.)

Dietl, Joseph (1804–78). Pathologist of Cracow. Described the episodes of pain of intermittent hydronephrosis—the so-called Dietl's crises.

dilate. Latin, dilatare, whence *dilatation*. The shorter 'dilation' is wrong.

Dormia, Enrico. Contemporary assistant Professor of Urology, Milan. Devised his basket for dislodging stones, and now celebrated for methods for dissolving calculi with continuous ureteric irrigation.

Ducrey, Augosto (1860–1940). Dermatologist of Rome. Described the *Haemophilus ducreyi* which causes soft chancre.

Duplay, Simon (1836–1921). Surgeon of Paris. Devised an operation for urethral stricture similar to that of Denis Browne. (See: Injuries and disease of the urethra *Int. Encycl. Surg.* (1886), **6,** 487.)

enuresis. Greek ένουρεῖν, incontinence of urine. Today generally applied to bedwetting, which should strictly be called nocturnal enuresis.

epididymis. Greek, ἐπι upon, and δίδυμοι twins (testes).

epispadias. Greek, ἐπι and σπάδον a rent or tear.

Escherich, Theodor (1857–1911). Paediatrician of Munich who described *Bacillus coli*, now named *Escherichia coli* in his memory.

extrophy. Greek ἐξ and τροφή, nutrition.

Fallopius, Gabriel (1523–62). Polymath of Padua, favourite pupil of Vesalius.

Fenwick, Hurry (1856–1944). Surgeon at St Peter's and The London Hospital. Introduced the new-fangled electric cystoscope to England, founded the International Society of Urology and pioneered retrograde urography.

Foley, Frederic Eugene Basil (1891–1966). Urologist of Minneapolis–St. Paul. Devised self-retaining balloon catheter and a method of pyeloplasty.

fossa. Latin, ditch.

Fournier, Jean Alfred (1832–1914). Venereologist and dermatologist at Hôpital St. Louis, Paris. Described Fournier's gangrene.

fraenum, fraenulum. From Latin, fraenum, a bridle.

Freyer, Sir Peter J. (1851–1921). Surgeon at St. Peter's Hospital. Brilliant Irish surgeon, won international fame by litholapaxy in children in India, later perfected the method of transvesical prostatectomy now named after him.

Fuller, Eugene (1858–1930). New York urologist. Made many contributions to urology including the transvesical operation. (See: *J. Cutan. Genit. Dis.* (1895) **13,** 229.)

fundus. Latin, bottom. The bottom or the part furthest from the orifice.

Gerota, Dumitru (1867–1939). Anatomist of Budapest, described the posterior fascia of the kidney. (See: *Arch. Anat. Leipsig* (1895) 265.)

Gersuny, Robert (1844–1924). Surgeon of Vienna: attempted to devise method of urinary bladder substitution using rectum for urine, and bringing faecal stream through anal sphincter (his case died).

Gibbon, Norman. Contemporary urological surgeon, Sefton Hospital, Liverpool: devised narrow plastic catheter for use in paraplegics.

Gil-Vernet, J.M. Contemporary Spanish surgeon of Barcelona. Devised extended pyelolithotomy through renal sinus.

Giraldes, Joachim (1808–1875). Professor of Surgery, Paris. (See *C.R. Soc. Biol. Paris* (1859) 123.)

Grawitz, Paul Albert (1850–1932). Pathologist of Greifswald. (See: *Virchow's Archiv.* (1883) **93,** 39.)

gum elastic. Catheters formerly made of silk, woven and impregnated with gum. Invented by Bernard (a Parisian jeweller) in 1779.

Guthrie, Sir George James (1785–1856). Hero of Waterloo and Surgeon to the Westminster Hospital. Pioneer of T.U.R.

Harris, Smuel Henry (1880–1937). Urologist of Sydney, Australia, who published first safe and antiseptic transvesical I-stage prostatectomy series. (See: *Brit. J. Surg.* (1933), **21**, 434.)

Helmstein, Karl. Contemporary Swedish urologist, Stockholm.

Henle, Freidrich (1809–85). Anatomist of Berlin.

Henoch, E. (1820–1910). Paediatrician, Berlin.

Hopkins, Professor Harry. Contemporary, Professor of Optics, University of Reading. Devised modern rod-lens system, and flexible fibre optic cable used throughout modern urology.

Hunner, Guy Leroy (1868–1951). Gynaecologist at Johns Hopkins Hospital, Baltimore. Described interstitial cystitis, 1914. (See Hunner, G.L. *Boston Med. Surg. J.*, 660.)

hyaline. Greek ὕαλος, glass.

hydatid. Greek ὕδωρ, drop of water.

hydrocele. Greek κήλη, swelling, like κοίλακος, belly: often misspelt hydrocoele from confusion with κοίλος, hollow, hence coelom: means watery swelling.

hypospadias. Greek ὑπο, below, σπάδον, a rent or tear.

Jaboulay Mathieu (1860–1913). Surgeon of Lyons.

Jacques, Frère Jacques de Beaulieu (1651–1714). Itinerant lithotomist through lateral approach. (See: Barrett (1949) *Ann. Roy. Coll. Surg. Eng.*, **5**, 275.)

Jaques, James Archibald (1815–1878). Works manager, William Warne and Co. Ltd., Barking, Essex. Improved and patented soft rubber catheter.

Johanson, Bengt. Contemporary surgeon. Stockholm. Pioneer of urethroplasty.

Kidd, Frank, S. (1878–1934). London Hospital surgeon. Invented the 'big-ball' diathermy cystoscope.

Klinefelter, E.W. Contemporary radiologist. Massachusetts General Hospital.

Kolff, W.J. Contemporary nephrologist: pioneer of first effective artificial kidney in Holland during Nazi occupation 1944. Now at Cleveland.

Leadbetter, Wyland (1911–1974). Distinguished urologist of Boston.

Leydig, Franz von (1821–1908). Anatomist and zoologist of Bonn.

litho. Greek λίθος, stone, *-tripsy,* Greek τρίβειν, wear away, τομή cut, - λάπαξις, evacuation.

Littre, Alexis (1658–1726). Anatomist of Paris.

Loewenstein–Jensen. Culture medium for tuberculosis. Ernst Loewenstein (1878) pathologist of Vienna and Carl Oluf Jensen (1864–1934) pathologist of Copenhagen.

Lowsley, O.S. (1884–1955). New York urologist.

McCarthy, Joseph Francis (1874–1965). New York urologist: inventor of the foroblique lens, and the 'panendoscope'.

malakoplakia. Greek μαλακός, soft and πλακεῖα, plaque.

Malécot, Achille Etienne (b. 1852). Described his winged self-retaining catheter in 1892. (See: Outwin, E.L., The development of the modern catheter. *J. Amer. Surg. Tech.* (1955), **1**, 8.)

Malpighi, Marcello (1628-94). Anatomist, physician, polymath of Rome and Bologna. Described just about everything.

Marchetti, A.A., see below.

Marshall, Victor F. Contemporary urologist at New York Memorial Hospital. (See: Marshall, V.F., Marchetti, A.A., and Krantz, K.E. (1949) The correction of stress incontinence by simple vesicourethral suspension. *Surg. Gynec./ Obstet.*, **88**, 509.)

Marion, Georges (1869–1960). French urologist of Paris, described many conditions, especially 'prostatisme sans prostate' i.e. bladder neck stenosis, which is sometimes called after him, though it was described by John Hunter, Morgagni, Valsalva and Ambroise Paré beforehand.

meatus (pl. meatus). Latin, a passage or channel.

micturition. From Latin micturire, derived from mingere to mix (originally meant the desire to make water, implying 'a morbid frequency in the making of urine: often erroneously the action of making water' O.E.D.).

Millin, Terence. Contemporary urological surgeon. Described retropubic prostatectomy. (See: *Retropubic Urinary Surgery,* E. and S. Livingstone, Edinburgh, 1947.)

Morgagni, Giovanni Battista (1682–1771). Anatomist and pathologist of Padua.

Morris, Sir Henry (1844–1926). Surgeon trained at Guy's Hospital, London, worked at the

Middlesex Hospital. Did the first deliberate removal of a calculus from the kidney. (See: *Invest. Urol.* (1973), **11,** 170.)

Müller, Johannes (1801–58). Physiologist of Berlin, described the paramesonephric ducts and the organs (Müllerian this and Müllerian that) which are derived from them.

navicularis. Latin, having the shape of a small boat.

Neisser, Albert Ludwig Siegmund (1855–1916). Dermatologist of Breslau. (See: *Centr. med. Wiss.* (1879), **17,** 497.)

neph. νέφρος, Greek, kidney; -ectomy, -itis, -stomy, etc.

nexus. Latin, a tying together (like connected, knitted, etc).

Nitze, Max. Professor of Urology in Berlin, invented the first incandescent lamp cystoscope in 1877.

nocturia. the discharge of an abnormally large quantity of urine at night.

Otis, Fessenden Nott (1825–1900). American urologist who devoted his life to the study of the urethra.

Paget, Sir James (1814–1899). Surgeon, St. Bartholomew's Hospital London. (see *St. Barts. Hosp. Rep.* (1874), **10,** 87).

Papanicolaou, G.N. (1833–1962). Greek pathologist working in New York. (See: Cytology of the urinary sediment in neoplasms of the urinary tract. *J. Urol.* (1947), **57,** 375.

papilloma. Latin papilla, a nipple, and Greek -oma, tumour.

Politano. Victor. Contemporary urologist, Miami, Florida.

Peyronie, François de la (1678–1747). Surgeon of Paris

Pfannenstiel, Hermann Johann (1862–1909). Gynaecologist of Breslau. Described the lower abdominal incision named after him.

polyuria. Greek poly, much, and uria. An increase in the amount of urine excreted, usually implies frequency.

Queyrat, L. Dermatologist of Paris. (See: Queyrat, L. (1911) Erythroplasie du gland. *Bull. Soc. Franç. Derm. Syph.* **22,** 378.) Described carcinoma *in situ* of penis, already described by Paget (1874).

Randall, Alexander (1883–1951). Urologist of Philadelphia: made many contributions including the description of the various lobes of the prostate and the 'bar at the neck of the bladder', as well as the Randall's plaques on the renal papillae.

Rehn, Ludwig (1849–1930). Surgeon of Frankfurt. Noticed workers in factory making fuchsin got bladder cancer.

Riches, Sir Eric. (contemporary Consulting Urologist: Middlesex Hosp.

Rovsing, N.T. (1862–1927) Prof. of Surgery, Copenhagen.

Scarpa, Antonio (1747–1832). Professor of Anatomy at Pavia, Italy.

Sertoli, Enrico (1842–1910). Physiologist of Milan.

Stewart, Henry Hamilton (1904–1970). Urologist of Bradford. One of the pioneers of punch resection in England; inventor of numerous ingenious plastic urological procedures for urethral stricture, hydronephrosis, etc.

strangury. From Greek στράγξ, drop squeezed out, and οὖρον, urine. Slow and painful emission of urine.

teratoma. From Greek τέρας, monster.

testis. Latin, witness.

Thompson, Sir Henry (1820–1904). Great stone-crusher. (See: *Invest. urol.* (1973), **11,** 263.)

Tiemann, G., and Co. Instrument makers of New York.

trichomonas. θρίξ, a hair, μόνος, unit (though it has 3 to 5 hairs!).

urethra. Greek, οὖρηθρα.

utriculus. Latin, small bag.

vas. A vessel, deferens, carrying.

verumontanum. Latin veru, a spit; montanus, mountainous.

vesicle. Latin, a little bladder.

vulva. Latin, a wrapper.

Wilms, Max (1867–1918). Surgeon of Heidelberg. Nephroblastoma was previously described by *Rance* (1814).

Wolff, Kaspar Friedrich (1733–1794). German anatomist and embryologist, working in St. Petersburg.

xanthogranuloma. ξανθός, Greek, yellow.

Young, Hugh Hampton (1870–1945). Urologist of Baltimore, inventor of the first cold punch, and a method of perineal prostatectomy.

Ziehl–Neelsen. Method of staining the tubercle bacillus, named after Franz Ziehl (1859–1926), physician of Lübeck, and Friedrich Karl Adolph Neelsen (1854–1894) pathologist of Dresden.

Zuckerkandl, Emil (1849–1910). Anatomist of Vienna.

Index

316

Index